ANIMAL GENETICS AND BREEDING

ANIMAL GENETICS AND BREEDING

Simone Bogoviz
Karl Cowell

Kruger Brentt
Publishers
2023

Kruger Brentt Publishers UK. LTD.
Company Number 9728962

Regd. Office: 68 St Margarets Road, Edgware, Middlesex HA8 9UU

ISBN: 9781787150515

For information on all our publications visit our website at http://krugerbrentt.com/

PREFACE

Animal Genetics and Breeding is the field of study that includes all the aspects of livestock genomics and breeding for better production of farm animals as well as the products from these animals (milk and milk products, meat, fibre, and eggs). Modern livestock and aquaculture production aims for the production of healthy and robust animals with improved animal welfare and preserving genetic diversity. Animal breeding plays an important part in progressing animal production systems, from conventional to organics. By improving the abilities of animals for certain traits entire populations can be enhanced, creating benefits for farmers, consumers, and the environment. Animal breeding can be explained as the selective crossing of domestic animals that have desirable qualities resulting in improved offspring. These 'qualities' are translated as breeding values for a number of interesting traits. A few examples could be, milk and meat production and quality, as well as disease resistance, robustness, fertility, longevity and the reduction of the impact in the environment (e.g. methane reduction and better use of feed resources). Balanced breeding means to find a compromise between the health and welfare of animals, their environmental impacts and the quality and the quantity of the production (milk, meat and eggs). Currently, pigs and poultry only need half of the feed than 40 years ago. And improving robustness and longevity of dairy, leg strength in both pigs and poultry, or reducing misbehaviour in pigs and osteoporosis in laying hens are some examples of breeding elements.

In the context of climate warming and biodiversity loss, the way we produce and consume must be reviewed. Animal breeding has a role to play to reduce the impact of animal production and to help farmers to become more sustainable. Improved animal welfare, a better use of resources, reducing impact in the environment by reducing GHG and ammonia emissions, disease resistance and more robust animals are some of the characteristics that breeders help to improve. They are essential to provide nutritious and safe food for populations. Animal breeders participate on this effort. Animal breeders collaborate to adapt breeding programs depending on the farming context. They also participate in the preservation and promotion of local breeds.

The present book contains twelve chapters covering all related disciplines. These chapters include Introduction to animal breeding, Introduction of DNA in animal breeding, Organization of breeding activities, Results of animal breeding, Negative effects of animal breeding, Basics of animal breeding, Challenges for animal breeding, Genetic models, Genetic diversity and inbreeding, Inheritance of monogenic, Selection and mating, Crossbreeding. This book is designed to provide in-depth information about applied breeding methods for different domestic animal species as currently implemented. It is written in a lucid style with theoretical discussions and being supplemented with illustrations, and tables for easy understanding of the subject. The book is also supported with a comprehensive glossary and index in the end. This book will serve as a valuable resource for graduate and postgraduate students' teachers, researchers of animal breeding.

We are grateful to all those persons as well as various books, manuals, periodicals, magazines, journals etc. that helped in the preparation of this book. In spite of the best efforts, it is possible that some errors may have occurred into the compilation and editing of the book. Further queries, constructive suggestions and criticisms for the improvement of the book are always welcome and shall be thankfully acknowledged.

Simone Bogoviz

Karl Cowell

CONTENTS

1

INTRODUCTION TO ANIMAL BREEDING

Farm animal breeding is the activity in farm animal production providing the next generation of farm animals. Animal breeding ensures a continuous improvement of farm animals, generation after generation. Different animal traits are measured and the best animals are used a parent-animals. In this way, breeders provide livestock farmers with a next generation of animals. Farm animal breeders have an essential contribution to a healthy and sustainable food supply chain.

The importance of selection by nature and important aspects of the domestication process will be described. Mankind started to create breeds accompanied with artificial selection 250 years ago.

Nowadays, breeding of high productive farm animals, like cattle, pigs and poultry is in the hands of multinational companies which invest a lot of money in state of the art breeding programs. The breeding of sheep, goats, horses and companion animals, e.g. the dog is based on individual breeders collaborating in the setting of a herd book or a breeder's association.

Animal breeding is aiming at the improvement of animals by changing their genetic abilities for important traits. These traits are determined by the requirements and wishes from the society which might change over time. Animal breeding is highly influenced by research and developments in population-, quantitative- and molecular genetics. Sometimes, unexpected negative effects of animal breeding are observed that require adequate corrections.

A breeding program will be presented here as a circular activity. Each generation, the program starts with formulating the breeding goal and ends with a critical review of the results obtained in the next generation.

The science of animal breeding is defined as the application of the principles of genetics and biometry to improve the efficiency of production in farm animals. These principles were applied to change animal populations thousands of years before the sciences of genetics and biometry were formally established. The practice of animal breeding dates back to the Neolithic period (approximately 7000 BC), when people attempted to domesticate wild species such as caribou, goats, hogs and dogs.

Domestication was performed through controlled mating and reproduction of captive animals which were selected and mated based on their behaviour and temperament. Judging from cave paintings that have survived, selection was also applied to some qualitative traits such as coat colour and the absence or presence of horns. Without written records, there is no certain knowledge of the evolution of animal breeding practices, but written documents dating back more than 4000 years indicate that humans appreciated the significance of family resemblance in mating systems, recognized the dangers of intense inbreeding, and used castration to prevent the reproduction of undesirable males.

Progress in the performance of domesticated animals through these selection practices was very slow; improvements were mainly due to animals adapting better to their environments.

Robert Bakewell, an English animal breeder of the 18th century, is considered the founder of systematized animal breeding. He was the first to emphasize the importance of accurate breeding records, introduced the concept of progeny testing to evaluate the genetic potentials of young sires, and applied inbreeding to stabilize desired qualitative traits. He also promoted concepts such as "like begets like,""prepotency is associated with inbreeding" and "breed the best to the best." Bakewell and his contemporaries in Europe pioneered the development of diverse breeds of beef cattle, dairy cattle, sheep, hogs and horses.

BREEDING

- Farm animal breeding includes all farmed animal species both on land and in water.
- Animal breeding and reproduction is at the top of the animal production pyramid and hence defines the quality of all animals used in agriculture.
- Farm animal breeders indirectly influence food safety and public health, product quality, efficiency, environment, animal health and welfare, and genetic diversity.
- Breeding is society sensitive because it drives changes in the genetic make-up of animals and the use of new technologies (e.g. genomics, computing sciences).

The need for animal breeding

Global demand for animal products is expected to double in the next decades due to an increasing global population and global wealth. Animal products from a great source of protein that are essential in a healthy and balanced diet. To fulfil this growing demand, global animal production should increase while taking into account issues of environmental sustainability, food safety, and animal welfare. The breeding sector can contribute to finding solutions that are cost and resource efficient, diminish or eliminate environmental pressure, are adaptive to climate change, are beneficial for animal health and welfare, improve food quality and safety, and that meet the needs of citizens, both today and in the future.

This requires healthy, robust and efficient animals with improved animal welfare.

TYPES OF ANIMAL HUSBANDRY

There are four major types of animal husbandry practised in the world today:

Dairy Farming

Dairy farming is the agricultural technique concerned with the long term production of milk, which is then processed to obtain dairy products such as curd, cheese, yoghurt, butter, cream, etc. It involves the management of dairy animals such as cows, buffaloes, sheep, goat, etc.

The animals are taken care of against diseases and are inspected regularly by veterinary doctors. A healthy animal is physically, mentally and socially sound.

These animals are milked by hand or by machines. The milk is preserved and converted into dairy products industrially, which are then used for commercial purposes.

Poultry Farming

Poultry farming is concerned with raising and breeding of birds for commercial purposes. Birds like ducks, chickens, geese, pigeons, turkeys, etc. are domesticated for eggs and meat.

It is very important to take care of the animals and maintain them in a disease-free environment to obtain healthy food from them. The eggs and meat are a rich source of protein.

Sanitation and hygienic conditions need to be maintained. The faeces of birds are used as manure to improve soil fertility. Poultry farming provides employment to a large number of people and helps in improving the economy of the farmers.

Fish Farming

Fish farming is the process of raising fish in closed tanks or ponds for commercial purposes. There is an increasing demand for fish and fish protein. Fish species such as salmon, catfish, cod, and tilapia are raised in fish farms.

Fish farming or pisciculture is of two types:

- Extensive aquaculture, based on the local photosynthetic production
- Intensive aquaculture, based on the external food supply given to fishes.

Bee Farming

Bee farming or apiculture is the practice of maintaining bee colonies by humans in man-made hives. Honey bees are reared on a large scale. The bees are domesticated for honey, wax, and to pollinate flowers. They are also used by other beekeepers for the same purposes. The place where bees are kept is known as an apiary or a bee yard.

ROLE OF ANIMAL HUSBANDRY IN HUMAN WELFARE

Animal husbandry is beneficial to human beings in the following ways:

Dairy Products

Animals such as cows, goats, sheep, etc. are the major source of milk and milk products such as yoghurt, cheese, butter, etc.

Meat

Animals such as cows, buffaloes, pigs, and goats are reared for their meat. Their meat is a rich source of dietary protein.

Land Management

The livestock is sometimes grazed to control the growth of weeds on agricultural land. The dry shrubs in the areas that are prone to wildfire are eaten by goat and sheep, which reduces the risk of fire.

Fibre

Animals also produce fibres or textiles such as wool and leather. For eg, sheep are reared for wool whereas leather can be obtained from camel.

Manure

The excreta, blood and bones of animals are used as manure. The manure is spread on the fields to increase the crop yields and **crop production**. It is also used as fuel for fires and as plaster for walls and floor.

Labour

Animals are a source of non-human labour. They are used for ploughing fields, transporting goods and military functions. For ag., horses, yaks and donkeys are used for such purposes.

THE IMPORTANCE OF ANIMAL HUSBANDRY – ALL YOU NEED TO KNOW

Animal rearing is important for humans as they attain a wide range of food products having high nutrient values. They meet the commercial requirements of high demand for food such as dairy needs from cows, goats, and buffaloes. They are called milch animals as they provide us milk which is full of protein and other vitamins and minerals.

The importance of animal husbandry further extends to another set of animals that are important to humans for eggs and meat such as hens, ducks, goose, goat, fish, etc. They are also bred for meat which is rich in protein, iron, fats, vitamin B_{12} and Zinc. All of these nutrients are essential to enhance metabolic rate, promote fullness, and reduce hunger. Marine animals like fish are also believed to keep a person happier and healthier as these have Omega-3 fatty acids, DHA, and vitamin D.

Animal husbandry takes care of the management and breeding of animals and is a large scale business. A farm or a specific region is built for providing shelter, food, and undertaking culturing processes. It also involves apiculture i.e. bee agriculture and aquaculture i.e. marine animals culturing.

ORIGIN OF ANIMAL DOMESTICATION AND HUSBANDRY - WORLD HISTORY

It has a long history when animals were initially domesticated during the Neolithic revolution. Earlier, cattle, goats, sheep, and pigs were raised on farms on a low scale. After the 18th century, agriculturalists rapidly took animal husbandry to the next level and yielded more meat, wool, and milk day by day. A wide variety of species like horses, rabbits, guinea pud, and water buffalo were also used in some parts of the world.

Aquaculture of molluscs, crustaceans, and fish was on the rise and insect farming was also adopted. Contemporary methods to define animal husbandry depend on the type of land available and production systems adapted to these. Intensive animal farming that involves maximum production with minimum cost has been adopted by the modern methods that make available thousands of chickens and high-density feedlots. This helps in increasing the yield per area of land with an investment of a good amount of money and labor.

Modern methods involve intensive animal farming which seeks maximum production at minimum costs. This has led to exploitation and growing vulnerability in the existing livestock resources.

ROLE OF ANIMAL HUSBANDRY IN AGRICULTURE

The role of animal husbandry in human welfare can be described as follows:

- Dairy products producing animals like cows, sheep, and goats are the major sources of milk and milk products including butter, cheese, yogurt, cottage cheese, etc.
- Many animals including chicken, goat, duck, pigs, and buffaloes are used for their meat because of their highly nutritious value.
- Livestock is used to control the growth of weeds on agricultural land as the dry shrubs that are prone to fire are eaten up by various animals. This reduces the risk and harm that can be faced with unprecedented situations. So, it is important for land management.
- Wool and leather are the fibre by-products from animals like sheep and camels. When these animals are reared in a vast number, the products can be obtained largely too.

- The importance of animal husbandry also lies in the fact that the excreta, bones, and blood of animals can be used as manure or fertilizers via composting. These can be spread on fields to enhance crop yield.
- Animals are helpful for ploughing fields, military functions, and transporting goods from one place to another. Example: Horse, yak, and donkey.

History of animal breeding

- Till 500 A.D. when the fall of Roman Empire began animal breeding was at its esteem. With the fall of Roman Empire for about 1000 years called Dark and Middle Ages, animal husbandry was at a still.
- From 1700 A.D., again there was an improvement. The beginning of modern animal breeding is to be found mainly in England and Europe.
- The British Royalty encouraged horse breeding especially for race horses. The Earls and Dukes imported bulls from Holland and bred their native stocks. Dutch cattle were introduced into Herefordshire that laid the foundation of the present Hereford cattle. By crossing the native and Dutch cattle and subsequent inbreeding, the British cattle were improved far beyond the best.

HERITABILITY AND ITS USE IN ANIMAL BREEDING

Heritability is the single most important consideration in determining appropriate animal evaluation methods, selection methods and mating systems. Heritability measures the relative importance of hereditary and environmental influences on the development of a specific quantitative trait. More specifically, it measures that part of the total variability of the trait caused by genetic differences among the animals on which the measurements were taken. Heritability, then, is a ratio of genetic variance (V_g) to total variance (V_p) (i.e., $h^2 = V_g/V_p$). Total variance (or phenotypic variance) includes variance caused by genetic and environmental factors (i.e., $V_p = V_g + V_E$).

The numerical value of the heritability estimate is given as a percentage or a decimal and should, of course, lie between 0 and 1. In some instances, the value falls outside this range. This is a chance occurrence caused by statistical manipulation.

A heritability estimate is a partial description of one trait in one group of animals at some particular time. It may vary (for each trait) during one time period from herd to herd, or it may vary in the same herd from time to time. This is natural because herds differ in genetic makeup and because there are many different environmental circumstances from herd to herd or within a herd from year to year. These genetic and environmental differences influence the size of the numerical value of the terms (i.e., genetic variance, V_g and total variance, V_p) used in the estimation of heritability.

The numerical value of a heritability estimate can be increased or decreased by changes in either of its component parts. An increase results from a reduction in the environmental variance or from an increase in genetic variance. Conversely, a decrease results from an increase in environmental variance or from a reduction in genetic variance.

A number of factors affect genetic variance. Introduction of new and unrelated animals into the herd may increase the genetic variance. Effective selection within a group of animals over a number of generations decreases the genetic variance. The use of inbreeding as a system of mating also reduces the genetic variance.

Any management practice that ensures uniform treatment of animals reduces environmental variance. For example, if you give each animal the same amount and quality of feed, you reduce environmental variance. When you make adjustments for any environmental differences, your objective is to remove performance differences that result because animals are "treated" differently.

Weaning weight provides an example. To get accurate figures, you make adjustments for the dam's age or the calf's season of birth to remove their effects on weaning weight. Effective adjustment also reduces total variance of weaning weight within individual herds. This reduction makes recognizing genetic differences among animals in the herd easier. When you adjust records and treat animals uniformly, you are attempting to reduce environmental variance so you can more easily recognize genetic differences.

Calculation of heritability estimates

The heritability estimates in Tables 1, 2 and 3 are average values based on many studies conducted at USDA research centers and college of agriculture experiment stations in many states.

Table 1 Heritability estimates of some important traits in beef cattle

Trait	Number of estimates	Average estimates
Reproduction Calving interval	3	0.08
Fertility		0.10
Growth		
Birth weight	75	0.45
Gain, birth to weaning	62	0.30
Weaning weight	83	0.24
Feedlot gain	43	0.34
Pasture gain	14	0.30
Final feedlot weight	36	0.46
Final yearling pasture weight	19	0.44
Conformation		
Weaning score	52	0.38
Final feedlot score	16	0.36

Yearling pasture score	12	0.30
Efficiency		
Feed efficiency	20	0.45
Height		
Weaning, shoulder, creep fed	6	0.82
Weaning, shoulder, non-creep fed	6	0..88
Weaning, hip, creep fed	6	0.82
Weaning, hip, non-creep fed	6	0.95
Carcass		
Grade		0.50
Dressing percent		0.45
Ribeyeareaperhundredweight		0.70
Fat thickness per hundredweight		0.45
Tenderness		0.60
Retail product, percen		0.30
Retail pounds Retail produc		

Trait	Average estimate
Reproduction	
Gestation length	0.45
Multiple birth	0.15
Growth	
Birth weight	0.30
Rate of gain	0.30
Weaning weight (at 60 days)	0.10
Weaning weight (100+ days)	0.30
Mature body weight	0.40
Conformation	
Weaning type score	0.10
Yearling type score	0.40

Trait	Average estimate
Fleece	
Face cover	0.56
Neck folds (at weaning)	0.39
Skin folds	0.40
Fleece weight, grease	0.38
Fleece weight, clean	0.40

Staple length (at weaning)	0.39
Staple length (at yearling)	0.47
Grade	0.35
Carcass	
Loineye area	0.53
Fat thickness over loineye	0.23
Weight per day of age	0.22
Length	0.31
Fat weight	0.57
Bone weight	0.30
Lean weight	0.39
Grade	0.12
Retail cut weight	0.50
Dressing percent	0.10

Table 3. Heritability estimates of some important traits in swine

Trait	**Average estimate**
Reproduction	
Number farrowed	0.10
Number weaned	0.10
Growth	
Birth weight	0.10
Weaning weight	0.15
Growth rate	0.30
Efficiency	
Feed efficiency	0.35
Carcass	
Meat tenderness	0.30
Meat color	0.30
Marbling (in loin)	0.30
Meat firmness	0.30
Backfatthickness	0.50
Trait	**Average estimate**
Loineye area	0.50
Length	0.60
Percent ham, chilled carcass weight	0.60
Percent fat cuts, chilled carcass weight	0.60
Percent lean cuts, chilled carcass weight	0.50

In general, each estimate of heritability is based on the degree of resemblance among related individuals vs. non-related individuals in some animal population. Family units most often used to evaluate degree of resemblance include parent and offspring; parents and offspring; full sibs (i.e., full brothers and/or sisters); and paternal half sibs (i.e., half brothers and/or sisters).

The statistical technique used in calculating heritability is chiefly dependent upon available records. One practical consideration is the kind of family units represented in the data. This may dictate the technique used. If you have a choice of techniques (for example, if more than one kind of family unit is represented in the data set), then you must consider which technique gives the least amount of bias from a variety of sources.

Complications in any technique arise most often when you try to account for the effects of environmental factors. You must equalize environmental factors as much as possible and adjust for other non-genetic factors that influence animal performance. For example, if you are evaluating resemblance between weaning hip heights of cows and their calves, you might make adjustments for differences in age at the time of measurement, age of dam, sex of calf, season of birth, and so forth.

If you fail to adequately account for environmental contributions, you will reduce the estimate of heritability. From a practical standpoint, this means you will be less able to recognize genetic differences among animals you are considering for breeding purposes.

One of the most common estimation techniques, and the one described here, is the paternal half-sib analysis of variance. With this method, the total variance is divided into two parts. In one, variation is attributed to differences among progeny of different sires. In the other, the variance is attributed to differences among offspring of the same sire. The analysis of variance is generally put into tabular form as follows:

Source of variance	Degrees of freedom	Mean squares	Expected mean squares
Total	N - 1		
Among sires	S - 1	M_1	$V_w + kV_s$
Within sires	N - S	M_2	V_w

Degrees of freedom is an awkward concept. In general, it is related to number of observations minus number of constraints. For example, N - 1 is the total number of measurements (observations) of a specific trait, such as hip height, minus 1.

Mean squares, M_1 and M_2, represent estimates of variances associated with "among sires" and "within sires" sources of variance.

Expected mean squares are theoretical components of their respective mean squares.

k is the weighted number of progeny per sire.

$\mathbf{V_s}$ is a measure of the resemblance among half sibs and is interpreted to be one-fourth of the genetic variance for the trait concerned.

V_w is interpreted to be three-fourths of the genetic variance and all of the environmental variance.

V_s is calculated from the mean squares (i.e., variances) associated with the "among sires" and "within sires" sources of variance as $(M_1 - M_2)/k$.

Heritability, h^2, is then calculated as:

$$h^2 = \frac{4V_s}{V_s + V_w}$$

Usefulness of heritability estimates

You can use heritability estimates to estimate progress and setbacks in different traits that you can expect from different matings. For example, a particular mating may bring improvement in rate of gain if the parents are genetically superior. If they are inferior, however, they may cause a decline in rate of gain in their offspring.

To illustrate how to figure expected progress from particular matings, assume you have a herd with an average daily gain in the feedlot of 2.40 pounds per day. From that herd, you kept bulls that gained 3.20 pounds and heifers that gained 2.80 pounds per day for breeding purposes.

How much gain in genetic improvement could you expect in the progeny of these selected parents?

To answer this question, first calculate just how superior these parents were to the average in the herd.

Calculate the superiority of the breeding animals as follows:

- Superiority of dams = 2.80 - 2.40 or 0.40 pounds per day.
- Superiority of sires = 3.20 - 2.40 or 0.80 pounds per day.
- Superiority of parents = (0.40 + 0.80) ÷ 2 = 0.60 pounds per day.

The next question is, "How much of this 0.60 pound advantage is transmitted to the offspring?" To answer, you must know the heritability of feedlot average daily gain. The average estimate for this trait is 0.34 (Table 1).

Expected genetic gain, then, is equal to the average superiority of the parents multiplied by the heritability (i.e., 0.60 x 0.34 or 0.20 pounds per day).

The herd average was 2.40 pounds feedlot gain per day. With all other things equal, you would expect the offspring of the selected parents to gain an average of 2.40 + 0.20 = 2.60 pounds per day. This is the average of the herd plus the genetic advantage transmitted by the parents.

The calculations above illustrate two important points. First, if the selected parents had not been superior in rate of gain over the average of the herd, there would have been no genetic improvement in rate of gain of their offspring, regardless of the degree of heritability of the trait.

Second, the amount of genetic progress is also dependent on how highly heritable a trait is. Though the parents had an advantage over the herd average of 0.60 pounds per day in gain, they would not have transmitted any of this advantage to their offspring if the trait had a herd heritability.

The general conclusion, then, is that the greater the superiority of the individuals selected for breeding purposes and the higher the heritability of the trait, the more progress will be made in selection.

A knowledge of the size of the heritability estimate is also important in deciding which animal evaluation method should be used. When heritability of the trait is medium to high (above about 0.30), selection based upon the individual's own level of performance allows a relatively rapid rate of improvement. When the trait has a low heritability, you should use other methods to identify genetically superior individuals. The "other" methods involve various schemes for including the level of performance of related individuals such as siblings or progeny.

You can make more improvement in low heritability traits by using mating systems that take advantage of heterosis (hybrid vigor). As a general rule, the lower the heritability of a trait, the greater the heterotic response from various outbreeding mating systems.

Low-heritable traits, such as those associated with reproductive efficiency, show the greatest benefit from using outbreeding mating systems. Highly heritable traits, such as carcass quality traits, show very little if any heterotic response from outbreeding mating systems.

An important difference lies between these two avenues of trait improvement. Improvement from selection schemes is cumulative over the generations. But improvement that comes from exploitation of heterosis is maximized in one generation and must be recreated each generation thereafter.

DOMESTICATION AND ANIMAL BREEDING

Domestication happens through selective breeding. Individuals that exhibit desirable traits are selected to be bred, and these desirable traits are then passed along to future generations.

Domestication is an evolutionary process by which animals are artificially selected and undergo huge phenotypic behavioral and physiological alterations. These transformations occurred at the same time in several regions with a tremendous impact on human societies (Neolithization). Domestication is well known not only for its slow course but also for its extreme techno-economic alterations, from hunting-gathering to food production. It depends on many important factors, such as strong demographic transition, cultivation, and husbandry of valuable domesticates, along with profound social and spiritual changes.

Dogs (*Canis lupus familiaris*) were the earliest species domesticated by Asian and European gatherers during the late glacial period approximately 17–15 thousand years (kyrs) before the present (BP) followed later by the domestication of livestock and crops. Interestingly, while in some species (dogs and cattle), domestication was a human-driven process, for other species (cat, rat, and house sparrow), it occurred naturally. Nowadays, several authors agree that there are approximately 40 animal species domesticated in different geographic areas.

Differences in morphological features and behavior of most domestic animals from their wild counterparts came about by controlling breeding and persistent animal husbandry. These practices also designed and shaped the diverse genetic makeup among different breeding populations.

The variation in the phenotypes of the domesticated animal led to the basis of the Darwinian evolutionary study, which highlighted several queries for further studies, namely: when, where, and how did the domestication of these animals start, and what are the genetic origins of domestication development.

Darwin's initial observations in "On the Origin of Species," and his variation under domestication began an essential debate for future works. Commonly, for different domestic animals, there are two evolutionary phases: an ancient domestication event where a wild ancestor become a domesticated species followed by a modern breeding process. Ancient domestication occurred approximately 12,000–14,000 years ago, during the agricultural surge of the initial Neolithic period, along with the domestication of major crops.

On the other hand, modern breeding occurred only in the past 300 years (since the eighteenth century) and started with the selection of breeding animals based on their demand by human societies.

In the current review, we try to summarize the existing information on domestication from the literature. We start by addressing the evolution of animal domestication through an evolutionary perspective. We address the roots, demographic history, and impacts on domestication, genetic architecture, and methodologies taken to monitor domestication procedures by selective pressures. We also conclude presenting the challenges to the research and a preview of future directions for this thematic.

Animal domestication is the process of a prompt, artificial, and intensive selection of wild animals that, over the last 11,500 years, has altered the Earth's biosphere, shaped human evolution, and influenced the size of the human population. The foundation of domestication is linked to the cultural progression from hunting to farming in ancient civilizations during the Neolithic period, possibly with the exclusion of dogs, which were the earliest domesticated animals (Savolainen et al., 2002) and diverge from other species regarding both location and timing of domestication.

The periods where animal domestication occurred were determined through archeological clues and reflected selection forces generated by human activities and by human-adapted environments. During the last years, several studies have focused on animal domestication, and nowadays, it is possible to establish a timeline for the domestication of several animals. Despite this, there are still several questions regarding the timing, location, and the evolutionary domestication process.

Since the Neolithic period, humans struggled to domesticate wild animals and use them as food sources (milk and meat), commodity manufacturers (silk and wool), protection, and transportation. There are three pathways described for domestication: commensal, prey, and direct pathways. In the commensal pathway, the wild animals were attracted to anthropogenic habitats, mainly for human food waste or small prey, establishing a commensal relationship with humans.

Dogs, cats, or chickens are some of the species that followed this pathway. In the prey pathway, humans start hunting some species like pigs and cattle for their meat in response to depletion of the local stock of these animals. Over time, these game management strategies developed into controlled breeding of these species. In the direct pathway, humans captured wild animals (horses, donkeys, and camelids) to obtain some resources by controlling their movements, their nutrition, and reproduction, which lead to a dramatic bottleneck.

Brief history of the major domesticated animals

Even though the decision to consider farmed or captive animals as domesticated is subjective and arbitrary, most authors agree that about 40 species around the world that directly or indirectly contribute to agriculture are domesticated; this number varies between 20 and 50 following the definitions used for a domesticated animal. Several of those domesticated species have a distinct scientific name than their wild ancestors.

For the five most valuable species, the domestication resulted in the creation of hundreds of breeds, particularly in the past centuries. In France, the article D.653.9 of the rural code defines breed for ruminant species as "a group of animals that share sufficient common features to be considered homogeneous by one or several groups of breeders that agree on the broodstock renewal and induced changes, including the international level".

Breeds have therefore both a biological sense (common features) and a social acceptance (group of breeders); the relative importance of the latter increased in the past years, for scientists as well as in the application of policies.

Cattle

The wild ancestor of cattle is a group of races of the now extinct aurochs *Bos primigenius*. The aurochs, the last specimen of which died in a Polish park in 1627, had a very wide geographic distribution, which extended from East Asia to Europe and North Africa. Traditionally, two major types of domestic cattle are considered: zebu (*Bos indicus*) which have a prominent thoracic hump and taurine (*Bos taurus*), which do not. However, these two species fully interbreed, and a meta-analysis of different microsatellite datasets revealed taurine-zebu admixture over Europe, southwest Asia, and Africa.

Molecular evidence suggest that these two species came from two independent domestication events: zebu cattle were domesticated in the Indus valley region ca. 8000–7500 B.P., whereas taurine cattle were domesticated in Anatolia 10,500–10,000 B.P. However, researchers recently suggested that only the latter was domesticated, while zebu may have resulted from the introgression of wild zebu populations into taurine cattle that were transported eastward.

During several millennia, extensive gene flow among different groups of domestic cattle, as well as with aurochs until its extinction, was possible, leading to relatively high effective population sizes and preventing genetic drift at the regional scale.

This might partly explain the relatively large cattle gene pool despite a likely bottleneck at the time of domestication. Besides, it is also possible that other species were crossed with cattle in some areas of the world, including the yak (*Bos grunniens*) in Nepal or banteng (*Bos javanicus*) in Southeast Asia and Indonesia, which also contribute to maintain or increase genetic variability.

The large size of cattle and its low growth, as well as the early use for milk or traction, imply relatively low levels of directed selection during millennia.

However, this situation changed dramatically about 200 years ago with the emergence of breed concept. The first cattle herd book was published in Britain in 1822. Since that time, stronger selection pressures have been applied to local populations followed by standardization of the desired conformation and performance, such as high milk yield for dairy cattle breeding programs. This led to an isolation of breeds from each other (ca. 800 are now recognized), which could have caused a genetic drift and inbreeding and perhaps a fitness decrease.

Nevertheless, gene flow between neighboring regions did not completely stop, as deliberate upgrading was realized in order to increase production characteristics by using bulls of other populations from the same or a different country. More recently, the number of males involved in reproduction schemes has drastically decreased with the expansion of artificial insemination, leading to another strong reduction of effective population size of breeds and inexorably to a genetic drift and loss of alleles.

For example, at the worldwide level, the Holstein cattle has an effective population size of about 50. This strong decrease of the effective population size might explain the strong reduction in fertility as well as the genetic diseases observed in this breed]. An even more extreme result was found in Japan, where the Japanese black cattle had an effective population size of 17.2 in between 1993 and 1997, despite a census size of 0.53 million reproductive cows. Another extreme case of low genetic variability is a feral British breed, Chillingham cattle, for which 24 out of 25 microsatellite loci were found homozygous. Inversely, numerous cattle breeds still have substantial nucleotide diversity, indicating a large ancestral effective population size. In the past decades, a few of the most productive breeds were imported throughout the world at the expense of local, apparently less productive populations.

Pig

The wild ancestor of domestic pigs is boar *Sus scrofa*. Wild boars occurred throughout Eurasia and North Africa. Multiple independent domestication events, mainly in Asia Minor, Europe, and East Asia, have probably occurred, starting approximately 9000 years ago; the earliest remains of domesticated pigs have been excavated at Çayönü in Southeast Anatolia. Chinese breeds originated in East Asia, whereas European breeds are believed to have originated in Southwest Asia. These domestication events were separated not only by thousands of kilometers but also by thousands of years.

During millennia, it is likely that out-crossing of domestic pigs with wild boar was common in traditional pig husbandry across Europe. By the late middle ages, European and Asian domestic pigs were genetically very different because they were based on wild boar populations that diverged around 1 million years ago, and for thousands of years, they were submitted to selection pressures on very different traits. By the late eighteenth to early nineteenth century, strict organized breeding was adopted to improve and develop livestock breeds, particularly in Britain, as a reaction to increasing demand for meat in the wake of the industrial revolution.

European breeders turned also their attention to Asia and imported Chinese pigs to improve their breeding stock. From the eighteenth century, pig breeds were selectively bred for specific production traits such as early maturation, rapid growth, and increased prolificacy. In addition, the coat color phenotype (which includes both skin and hair pigmentation) was another morphological trait often used during the selective breeding process. Substantial changes (body size, color, body shape, skull morphology, ear carriage, behavior, prolificacy, teat number, and other traits) occurred in breeds over a short period of time, resulting in the development of numerous distinct pig breed phenotypes.

From the twentieth century, with the recognition of the benefits of genetic improvement and changing consumer preferences, certain pig breeds experienced further strong selection for lean meat content, muscularity, and enhanced reproduction. To date, there are likely over 730 pig breeds or lines globally of which two thirds are in China and Europe and over 270 are considered as endangered or critical. Currently, 58 pig breeds are recorded as "transboundary" (occurring in more than one country) including 25 regional transboundary breeds and 33 international transboundary breeds. The worldwide distribution of pigs is dominated by five international transboundary pig breeds from the United States (USA) or Europe, i.e., Large white (117 countries), Duroc (93 countries), Landrace (91 countries), Hampshire (54 countries), and Pietrain (35 countries).

Sheep

The wild ancestors of the domestic sheep are probably the mouflon (*Ovis musimon*) and the urial (*Ovis orientalis*). Both archaeological and genetic data spot the domestication center of sheep in eastern Anatolia and North-West Iran between 8500 and 12,000 years ago. The sheep mitochondrial DNA polymorphism diversity and single-nucleotide polymorphism (SNP) diversity seem to support an absence of a genetic bottleneck, and thus domestication occurred from a broad genetic base.

Sheep were first farmed for access to meat before human-mediated specialization for wool and milk commenced ca. 4000–5000 years ago. It has recently been shown that particular regions of the genome contain strong evidence for accelerated change in response to artificial selection, such as the removal of horns, likely to be one of the oldest morphological modifications that accompanied domestication and a trait now common across many modern breeds.

Furthermore, other genomic regions under selection in sheep contain genes controlling pigmentation, reproduction, and body size. In the last few hundred years, the division of animals into breeds, followed by the identification of superior rams and their disproportionate genetic contribution via artificial insemination, has lifted the pace of genetic gain for production traits. Extensive haplotype sharing and generally low divergence time between breeds reveal that frequent genetic exchange has occurred during the development of modern breeds.

Approximately 75% of modern sheep breeds have retained an effective population size in excess of 300. The number of breeds is comprised between 850 and 1409. Yet, many sheep breeds originally selected for good performance in a specific, sometimes isolated, geographical area (e.g., the Shetland, Soay, or Herdwick breeds) are now considered rare. With generalist-type sheep taking over the larger part of intensive sheep production, maintaining genetic diversity by conserving these traditional breeds has become a challenge.

Goat

The wild ancestor of goat is the bezoar, *Capra aegagrus*. The first archaeological evidence of goat domestication traces back in the Fertile Crescent about 10,000 years ago. A large-scale analysis of current bezoar mitochondrial DNA (mtDNA) polymorphism over its whole geographic distribution suggested that the domestication process occurred over a very large area encompassing eastern Anatolia and North-West Iran.

Additional primary centers of goat domestication, including the Indus Valley, Southern Levant, and China, have not been convincingly demonstrated yet. Analysis of the goat mitochondrial DNA polymorphism of the main haplogroup (representing more than 90% of the haplotypes) strongly supports the absence of bottleneck at the domestication time in goats. Besides, goat mtDNA polymorphism also suggests high historical gene flow among continents, which already occurred during the Neolithic expansion into Europe. The extraordinary adaptability and hardiness of goats favored their rapid spread over the Old World.

Goats have successfully adapted to desert, mountainous, and tropical areas where other livestock species would not thrive. Between the fifteenth and eighteenth centuries, goats were transported to America and Oceania. Over the course of domestication, several morphological traits were modified, such as horn and ear shapes, the presence of wattles, long hair, and coat colors, which were driven probably by intentional selection as well as by genetic drift, isolation, and founder effects. Throughout the ages, goats have been raised for milk production and cheese, meat, and skin and fiber commodities such as leather, mohair wool, and cashmere hair.

Breeds also show strong differences in their physiological capacity of adaptation to extreme conditions of temperature and humidity and differ in feed efficiency, behavior, and resistance to infectious and parasitic diseases. Today, Asia and Africa contain 58.2 and 36.2%, respectively, of the 1 billion goats worldwide with much smaller populations in Europe (1.7%), America (3.5%), and Oceania (0.4%). China (187.8 million heads), India (133 million heads), Nigeria (71 million heads), Pakistan (66.6 million heads), and Bangladesh (55.9 million heads) are the top five goat producers. In most countries, the sustained growth of the world goat population during the last 50 years (from 368 million heads in 1964 to 1006 million heads in 2014) has not involved a general improvement of the production and reproduction techniques associated with their management.

Well-organized selection programs are in contrast restricted to a few highly productive dairy breeds from Europe, North America, and Australia. Despite its low caprine census, Europe produces 17.5 and 42.5% of the goat milk and cheese, respectively, consumed around the world, reflecting the benefits of raising highly selected dairy breeds such as the Saanen, Alpine, and Toggenburg under semi-intensive or intensive conditions.

The main traits under selection are milk production, protein and fat contents, somatic cell count, and udder morphology. Globally, it has been proposed that 500–600 goat breeds exist; yet it is difficult to establish a reliable figure because several local populations are not managed via phenotypic standardization, herd book registration, and controlled reproduction. Among these breeds, 86 have spread beyond their countries of origin and are considered cosmopolitan or transboundary breeds, whereas 19 have become extinct, and about 90 are critically endangered or just endangered (such as Arapawa, Bagot,

Golden Guernsey, San Clemente, and Mallorquina), whereas 157 are not at risk.

Population decline of local goat breeds is mostly due to their replacement or uncontrolled crossbreeding with more productive foreign varieties, the progressive abandonment of low income rural activities, and the lack of genetic conservation programs. Some goat populations have escaped from captivity and became feral.

Horse

The wild ancestor of domestic horse is the now extinct, *Equus ferus* from central Asia. The Asian wild horse, *Equus przewalskii*, also significantly contributed to the genetic makeup of domestic horses. Even though there have been no confirmed sightings of wild Przewalski's horses since 1966, the species has been maintained in captivity for the last 90 years. In addition to Przewalski's horse, a third divergent lineage corresponding to a wild population that inhabited the Holarctic region has also contributed to the genome of modern domestic horses. Both archaeological and genetic evidence strongly support the onset of domestication of horse in the western Eurasian Steppes of Ukraine dating to 5500 years ago. Over the course of domestication, it has been argued that difficulties in maintaining domestic horse herd sizes during pastoral migrations led directly to restocking through the capture of wild females.

Horses were not only used as a source of meat and milk; their stamina and quickness provide humans with rapid transportation, which has considerably changed the speed and magnitude of the circulation of goods and people, as well as cultural exchange, including the spread of Indo-European languages, religions, science, and art, and diseases. With the introduction of the horse collar and horseshoes in agriculture, the horse was increasingly used for tilling soils, incrementing farmland productivity in medieval Europe, and remains today a crucial asset to the agriculture of the least-developed countries. With a few notable exceptions, such as the Arabian, Mongolian, and Icelandic horses, breeds have been created in the last two centuries. The earliest horse studbook, that of the Thoroughbred racing horses, was created in 1791.

The population structure resulting from selective breeding is characterized by high interbreed and low intrabreed genetic diversity. Domestic horses exhibit remarkable variation in coat coloration, including the bay or bay-dun wild-type phenotypes, other basic colors like chestnut and black, as well as dilution (e.g., cream and silver), and spotting patterns (e.g., leopard complex, tobiano, and sabino).

Horse locomotion has also been recurrently selected, including their ability to perform alternate gaits, such as four-beat, lateral, or diagonal ambling. Although some horse breeds, such as the Thoroughbred racing horses, are still extremely popular, a significant part of this great diversity is currently endangered: 87 horse breeds are already extinct, and among the remaining 905, almost a quarter are categorized as at risk.

GWAS, NGS, Microarray, and mtDNA

In domestic animals, the genome-wide association studies (GWAS) has become an important method to study the genomic regions involved in traits of concern with the sequencing of the pig, cow, and dog genomes. This method investigates the likelihood of the association of the genetic markers with a specific trait in domestic animals. The variation in these traits is due to intensive selective pressure elucidated by a small number of loci in these species. Consequently, in several domesticated species, GWAS have effectively recognized contributing genes both for complex traits and Mendelian traits controlled by loci with big influence size. The use of genome-wide methods initiated the microarray gene expression studies in the search for a group of genes or gene linkages involved in composite phenotypes in domesticated animals.

However, the use of microarray techniques is narrow due to their dependencies on the use of identified probes, needing species-specific markers for the most precise results. The introduction of next-generation sequencing (NGS) technologies has revolutionized the gene expression research by removing the need for prior probes for transcripts. RNA-seq or RNA sequencing requires the high-throughput reads generated by NGS to characterize the whole transcriptome: in other words, all transcripts generated in a tissue sample plus novel isoforms and formerly uncharacterized recorded sequences. RNA-seq is generally used for a range of applications, such as to compare the group of differentially expressed genes in tissue samples or samples from different experimental groups or populations.

Based on NGS or RNA-seq data, the individuals can be grouped into healthy or diseased by identifying the gene linkages associated with hereditary diseases or other genetic traits or by mapping various genetic loci. Furthermore, mtDNA technology was used to recognize the genomic regions associated with important phenotypic traits as well as to identify the evolutionary history and the origin of domestication in animal species as compared with nuclear markers. Since 2000, sequences of mtDNA fragments such as D-loop and cytochrome b regions have been used to study distribution of different domesticated animals, including dogs, sheep, pigs, goats, horses, chickens, donkeys, and cats, as well as those with more restricted dispersals, such as water buffalo, and zebu cattle. mtDNA research has provided a viewpoint, at least from the parental side, as to the probable ancestors and candidate pedigrees involved in the domestication of species.

Understanding the genetic basis of phenotypic variations is the major aim of genetics. Domestic animals offer a subjective opening for making significant improvement toward the goal of minimizing the gap between human biology and traditional model species. The continuous progress of high throughput sequencing technologies and modern bioinformatics approaches provide the complete genetic variation map of an individual, and it is now likely to test for phenotypic variation caused by single nucleotide polymorphisms (SNPs).

The genome-wide association studies (GWAS) and candidate gene approach are two primary methods that are currently followed to recognize genomic regions or genes affecting the particular trait. Population genomics has presented a new model for linking DNA with a phenotype that has been revealed as a selection signature analysis. This is a genome to phenotype method that includes the statistical assessment of population genomic data irrespective of phenotype to find out targets of the previous selection.

Selection analysis can be employed in the natural population so numerous species for which a high-density genetic record is available. An additional benefit is that it can detect selection if the preferred allele is previously fixed, while GWAS fails in such a condition.

SNP Chip

In modern researches, through using recent genomics technologies, it has become likely to explore the micro-evolutionary developments underlying animal domestication at the molecular level. In this regard, various studies that have been done to produce domestic red fox, silver foxes (*Vulpes vulpes*), and rats (*Rattus norvegicus*) have provided valuable understandings that were introduced during the middle of the twentieth century.

Furthermore, functional genomics, quantitative real-time PCR, microarray and reverse transcription studies of brain tissues from domestic dogs and wolves, transcriptional profiling through RNA-sequencing of rat brains combining genome mapping studies have identified numerous candidate genes and putative regulatory regions that have influenced docility and viciousness in animals. It is necessary to annotate that the acute changes in gene expression linked to domestication possibly affect the growing stages in a specific tissue and will require extensive work to be conclusive.

Gene enrichment analysis recognized that neurobiology is affected by the loci of those genes that were over-represented and targeted by directional selection, and principle functional analyses exposed that derived single nucleotide polymorphisms in developmental genes (*PAX2* and *SOX2*) were possible to be fixed within, or close to, regulatory sequences. Most remarkably, it was concluded that domestication was predominantly associated with selective sweeps causing genetic variations on regulatory regions throughout the animal genome, therefore indicating micro-evolutionary developments during the initial periods of domestication of vertebrate species.

Understanding the significance of single disease-associated SNP alleles itself is neither necessary nor enough in causal of a disease. Rather, it is possibly the collective consequence of a set of SNP alleles enclosed by key genes, plus environmental factors that jointly conclude whether an individual experiences a certain disease.

The association study process includes the frequency determination of test factor (e.g., an SNP allele) among several patients and in the race and age-matched controls. The determination of the validity of this test crucially depends on appropriate patient-to-control matching (population stratification).

Another way of performing association studies more efficiently is by limiting the SNPs through pre-selection by testing the pathogenic effects of SNPs. For the betterment of association studies design, one way is to exploit pathogenic allele's linkage disequilibrium. When there is strong linkage disequilibrium among the SNP marker and an unknown pathogenic allele, both can show a parallel association with the disease.

Nuclear Genes Epigenetics

More recently (since 2006), "next-generation sequencing" (NGS) technologies allowed access to the whole-genome sequences and gained new information about timing and location of domestication. These approaches expanded the scope of comparative genomics from single genes to gene families and entire genomes. Mutations in DNA can vary from a single polymorphism to gene duplication or even complete genome duplication leading to many consequences, including phenotypic alterations.

Additionally, a single gene can be involved in multiple, unrelated phenotypes, and genes of polygenic traits can act in combination to produce a single phenotype. The variations within the gene could be triggered by nucleotide exchange (non-synonymous or synonymous) or indels, which can generate adaptive, negative, or neutral alterations in the gene.

More recently, these approaches allowed the availability of genomes for several species and permitted the association of genes to specific traits of domestication in cattle, rabbits, sheep, pigs, horses, dogs, and ducks. Several other studies focus on the search for signatures of selection in those genes already described as important for the domestication process.

Paleogenomics, also known as genome-wide ancient DNA (aDNA) analysis, gives valuable information and has been crucial to investigate when, where, and how rapidly adaptive alleles spread in the populations. Indeed, recent studies using this approach provide new insights into the evolution and history of the cave bear and horses.

In livestock, biotechnology and conservative tools have contributed considerably to improve productivity, preserve genetic diversity, and enhance the adaptation to the environment. Furthermore, functional genomics, quantitative real-time PCR, microarray, and reverse transcription studies identified many candidate genes and putative regulatory regions that have influenced docility and viciousness in animals.

With these advances in technology, the genetic architecture of domestication and the domestication process in some species became clearer. For example, it was possible to discover that pig populations were domesticated in one place and then moved to new areas successively gained the mitochondrial signature of native wild populations. The same applies to other taxa. These new approaches also allowed to verify that African cattle are mixtures of "taurine" and "indicine" that possess both Y-chromosome signature and mitochondrial signals.

GENOMICS AND THE DOMESTICATION PROCESS

The development of genome technologies such as genome assembly by sequencing, whole-genome shotgun (WGS) method, NGS, and third-generation single-molecule sequencing tools are outstanding approaches are advancing our understanding to study animal domestication.

Genome sequencing of domesticated species not only provides important resources to answer the queries raised by Darwin but also provides prospects to discover the genetic origin of profitable traits in domesticated species.

The current information on genome projects highlights the demographic history, origins, and the artificial selection of domesticated animal species. Additionally, it was determined with a preview of future guidelines for animal domestication. Various techniques were established to allow the *de novo* assembly of genomes during the human genome project. The most effective technique was WGS sequencing, along with the building of physical maps. By 2009, four domesticated animals (horse, cat, dog, and taurine cattle) genomes and one wild species genome (the red jungle fowl) were sequenced and assembled based on this method.

The domestication process is demonstrated through the detection of selection at a very large number of genomic loci that have likely evolved by natural and artificial selection.

Recently, it has become possible to explore the domestication process by complete genome sequences analyses at high resolution to define how it has formed modern domestic animal. Several genomic loci such as the *DGAT1* gene that is associated with lactation traits comprise a major quantitative trait nucleotide has been identified putatively under the selection through genome-wide comparisons of data from modern taurine and indicine cattle.

Furthermore, 106 candidate genes were found under selection using population genomics approaches that were particularly involved in muscle development, growth, function, and immunity. This first genome-wide selection analyses detected genes that are considered as important candidates of domestication.

However, many methods are available to retrieve and sequence genomes routinely and recognize hundreds of genomic loci under selection through genotyping. It is revealed that paleogenomics techniques will be used to investigate when, where, and how rapidly adaptive alleles spread at the population in domestic animals.

Several arithmetical methods have been established by scientists to reveal diverse features of how to accomplish variations from and what is anticipated with respect to genetic differences in the neutral model. While all statistical methods are based on neutral genomic differences, not all of them are based on similar information. Most of the methods were established for complete sequence data and not for genome-wide pools of predetermined SNPs, which are presently accessible in few livestock species.

EPIGENETICS IN THE EVOLUTION OF THE DOMESTIC TRAITS

Evidence illustrates that in addition to genetic factors, epigenetic factors can affect the behavioral phenotypes as well as other traits within breed or species. For example, the difference in the behavior of the great tit is statistically linked to the DNA methylation at dopamine receptor genes.

Similarly, maternal behavior affects the DNA methylation of the hippocampal glucocorticoid receptor gene in rats. In domestic chickens, variances in DNA methylation are linked to disease exposure, immune reactions, metabolism, and growth.

Furthermore, epigenetic changes can occur just after individuals are exposed to various rearing environments. Although cell division maintains the DNA methylation patterns, sometimes these could be regulated by external stimuli.

The DNA methylation changes that are controlled by the environment can be transferred through the germline and remain unchanged over generations in somatic tissues. Somatic epigenetic changes can affect phenotypic traits, whether selected deliberately or involuntarily or formed by the environment.

Therefore, mechanisms of epigenetic changes could be an essential factor in the development of prompt phenotypic variations that arise during domestication. For example, these methylation changes are controlled by substantial hyper-methylation in domestic white Leghorn chickens as compared to the red jungle fowl, in pedigree dogs compared to wolves, and in domestic compared to wild worms.

Domestication Genes

As described above, selection played a crucial role during domestication accelerating phenotypic variations. Skin and coat color are considered the only domestic traits subject to early selection by humans, thus becoming an essential genetic marker. Coat color can have patterned (spotted, striped) and non-patterned (solid colors) phenotypes that are defined by the proportion of two pigments: eumelanin (black/brown) and pheomelanin (red/yellow). During the past years, this has been a central question in domestication studies, and *MC1R*, *ASIP*, *TYRP1*, *CBD103*, *KIT*, and *PMEL17* genes were associated with different traits in several species. A variety of mutations, including single nucleotide polymorphisms (SNPs), insertions, deletions, and duplications are responsible for coat color discrepancies in both domestic and wild populations.

ORIGIN OF ANIMAL BREEDING

The practice of animal breeding dates back to the Neolithic period (approximately 7000 BC), when people attempted to domesticate wild species such as caribou, goats, hogs and dogs. In Europe, the origin of animal breeding lays in the United Kingdom. It was Sir

Robert Bakewell (1725-1795) who introduced keeping accurate records of performance of animals so that objective selection became possible.

He used inbreeding (mating of related animals with similar traits) to fix certain characteristics in animals and he also introduced *progeny testing*: the method of evaluating performance of the first (small) group of progeny and use that information to select the best father of future progeny.

He promoted the idea to 'breed the best to the best'. Bakewell developed the New Leicester sheep from the old Lincolnshire breed. The New Leicester had good quality fleece and a good fatty shoulder that was popular at the time. Bakewell also noticed that Longhorn cattle were growing well and used less feed compared to other cattle. So he developed that further in order to grow more meat efficiently. It is amazing he did this without knowing anything about genetics.

Selective Breeding

Selective breeding is evolution by human selection. As nineteenth-century British naturalist Charles Darwin noted in *Variation of Animals and Plants under Domestication,* selective breeding may be methodical or unconscious. Methodical selection is oriented toward a predetermined standard, whereas unconscious selection is the result of biases in the preservation of valuable individuals. Methodical selection requires great care in discriminating among organisms and is capable of rapid change in specific traits, such as milk production or silk color. Unconscious selection, more common in ancient times, resulted in grains and seeds such as wheat, barley, oats, peas, and beans, and in animal traits such as speed and intelligence.

Selective Breeding Vs. Natural Selection

Like natural selection, selective breeding requires genetic variation on which to act. If the variation in a trait is strictly environmentally induced, then the selected variants will not be inherited by the next generation. Selective breeding also requires controlled mating. Thus, animals that are social and easily manipulated, such as **bovids** , sheep, and dogs, were easier targets for selective breeding than territorial species, such as cats and other carnivores. Cultures without a strong concept of property rights, such as those of pre-Columbian South America, were less likely to domesticate species because of their difficulty segregating different breeds. A short generation time also facilitates selective breeding by speeding up the response to selection. For example, most plants with multiple breeds (races) are annuals or biennials.

Selective breeding differs fundamentally from natural selection in that it favors **alleles** (forms of a gene) that do not contribute favorably to survival in the wild. Such alleles are usually **recessive** , for otherwise they would not persist in wild populations. Selective breeding is essentially a process of increasing the frequency of rare, recessive alleles to the point where they usually appear in homozygous form. Once the wild-type alleles are eliminated from the population, the process of domestication has become irreversible and the domestic species has become dependent on humans for its survival.

There is abundant evidence of the effectiveness of selective breeding. In general, there is more genetic variation among breeds of the same species for valuable traits than for others. For example, tubers are diverse among potatoes, bulbs are diverse among onions, fruits are diverse among melons. The implication is that selective breeding for valuable traits has created the diversity.

2

INTRODUCTION OF DNA IN ANIMAL BREEDING

INTRODUCTION

Genetic engineering is the name of a group of techniques used for direct genetic modification of organisms or population of organisms using recombination of DNA. These procedures are of use to identify, replicate, modify and transfer the genetic material of cells, tissues, or complete organisms. Genetic engineering in animal production has a growing number of practical benefits, such as in the production of transgenic animals resist to disease, increasing productivity of animals, in the treatment of genetic disorders and in the production of vaccines. This technology will supply various applications in biomedicine that are rather impossible without it. Away from economic constraints, there are concerns of well-being and ethics as introduction of genes from one organism to another may create alteration of the natural genetic balance and lead into unwanted consequences.

Although the existing limitations, the application of this radical technology to increase livestock productivity could be not satisfying in the Ethiopian context. The technology should also be sophisticated in a way to minimize well-being and ethical concerns. Different genes are responsible for the various characteristics and properties of a living organism. To change part of an organism's genome to create some desired or beneficial trait we use genetic engineering. Now it is possible to directly alter a genome and insert or remove a chunk of DNA to create something beneficial the rapid developments in the field of genetic engineering have given a new movement to biotechnology.

This introduces the possibility of dress making organisms to optimize the production of established or novel metabolites of commercial importance and of transferring genetic material from one organism to another. In order to achieve potential benefits of genetic engineering the only need is to develop perfect tools and techniques. Once it has been perfected, all the problems associated with food production can be solved, the world environment can be restored, and human health and lifestyle will be improved beyond imagination. No doubt that there are almost no limits to what can be achieved through responsible genetic engineering.

For that reason, the general objective of this review focuses on the application of genetic engineering to animals for genetic improvement of animal breeding, including a description of the methods, their potential and current uses, and ethical issues.

Until 1953, scientists used statistics and presumed mechanisms to make predictions about inheritance. Nobody knew what exactly was the mechanism behind it. But in 1953 Watson and Crick, using research results from Wilkins and Franklin, discovered the double helix structure of DNA and together they won the Nobel prize for their discovery. Since the discovery of the DNA structure a lot has happened. In the beginning studying the DNA was very labour intensive and thus also very costly.

Nowadays robots can perform large scale genotyping e.g. of more than 60,000 genetic markers on thousands of individuals within very limited amounts of time. A genetic marker can be considered a kind of 'flag' on the genome. Its location and composition ('looks') are known. These genetic markers can, for example, be used to compare animals based on the looks of the various flags.

Main idea behind genomic selection is that the association between the DNA make-up and performance of animals can add to the estimated breeding value, or even replace it. Because you don't have to wait until the phenotype can be measured on the animals anymore as you have the associated DNA information, you can select animals already at very early age and you don't have to wait until they become adult. You can also use this, for example, for traits that are difficult to measure such as disease related traits. The aim would be to prevent diseases in as many animals as possible.

It would be highly desirable if you would only need to infect a limited number of animals and measure their response to the infection, link that to their DNA, and use that estimated link to predict the sensitivity of other animals to that disease based on their DNA, without having to infect them. More about genomic selection later in this book. Meuwissen and Goddard (and co-workers) even take it a step further and already work on methods to incorporate full genomic sequences (all DNA in an individual) in estimating genomic breeding values. But large scale availability of full sequences is still something of the future, as that is currently still too expensive. But developments go fast you have to be prepared for the future.

GENETIC ENGINEERING: CONCEPTS

Genetic engineering is the name of a group of techniques used to identify, replicate, modify and transfer the genetic material of cells, tissues or complete organisms. This biotechnology of gene therapy, scientists are making efforts at curing genetic diseases by attempting to replace defective genes with the correct version and also used to produce more effective and efficient vaccines, therapeutic antibodies, antibiotics and other pharmaceuticals.

There are more than 370 drug products and vaccines obtained through biotechnology currently in clinical trials, targeting more than 200 diseases including various cancers, Alzheimer's disease, heart disease, diabetes, multiple sclerosis and arthritis. Animal breeding operates through the selection of genetically superior animals as parents for subsequent generations. So far artificial selection could therefore only be applied to traits which are "naturally" exhibiting genetic variation in the selected populations, i.e. traits characterized by some degree of "heritability".

The rate of genetic progress or of response to selection is a function of the accuracy of selection, i.e. the precision in the identification of genetically superior animals; the generation interval, the shorter the generation interval, the faster the genetic progress; the selection intensity, i.e. the more the future parental individuals deviate from the average breeding value of their contemporaries, the higher the genetic improvement they will cause.

Biotechnology is being applied to enhance genetic progress through these four factors: increase genetic variation (or the molecular substrate of breeding programmes), increase the accuracy of selection, and reduce the generation interval and to increase the selection intensity. Three major topics can be distinguished in the area of biotechnology applied to the genetic improvement of livestock: reproductive technologies, livestock genomics and marker assisted selection (MAS), and livestock transgenics

DNA AS CARRIER FROM GENETIC INFORMATION PASSED TO NEXT GENERATION

As a breeder you want to transfer the best genetic material you can get from the present to the next generation of animals. This genetic material is stored in the chromosomes in the nucleus of all cells of the animals that may be selected as parents for the next generation. This transfer process takes place with the transfer of chromosomes containing the genes via the creation of sperm cells and oocytes in the gonads.

The combination of a sperm cell and an oocyte into a zygote is the starting point of a new animal with a unique genetic composition. In the transfer of chromosomes from parents to offspring the meiosis plays an important role. It causes that the transfer is determined to some extend by laws, recognized by Mendel and to some extend by random processes. The laws connect genetically relatives, e.g. parents and their offspring: the parents each share for 50% the same chromosomes, the same DNA and thus the same genetic value with their offspring. Therefore phenotypic traits of parents, can be found in the phenotypic traits of their offspring, based on the genes they got from their parents. In conclusion: offspring and parents and more in general related animals share a part of their DNA; they have a genetic relationship.

Chromosomes as units of DNA

Body cells of mammals and birds have a nucleus where pairs of chromosomes (units of DNA) are found. Each species has a specific number of chromosomes as is illustrated in the table below:

Number of chromosome pairs for different species

Species	Number of chromosome pairs
Man	23
Cattle	30
Horse	32
Pig	19
Sheep	27
Goat	30
Rabbit	22
Chicken	39
Duck	40

GENETIC ENGINEERING AND ITS APPLICATION IN ANIMAL BREEDING

Genetic engineering is the name of a group of techniques used for direct genetic modification of organisms or population of organisms using recombination of DNA. These procedures are of use to identify, replicate, modify and transfer the genetic material of cells, tissues, or complete organisms.

Genetic engineering in animal production has a growing number of practical benefits, such as in the production of transgenic animals resist to disease, increasing productivity of animals, in the treatment of genetic disorders and in the production of vaccines. This technology will supply various applications in biomedicine that are rather impossible without it. Away from economic constraints, there are concerns of well-being and ethics as introduction of genes from one organism to another may create alteration of the natural genetic balance and lead into unwanted consequences.

Although the existing limitations, the application of this radical technology to increase livestock productivity could be not satisfying in the Ethiopian context. The technology should also be sophisticated in a way to minimize well-being and ethical concerns. Different genes are responsible for the various characteristics and properties of a living organism. To change part of an organism's genome to create some desired or beneficial trait we use genetic engineering. Now it is possible to directly alter a genome and insert or remove a chunk of DNA to create something beneficial the rapid developments in the field of genetic engineering have given a new movement to biotechnology. This introduces the possibility of dress making organisms to optimize the production of established or novel metabolites of commercial importance and of transferring genetic material from one organism to another.

In order to achieve potential benefits of genetic engineering the only need is to develop perfect tools and techniques. Once it has been perfected, all the problems associated with food production can be solved, the world environment can be restored, and human health and lifestyle will be improved beyond imagination. No doubt that there are almost no limits to what can be achieved through responsible genetic engineering. For that reason, the general objective of this review focuses on the application of genetic engineering to animals for genetic improvement of animal breeding, including a description of the methods, their potential and current uses, and ethical issues.

GENETIC ENGINEERING: CONCEPTS

Genetic engineering is the name of a group of techniques used to identify, replicate, modify and transfer the genetic material of cells, tissues or complete organisms. This biotechnology of gene therapy, scientists are making efforts at curing genetic diseases by attempting to replace defective genes with the correct version and also used to produce more effective and efficient vaccines, therapeutic antibodies, antibiotics and other pharmaceuticals.

There are more than 370 drug products and vaccines obtained through biotechnology currently in clinical trials, targeting more than 200 diseases including various cancers, Alzheimer's disease, heart disease, diabetes, multiple sclerosis and arthritis. Animal breeding operates through the selection of genetically superior animals as parents for subsequent generations. So far artificial selection could therefore only be applied to traits which are "naturally" exhibiting genetic variation in the selected populations, i.e. traits characterized by some degree of "heritability".

The rate of genetic progress or of response to selection is a function of the accuracy of selection, i.e. the precision in the identification of genetically superior animals; the generation interval, the shorter the generation interval, the faster the genetic progress; the selection intensity, i.e. the more the future parental individuals deviate from the average breeding value of their contemporaries, the higher the genetic improvement they will cause.

Biotechnology is being applied to enhance genetic progress through these four factors: increase genetic variation (or the molecular substrate of breeding programmes), increase the accuracy of selection, and reduce the generation interval and to increase the selection intensity. Three major topics can be distinguished in the area of biotechnology applied to the genetic improvement of livestock: reproductive technologies, livestock genomics and marker assisted selection (MAS), and livestock transgenics

TYPES OF GENETIC ENGINEERING APPLICATIONS IN ANIMAL BREEDING

Genetic engineering applications in animal breeding includes a description of the methods, their potential and current uses and ethical issues. Genetic engineering is the name of a group of techniques used to identify, replicate, modify and transfer the genetic material of cells, tissues or complete organisms. The important applications of genetic engineering in animal breeding are as follows:

Marker-assisted Selection (MAS)

The objective of this technology is to increase disease resistance, productivity and product quality in economically important animals by adding information of DNA markers to phenotypes and genealogies for selection decisions.

Transgenesis

The direct transfer of specific genes/alleles between individuals, species, or even Kingdoms, in order to change their phenotypic expression in the recipients. Compared to the 'traditional' improvement techniques based on phenotypic information only, these gene-by gene techniques allow theoretically a more complete management of animal genomes for animal breeding.

The MAS method is fruitful for traits with a simple genetic determinism but delivers unsatisfactory outcomes in many more complex conditions. The two key causes for this low productivity were the limited part of the genetic variance and also the low association between markers and QTL at population level. Another limitation of MAS is the expensive cast of genotyping of selection candidates, due to the benefits of MAS in commercial breeding programs.

GENOMIC SELECTION IN RUMINANTS

The objective of dense arrays for detection of SNPs has different implications according to the species of interest. In dairy cattle, it has been used to discover markers that will improve the reliability of traits associated with milk production, cow health, and cow conformation. Australia is the leading country in identifying genomic regions associated with milk production and several studies have also been completed in the United States, Canada and some other countries. Application of genomic estimation has caused significant changes in dairy cattle breeding; the reliability of genomic prediction in dairy cattle exceeds 0.8 for production traits and 0.7 for fertility and other traits.

The genotyping of young bull increased the genetic gain and also significantly lowered the cost compared to the genotyping of heifer calves. The lower cost of genomic selection compared to traditional methods has made an incredible impact on the development of dairy industry genomic selection could principally benefit more the beef cattle industry paralleled to dairy because beef cattle have long generation interval. Snags of saving phenotype data of satisfactory value and size hamper tradition methods for conventional evaluation; consequently, genomic selection has the efficiency to significantly improve the genetic gain by increasing selection reliability at an early age.

Techniques of Genetic Engineering

Exogenous pronuclear DNA Micro-injection in zygotes

Micro-injection is the first successful approach for the creation of transgenic animals based on the injection of a foreign DNA construct into a fertilized oocyte. The construct integrates randomly into the host oocyte genome, subsequently the zygote continues embryonic development and the embryo is transferred to a foster mother and eventually develops to a transgenic animal. However, this method has strong limitations: on average, less than 1% of embryos injected and 10% of animals born are transgenic, genes can only be added, not replaced or deleted, and multiple copies of the transgene are inserted at random, hindering the correct regulation of gene expression and possibly interfering with endogenous gene function. This requires large amounts of oocytes to be injected, as the overall efficiency of the process is very low.

Injection of genetically modified embryonic stem (ES) cells into blastocysts

Embryonic stem cells are derived from embryos at a very early stage (the blastula) and possess the important characteristics of pluripotency. Pluripotency is the ability of these cells to differentiate to any of the cell types and tissues found in the adult organism. Embryonic stem cells can be grown in culture for many passages and can be subjected to transformation with transgene constructs, resulting in modifications of their genome. The constructs used not only permit the selection of successfully transformed cells, but also allow gene targeting to be accomplished. Thus, genes can be specifically introduced, replaced or deleted (so-called knock-ins and knockouts). Injection of genetically modified embryonic stem (ES) cells into blastocysts, mainly through the feature of gene targeting, allows a broad variety of genetic modifications to be introduced. For many years, several laboratories worldwide have tried to produce ES cells from farm animals, and although some succe has been claimed, no robust and reproducible method has been published. Indeed, even in mice the production of ES cells is a costly and labor-intensive technology.

Retrovirus mediated gene transfer

Transgenes is may also be accomplished by employing virus derived vectors; namely, vectors based on the retrovirus-class of lenti viruses. Genes that are essential for viral replication are deleted from the viral genome, maintaining only the capacity for integration of the viral genome into the host genome. The parts of the viral genes can replaced by the transgene of interest, then viruses carrying the modified gene are produced in-vitro and subsequently injected into the perivitelline space of the zygote, resulting in infection of the zygote and integration of the viral genome into the host genome. Transgenesis rates reaching up to 100% of injected embryos have been described. Major drawbacks of this method are a limited transgene size and random transgene integration. Random and possibly multiple transgene integration may lead to position effects, disturbance of the host genome and dose effects, as is the case with pronuclear injection. Solving these problems holds great promise for the further development and application of lenti viral vectors.

USES OF ANIMAL GENETIC ENGINEERING

Increase animal disease resistance

Genetic engineering of agricultural animals has the potential to improve disease resistance by introducing specific genes into livestock. Identification of single genes in the major histo compatibility complex (MHC), which influence the immune response, was instrumental in the recognition of the genetic basis of disease resistance/susceptibility.

Animal biotechnology offers a number of approaches to fight diseases in animals. Firstly, through genetic selection, livestock producers can select for certain traits that are associated with disease resistance and populations of animals that are less vulnerable to diseases could be developed. Secondly, through genetic engineering, breeders can integrate disease resistance genes from new sources, allowing for improved animal health. Disease resistance benefits not only livestock producers and their animals, but consumers also benefit as a result of safer animal products in the market, and a reduction in the incidence of human-transmissible diseases such as avian influenza. Increased disease resistance can be achieved by introducing resistance-conferring gene constructs into animals or by depleting a susceptibility gene or locus from the animal. Hence, gain of function (additive) as well as loss of function (deletive, knock-out) gene transfer experiments can be used. Gene transfer experiments are often hampered by the lack of identified major genes or loci responsible for resistance.

Increase meat and milk production

The application of genetic engineering to increase milk and meat is a "value-added" opportunity in animal agriculture as it increases the concentration of existing proteins or producing entirely new proteins. Genetic engineering is important to increase milk and meat production of animals for the ever increasing human population in global. The production of human lysozyme in milk of transgenic mice also increased the antimicrobial properties of the milk, which in cows could reduce infections in the mammary gland and perhaps eliminate undesirable pathogens in the gut of humans who consume the milk.

Cattle are known as the best animals for producing large amounts of milk and/or meat and are regarded as a valuable protein resource. Evidences showed that the presence of 10 to 20% altered casein in milk produced by a transgenic cow could increase proteolysis and thereby promote the faster ripening of cheese. Results of experiments with transgenic mice illustrated the positive effects of adding genes such as the casein gene or human lysozyme gene to the milk protein system. The effects of genes encoding growth hormone- releasing factor (GRF) or insulin-like growth factor I (IGF- I) were reported in growth studies in mice and sheep. In pigs, there are evidences of transgene effects that reduced body fat and increased muscle fiber diameter by increasing IGF-I levels and growth hormone with no serious pathological side effects.

Improve wool production

The control of the quality, color, yield and ease of harvest of hair, wool and fiber for fabric and yarn production has been an area of focus for genetic engineering in livestock. The manipulation of the quality, length, fineness and crimp of the wool and hair fiber from sheep and goats has been examined using transgenic methods. The objectives aimed to improve sheep for wool production and to modify the properties of the fiber. Because cystein seems to be the limiting amino acid for wool synthesis, the approach is to increase its production through transfer of cystein biosynthesis from bacterial genes to sheep genome. Transgenic methods also allow improvements to fiber elasticity, surface and strength. Decreasing the surface interactions between fibers could decrease shrinkage of garments made from such fibers.

Vaccine production

Vaccination generally involves injecting weak live, killed, or inactivated forms of viruses or their toxins into the animal being immunized. Most conventional vaccines are killed microorganisms, inactivated bacterial toxins or live attenuated organisms. However, because the immune system acts only on a few protective immunogens, most molecular components of killed vaccines are redundant and or can cause adverse effects. To reduce these effects, nowadays, new technologies offer alternatives to classical vaccines. Most vaccines are now genetically modified. Genetically, engineered viruses are being developed that can still confer immunity, but lack the infectious sequences.

LIMITATIONS OF GENETIC ENGINEERING

Religious, cultural and ethical Issues

The current and potential impact of rapid developments in biotechnology to effect new innovations in medicine and drug development, as well as such diverse areas as crime detection, agriculture, pollution control and industrial processes, brings into question how these techniques can be used constructively without damaging the cornerstones of religious ethics like respect for human life. Revolutionary innovations in genetic engineering, the decoding of the human genome now make it possible for vegetables in our food chain to bear animal transgenes.

Economic constraints

The requirement of adequate infrastructure is a critical factor for the establishment of biotechnology companies. While research and development budgets for biotechnology research are only beginning to pick up in developing countries, start-up funding for biotechnology companies is still very rare to come by financing early stages of business development could be achieved through seed funding, easier access to loans and venture funds.

Antibiotic resistance

The major concern with the use of antibiotic resistance marker genes is that they will diminish the efficacy of antibiotics in humans and animals. The large presence of antibiotic resistance genes in the environment and soil, as well in the food eaten by animals and humans, could pass the trait of antibiotic resistance rapidly and widely. This can occur through a transfer of antibiotic resistance marker genes to bacteria in the guts of animals or humans, or to bacteria in the environment. Many bacteria have the ability to pick up genes from their surroundings and to pass these genes on to other species of bacteria including antibiotic resistance marker genes. Such genes might eventually find their way into diseasecausing bacteria, resulting in antibiotic resistance and therefore making treatment more difficult.

CONCLUSION

Genetic engineering in animal production has a growing number of practical benefits, such as in the production of transgenic animals resist to disease, increasing productivity of animals, in the treatment of genetic disorders and in the production of vaccines. This technology will provide various applications in biomedicine that are rather unthinkable without it. Apart from economic constraints, there are concerns of well-being and ethics as introduction of genes from one organism to another which may create alteration of the natural genetic balance and leads into undesirable consequences.

3

ORGANIZATION OF BREEDING ACTIVITIES

VETERINARY INSTITUTIONS

A net work of Veterinary Hospitals and Dispensaries manned by qualified Veterinarian have been established. These hospitals and dispensaries, besides undertaking treatment of ailing animals and birds, are taking preventive measures through immunisation for controlling specific diseases. To extend better health care service, Dispensaries and Veterinary Aid Centres have been established at convenient locations and are manned by suitable technical staff. Besides, there are Mobile Veterinary Dispensaries and Vigilance Units manned by the qualified Veterinarians to extend the facilities of animal health care etc. More new dispensaries and hospitals are being established to serve the people better. Action has also been taken to upgrade all the Aid Centres to Dispensaries.

CATTLE DEVELOPMENT

For all round development of Cattle wealth in the different parts, various development programmes such as Cattle Breeding Farms for producing inputs for distribution. Intensive Cattle Development Projects for cross breeding and upgradation programme have been taken up by the department. For peoples participation in production, incentives in the form of Grant in Aid and Subsidies are provided so that production status is enhanced to meet the demands.

CATTLE BREEDING FARMS

Four Cattle breeding farms - e.g. Indo-Danish Project, Upper Shillong, (East Khasi Hills); Regional Cross Bred Cattle Breeding Farm, Kyrdemkulai (Ri Bhoi District); Cattle Farm, Khliehtyrshi, (Jaintia Hills District) and Livestock Farm, Rongkhon (West Garo Hills) have been established to produce improved breeding stock for development of cattle in the State to boost up production of milk, Apart from this, these farms supply wholesome milk to the neighbouring urban areas and serve as the visual demonstration units in scientific method of rearing, feeding and management of cattle which includes fodder cultivation. One Buffalo Farm has also been established at Songsak (East Garo Hills) to initiate Buffalo Breeding Programme.

INTENSIVE CATTLE DEVELOPMENT PROJECT

The Intensive Cattle Development Project, one at Upper Shillong and the other at Tura, have been established in the State to take up an integrated approach in development of cattle breeding, fodder development etc. The objective of the project is to upgrade the local cows through introduction of better germplasm of the exotic Fresian and Jersey breeds and to induct the local tribal breeders to adopt modern scientific techniques in Animal Husbandry. The project also help to educate and encourage the farmers about requirement of feed and fodder. Subsidy for growing of fodder is also provided by the project. The activities of the project is discharged through a network of Stockman Centres established in different parts of the State. At present, Frozen Semen Technology is being used for artificial insemination service which are provided at the farmers door step. Two Liquid Nitrogen Plant has been installed in the state for the purpose.

Poultry Development

Poultry keeping is very common as a subsidiary occupation of the large section of the population both in the rural and urban areas. The general mass who cannot indulge in other Lucrative business, requiring very high capital, usually prefer this industry as the capital investment is very low and return anticipated within a short period of time. But in general poultry rearing is continuing in the traditional way as practiced earlier except in a very few cases, where improved types of birds are maintained in scientific manner. The open or free range system is the common practice of rearing poultry and ducks all over the State, whether in the rural or in the urban areas.

Proper housing, management, feeding and breeding for local poultry are not cared for in general. The birds which include chicks, adults and growers are let loose in search of feed and water from the field. Ducks rear in the ponds and other water logged areas. So the local poultry of the State, in general, has very low productivity yielding on an average a maximum of 105 eggs per layer in comparison to the improved birds yielding 200-230 eggs per layer or even more. The Poultry Development Programme of the State has, therefore, been directed towards increasing productivity of the poultry of the State by introducing improved breeds.

Efforts are also underway to put the Poultry Industry on a commercial footing by providing easy marketing facilities to poultry farmers. The Department has set up 10 Poultry Farms. One of these farms is the Regional Poultry Breeding Farm, Kyrdemkulai and the rest are the District Poultry Farms. The objective of these farms is to serve the purpose of experimentation, demonstration and production of eggs beside the main purpose for rearing chicks for distribution amongst the poultry rearers. One Broiler farm has been set up at Kyrdemkulai to produce one lakh broiler chicks annually for distribution to the District Poultry Farms and private farmers to meet the requirement of broiler meat in the State. Considering the requirement of poultry meat and eggs as well as the high cost of poultry feed ingredients the department have introduced low input breed of birds which can thrive well under the Meghalaya village conditions with a good return. This breed of bird is very much resistant to diseases and hence very much preferred by the villagers as economic loss is negligible. At present Poultry Farm Umsning and Rongkhon are producing low input breed of chicks and supplying to the farmers. Another such Farm is being established at Jowai.

Piggery Development

Pig rearing is an integral part of rural life in Meghalaya. The pig is an amazing creature for the service of mankind. Its high adaptability to a wide range of environments, resistance to diseases, high reproductive efficiency and adjustable feeding habits makes the pig the ideal meat animal of choice for the North Eastern States like Meghalaya.

It is this pig which can meet the challenge of Protein Hunger of the State. Given the adequate environment including housing, feeding, management and disease control, rearing of pigs throughout the State would be ideal as is already noticed in the State Pig Farms particularly the one at Kyrdemkulai. Departmental efforts in future plans would be directed to extend supply of quality pigs along with infra-structural support for input supplies, services, disease control and marketing in all the villages covering all the blocks in the State in a phased manner. In fact, Piggery development in Meghalaya demands a massive effort on PRIORITY basis.

It is here the State can build an all-India reputation which no other livestock in the State can ever match. At present the department have introduced Hampshire, Saddle Back and other Cross Breed Pigs for producing inputs for supplying to the farmers for upgradation of local indigenous stock so that production level is enhanced.

Sheep, Goat and Rabbit Development

Though the climatic situation is not very much conducive for sheep rearing, goats constitute a member of the rural family and more than 1.09 Lakhs Sheep and Goats are slaughtered annually producing about 1092 MT of meat per year. Khasi Hill Goat is a recognised breed of goats, which is on the verge of extinction. Steps are, therefore being taken to conserve and increase its population through selective breeding in State Farms. Goat keeping is also a commercially viable proposition and its development to the desired level is called for, Rabbit production has a good potentiality in the State. Initial trial has been made by the State Department as an introduction to the people in the State which shows promise for further initiative in this direction.

Feed and Fodder Development

Application of new technology supported by good management and health care, can produce a potential high yielding animal but without sustained supply of required level of nutritious feed such stock will not prove its worth. It is, therefore, essential that attempt should be made for ensured supply of feed. Feed is generally divided into (a) Concentrates, and, (b) Roughages. In concentrates, the D.C.P : T.D.N., ratio is narrow but well balanced and its requirement is much less as compared to roughages and it bridges the gap between the demand and availability of nutrition from roughages.

Roughages are bulky but cheap and normally available locally as by-products of agriculture specially cereal crops. Though remarkable advancement has been achieved in agricultural production, little attempt has been made towards development of animal feed whereas more and more land has been brought under plough ignoring the land capability and encroaching upon forest and grass cover. The shrinkage of forest and grass cover has been reflected in shortage of fuel wood and fodder. Realising such a situation all over the country afforestation programmes have been taken up with fodder development as a joint effort of the Forest and Animal Husbandry Departments.

Setting up of Agro-Forest/Silviculture/Social Forestry always incorporate grassland and fodder farming as components. Paucity of feed ingredients are one of the hurdle faced by the Livestock and Poultry rearers in the state. Most of the ingredients are to be imported from other states and therefore the cost of mixed feed is very high and not affordable to the poor farmers of the state. Effort are on to overcome such problem so that Animal Husbandry activities get a boost and thereby improves the rural economy.

DAIRY ACTIVITIES

Under Dairy Development, the main objective of the schemes are for overall development of Dairy Sector like supply of wholesome milk to consumers. Generally, milk is procured from different Dairy Co-operative Societies and farmers where it is being brought to the different Dairy Plants for pasturing the same before distribution to the consumers. The different schemes implemented under this sector are :-

- Cattle Cum Dairy Development Project
- Dairy Plants
- Rural Dairy Extension Centres
- Creamery and Ghee Making Centres
- Chilling Centres
- Schemes for Employment Generation for Educated Un-employed Youth
- Establishment of Marketing Packaging Centre
- Integrated Dairy Development Project under non operation flood for Hilly and Backward areas

BREED IMPROVEMENT PROGRAMME USING SUPERIOR GERMPLASM

Objectives:

- Progressive genetic improvement for milk production in important breed/type of cows and buffaloes by following scientific methods.
- Production and distribution of superior pedigreed bulls for use in Cattle and Buffalo Breeding Programme.
- Conservation of Indigenous Cattle Breeds germ-plasm.
- Upgrading non-descript low productive cattle by crossbreeding
- To bring non-productive/ infertile animals into production by making them fertile through infertility camps
- Making non-descript scrub bulls/calves sterile by castration for preventing breed deterioration

Indigenous Cattle & Buffalo Breed Improvement Programme

To preserve and develop the well recognized indigenous breeds of cattle of the state, the indigenous breed improvement programme is being operated in the native tract of cattle breeds viz. Gir (Jaipur, Sikar, Alwar, Dausa, Jhunjhunu, Ajmer, Bhilwara, Tonk, Udaipur, Chiitorgarh, Dungerpur, Banswara, Rajasamand, Pratapgarh, Kota, Bundi, Jhalawar, Baran, Bharatpur, Karauli, Swaimadhopur, Dholpur), Tharparkar (Jaipur, Sikar, Alwar, Dausa, Jhunjhunu, Nagour, Jodhpur, Pali, Jaisalmer, Barmer, Bikaner, Churu, Ganaganagar, Hanumangarh); Rathi (Bikaner, Churu, Ganaganagar, Hanumangarh), Kankrej (Sirohi, Jalore) and Nagauri (Nagaur district) & Buffallo breeds Murrah (for all state) and Surti(for Udaipur Division)

The frozen semen of the selected bulls of these breeds is provided for artificial insemination in animals of the respective breeds and genetic improvement is achieved by selective breeding / up gradation of the animals in the respective breed tract.

Goat Development Programme

Rajasthan is having 3 well known breeds of goats viz.: Jakharana, Sirohi, and Marwari breeds. The goat population of Rajasthan is more than 216 millions.

The programme for goat development is mainly aimed to help in improving the weaker sections of society. There are goat farms of the department working at Ramsar in Ajmer district, Cattle Breeding Farm, Nagaur and Kumher at Bharatpur District. Goat development programme is aimed to develop Sirohi goats in ten districts of South-Western regions of the State viz.: Ajmer, Pali, Sirohi, Bhilwara, Rajasmand, Chittorgarh, Dungarpur, Banswara, Nagaur and Udaipur. Sirohi breed kids of about 4-6 months age are selected from the home tract and are reared at Ramsar farm Ajmer and Cattle Breeding farm, Nagaur. The bucks of Jamunapari breed of goat are being reared at Cattle Breeding farm, Kumher, in Bharatpur District. These bucks are distributed in Bharatpur, Dholpur, Karauli, Alwar and SawaiMadhopur Districts.

These elite Sirohi/Jamunapari bucks after attaining breeding age are distributed to goat breeders @ Rs.1200 to BPL /ST/SC families and to others @ Rs. 1600 per Buck.

Sheep Breeding Programme

To improve the sheep population of the state genetically by providing superior breeding males (rams) to the sheep breeders, Department is running a Sheep Breeding Farm. According to the departmental sheep breeding policy, the indigenous pure breed Ram (Chokala, Nali and Marwari) of the farm has been distributed to sheep breeders @ Rs. 50/- per Kg live weight. In the year 2018-19, the farm has distributed 243 proven Rams at subsidized cost to sheep breeders.

Pig Breeding Programme

The pig is one of the most efficient animals having great food conversion efficiency among domesticated livestock that can play an important role in improving the socio-economic as well as nutritional status of the weaker sections of the society. The Department has established one Piggery Development Training Centre at Alwar where 3 days training programme is being conducted free of cost. Five batches of 25 pig farmers each training programs has been conducted in 2018-19. A pig breeding farm is maintained at Alwar. The large white Yorkshire pigs are provided to pig breeders for scientific breed improvement. Unit of pig (3 male + 1 female) is being supplied in the state especially to the Schedule Caste, Tribes and marginal farmers. This Pig unit (3+1) is being distributed to the Socially Backward Classes on subsidized rates i.e. @ Rs. 5000 per Unit.

VETERINARY HEALTH CARE & DISEASE CONTROL PROGRAMME

The veterinary health coverage programme is the most vital input for the livestock production programme. The genetic traits of the superior exotic and crossbred livestock cannot be exploited fully unless they are provided specialized health care and management as they are highly susceptible to the diseases. There has been continuous increase in the number of Veterinary Institutions in the State.

a. **Veterinary Health Care Programme:**- The health of the animals of the state is being taken care of by 7897 veterinary institutions comprising of 35 Polyclinics (VPC), 785, First Grade Veterinary Hospitals (VHF), 1710 Veterinary Hospitals (VH), 198 Veterinary Dispensaries, 5067 Sub-Centers (SC),102 District Mobile Veterinary Unit(DMVU). These institutions are situated in far flung areas of the state. The sub-centers and dispensaries are headed by technical subordinate staff i.e. Livestock Assistant (LSA) & Veterinary Assistant (VA), respectively. Whereas the VH, VHF & VPCs are headed by the state officer cadre staff i.e. Veterinary Officer

(VO), Senior Veterinary Officer (SVO) and Deputy Director (DD), respectively. All these institutions are stationary with working jurisdiction of villages falling in their 8 Km radius area.

b. **Disease Control Programme:-** The animals are vaccinated regularly against many fatal diseases viz. Haemorrhagic Septicaemia (HS), Black quarter (BQ), Enterotoxaemia (ET), Sheep Pox, Foot & Mouth Disease (FMD), PPR, Brucella and Rabies.

   The vaccination is done at a nominal cost i.eRs. 1.00 per dose for HS/BQ, Rs. 0.50 per dose for ET/Sheep Pox. Registration fee of Rs. 2.00 is charged for PPR, FMD, Brucella..

c. **Biological Production Unit (B.P.Lab):-** State Biological Product Laboratory, situated at Agra Road, Jamdoli Jaipur-302007, is producing various types of vaccines viz. Haemorrhagic Septicemia (HS), Black quarter (BQ), Enterotoxaemia (ET) etc. for effective control of diseases in the state.

d. **Disease Diagnostic Centres:-** Department is providing animal disease diagnostic facilities through One State Disease Diagnostic Centre, 6 Regional Disease Diagnostic Centres and 27 Disease Diagnostic Laboratories at District headquarters to the vast livestock population. For effective control of diseases in animals, the department is running a programme under Assistance to States for Control of Animal Diseases (ASCAD)

e. **Assistance to States for Control of Animal Diseases (ASCAD):-** This is a scheme of Government of India. Under this component, assistance is provided to State Governments for control of economically important diseases of livestock and poultry by way of immunization, strengthening of existing State Veterinary Biological Production Units, strengthening of existing Disease Diagnostic Laboratories, holding workshops/seminars and in-service training to Veterinarians and Para-veterinarians to carry out Disease Investigation work in the state through a network of Laboratories located at Capital, various Divisional & District places.

   1. State Disease Diagnostic Centre Jaipur.

   2. Regional Disease Diagnostic Centres Kota, Ajmer, Udaipur, Jodhpur, Bikaner & Bhagalpur.

- State Disease Diagnostic Centre, Jaipur:- The lab is controlled by Joint Director. All other disease d iagnostic laboratories of the districts except Jaipur are under the administrative control of their respective district Joint Directors, while technically these are controlled by Joint Director, SDDC Jaipur. SDDC acts as a referral unit for diagnosis and extends expert opinion to various departmental institutions like RDDCs, DDLs, Veterinary polyclinics, Veterinary Hospitals, Veterinary Dispensaries etc. Besides this it also conducts routine diagnostic work on the material received from the field Institutions. SDDC is recently upgraded to BSL –II, with this status centre equipped and authorized to screen Avian Influenza in the State.

- Regional Disease Diagnostic Centre Kota, Ajmer, Udaipur, Jodhpur, Bikaner &Bhagalpur: - The lab is controlled by Deputy Director. All regional disease diagnostic centres are under the administrative control of their respective Additional Director (Range), while technically these are controlled by Joint Director SDDC Jaipur. RDDC acts as a referral unit for diagnosis and extends expert opinion to various departmental institutions like, DDLs, Veterinary polyclinics, Veterinary Hospitals, Veterinary Dispensaries etc besides this it also conducts routine diagnostic work on the material received from the field Institutions.
- District Disease Diagnostic Laboratory- The Laboratory functions as a Disease investigation unit for diagnosis and extending expert opinion to various departmental Institutions at district level. Besides this it also conducts routine diagnostic work on the material received from the field Institutions.
- Poultry Disease Diagnostic Laboratory- One Poultry Disease Diagnostic Laboratory headed by a Deputy Director under the control of Joint Director SDDC Jaipur is working at Gandhinagar, Jaipur.
- Facilities available: - Routine pathological examination like Blood and Faecal examination, Screening of dairy animals for Brucella, Tuberculosis & Johne's Disease, Screening of Poultry farms for important diseases like Salmonellosis. Lab to Land Programme, Collection of sample of different Disease e.g. FMD, PPR, IBR, Swine Fever, Glander, Rabies & other disease.

Important Achievements

- The labs have completed the National Programme on Rinder-Pest Eradication successfully as per the O.I.E. mandate.
- Elisa Labs have been started at Jaipur, Jodhpur, Kota and Udaipur.

a. **Animal Disease Control:-** For surveillance & monitoring of disease there is extensive network of disease surveillance in the department. The Animal Disease Control Section responsible for monitoring & control of outbreaks of animal diseases and its containment.

   Simultaneously it also helps in containment of zoonotic diseases of public health importance. For any outbreak the veterinary hospital at field level, Joint director at district level and Joint director ADC, can be contacted at Directorate level.

b. **Anti Rabies Unit:-** In the state at Jaipur & Ajmer two units are functioning for control of rabies, under the scheme mass vaccination of pet dogs are performed through routine OPD services in respective policlinics.

EXTENSION ACTIVITIES

a. **Poultry Development Programme:-**A major breakthrough has been made in the field of development of high producing strains of layer stock in the State. One state level poultry farms is situated at Khatipura, Jaipur and a State disease diagnostic laboratory of poultry is also functioning at Gandhinagar, Jaipur.

b. **Livestock Marketing:** - Rajasthan is the home tract of various breeds of different livestock species. With a view to encourage the livestock farming and to maintain these important famous breeds of the livestock, 10 state level cattle fairs are organized every year by the department in the different parts of the State. The Animal Breeders earn about Rs. 25-30 Crore annually through the sale of the animals. Besides these state level cattle fairs, nearly 240 cattle fairs are also organized by different agencies like Panchayat Samities, Nagar Palikas etc. in the State.

c. **State Level Cattle Fairs:**- The heritage of Rajasthan and its cultural diversities is well projected in the various state level fairs conducted by the state Animal Husbandry department. These fairs are conducted with an aim to draw their attention to the scientific and technical developments in the Animal Husbandry sector and to motivate them for developing and rearing elite animals. These fairs are an appropriate source for sale and purchase of livestock adding to the income of livestock owners / breeders.

d. **Fodder Development:** - Balanced feeding is essential to fully exploit the genetic potential of livestock. In the State, fodder production is still deemed ancillary to agricultural production. Crop residues mainly sorghum, maize, Wheat and Bajra straws that are poor in nutritive value constitute the major fodder for livestock. If the animals are not properly fed the overall effects will be negative as far as breeding and management is concerned. Better feeding alone can bring about an increase of 30% in milk production.

   The green fodder availability is restricted to selected areas and seasons. High population pressure on grazing lands has led to depletion and over exploitation of available grazing lands. In addition, rapid urbanization has led to shrinking of grazing lands. Moreover, with the increasing pressure on land for growing food grains, oil seeds and pulses and diversified use of agriculture residues, the gap between the demand and supply of fodder is increasing.

   Presently under National Livestock Mission Programme fodder production from non forest/wasteland/grassland/non-arable land is running in four departmental farms.

e. **Goshala Development Programme:** - Under the Rajasthan Goshala Act 1960 till now 2727 Goshalas has been registered. These Goshalas have been established by the public trusts for maintaining old, infirm, unproductive cows and its progeny. Goshalas may be used for preservation & conservation of indigenous breeds. The central government as well as state government is also assisting these Goshalas for cattle development. For details contact to Joint Director, Goshala, Directorate of Animal Husbandry, Rajasthan, Jaipur.

f. **Training Programme:-**

1. **Poultry Training Programme** **15days poultry training programme for Veterinary Officer & paravets ** one month training programme for Poultry breeders Ajmer & Jaipur

2. **Three days Piggery Training** Alwar
3. **15 days A.I. Training Programme** KVS – Jaipur & Jodhpur
4. **3 days, 7 days & 15 days Refresher Courses for Veterinarians:** RSLMTI, Jaipur

e. **Sheep Migration:-** Migration of sheep is a regular feature of sheep rearing in the western parts of Rajasthan. Sheep from southern parts of Jodhpur-Jaisalmer pass through Bali, Abu-road through Palanpur, reach up to river beds in Baroda, and Surat where they spend about two months. Similarly sheep from northern parts of these regions go through Sawai-Madhopur or Hindauncity to river bank in Mathura. Usually, the farmers set out on their journey in winter and return to their homes in early monsoon. In Churu, Jhunjhunu and Sikar districts the flocks are relatively stable and they migrate for short period from their home village to grazing areas in neighboring villages when the local pastures are exhausted.

FUTURE ROLE OF BIOTECHNOLOGIES IN THE CONSERVATION AND IMPROVED USE OF ANIMAL GENETIC RESOURCES

Over the past decade there has been widespread concern about the loss of valuable animal genetic resources through indiscriminate crossbreeding, breed replacement and neglect. The concern has intensified over time despite the potential of new techniques to artificially generate new genetic variation. So why all the concern? In short, the elegance, sophistication and subtlety of nature is still poorly understood. Much remains to be learnt about the creation, maintenance and evolutionary role of natural genetic variation before man can sensibly devise ways for its more effective utilization in a sustainable manner. For this reason alone, protection of the world's genetic resource base is a high priority.

The purpose of this paper is to discuss how DNA based technologies can contribute to the conservation and utilization of animal genetic resources. Three main areas have been addressed. These are the storage of DNA from threatened breeds/strains, the analysis of population structure to prioritize breeds for conservation and the mapping of genes unique to adapted breeds. Ways of measuring genetic variability at the DNA level will also be considered since they are central to more effective use of genetic resources.

Collection and storage of DNA

The genetic information essential for the development, growth and efficient functioning of animals is housed within the DNA molecule. In higher mammals, around 3000 million individual bits of information are stored in each of the billions of cells that make up the entire organism.

When conservation of this genetic information is considered, it is essential to preserve a sample that is representative of the organism, to purify and preserve it in a way that maintains the basic structure of the DNA molecule, and to store the DNA in alternative forms that allow easy access to the genetic information. Biochemical methods are available to meet these requirements.

Structure and Properties of DNA

Fortunately DNA is a very resilient molecule. The four basic nucleotides are linked by a sugar-phosphate backbone forming a long molecule (e.g. a chromosome) that may be up to 100 million nucleotides in length. Two complementary strands are combined in a double helix formation held together by hydrogen bonds. In cattle, the entire genetic information content is found within sixty chromosomes in the nucleus of each cell.

To attain the high degree of condensation that is required to allow such large DNA molecules to be physically housed in the cell nucleus, the DNA is wound around protein molecules and stacked in highly space efficient tertiary structures.

It is the extraordinary length of the DNA molecules together with their highly ordered packing that imparts mechanical and chemical stability.

DNA can be treated with organic solvents, exposed to natural enzymes, heated to 75°C, desiccated and stored for thousands of years and its basic structure can still remain intact. It is however not totally impervious to damage. To be conserved efficiently it must be collected and stored with care.

Harvesting DNA

DNA is present in virtually every mammalian cell type. Any tissue, therefore, is a source of DNA. The ease of extracting the DNA is usually dependent on the tissue type. In dense tissues such as skin and tendon, DNA is difficult to obtain as the cells cannot be dissociated easily. Blood, however, provides an excellent source of loose cells and accessible DNA. A variety of DNA extraction procedures exist each of which incorporate the same basic principles. The cells must be ruptured, endogenous DNA degrading enzymes denatured and removed, the DNA packing protein removed, all lingering traces of any organic solvents removed, and the DNA re-solubilized in a stable buffer. These procedures apply to specialized organelle DNA such as mitochondrial DNA, as well as nuclear genomic DNA. Care must be taken to minimize the physical breakage of DNA, as large molecular size is essential for some analytical procedures.

Storage of DNA

DNA can be stably stored in a variety of ways. The method of choice often relates to the quantities of DNA required and to its intended use.

Tissue

The most basic storage form is frozen whole tissue. In this form, large amounts of DNA and RNA can be maintained with little preparation. The feasibility of this procedure is evident in the ability to recover DNA from whole mammals that have been entombed in glaciers for several thousand years. The key to the success of this method is rapid freezing of the tissue, and constant low temperature during the storage. RNA is not as well suited as DNA to long term storage in this form. An obvious drawback is the potential bulk of the tissue samples, with the exception of frozen semen. Semen samples have a high concentration of DNA and represent a convenient tissue for collection as well as long term storage. In addition, use can be made of existing artificial breeding infrastructures.

Cells/nuclei

Tissue bulk can be minimized by reducing the tissue to a whole cell or cell nuclei preparation before freezing. By removing the cellular cytoplasm in the nuclei preparation, the potential for autolysis by endogenous nucleases is also reduced. An alternative to dead cell storage is the generation of cell cultures from tissues such as skin or lymphocytes. This provides a pure, dissociated cell type that can be multiplied before harvesting the cells for storage as intact cells or as cell nuclei. The cell lines can also be stored live by freezing in liquid nitrogen, stored, and then revived and re-multiplied as necessary. However there is a risk of somatic mutations occurring as the cell line multiplies, thus creating material that is not identical to the original animal source.

Pure DNA

Purified DNA is certainly the preferred choice for the long term stable storage of DNA. Once dissociated from all protein, and free from bacterial or fungal contaminants, DNA can be stored indefinitely at - 20°C. A 10ml/10mg quantity of DNA extracted from any tissue and distributed in a number of "banks" could provide the basic resource from the conservation of the entire genetic information from a representative individual.

Libraries

Within the context of genetic conservation, there not only needs to be a means of storing a genetic resource; there also needs to be a method by which the information stored can be retrieved, studied and if necessary reused. The cloning of DNA into "libraries" can achieve this. A gene library is a representative portion of the genomic DNA that has been inserted into a "vector". Amplification of a library allows any single DNA fragment to be multiplied many times in number thereby facilitating analysis. Libraries can also be derived from an RNA rather than DNA source. Such libraries contain the genes that were transcriptionally active in the original tissue. Both RNA and DNA libraries can be used as a storage source of genetic information. However the biological limitations of cloning mean that libraries are not always fully representative. These libraries do, however, offer the only means to identify and isolate entire genes, and as such offer an opportunity to investigate important production characteristics found in exotic and threatened domestic animals.

DNA and RNA Storage in Conservation Programmes

At the present time, live animals cannot be regenerated from isolated DNA. Therefore DNA storage is complementary rather than an alternative to cryopreservation of semen and embryos and the in situ preservation of animals. DNA does contain the essential genetic information that allows each animal to express its particular phenotype. It is therefore a crucial resource in investigating the function of each gene. As the function of newly discovered genes are elucidated, their role in animal growth development and survival can be determined. DNA cloning together with gene transfer technologies allow single genes, modified genes, or gene systems to be expressed in novel genetic backgrounds. These technologies make very effective use of stored DNA. A situation can be envisaged where a desirable production gene is identified using DNA marker analysis on stored DNA samples of a particular breed, the gene is isolated from a DNA or RNA library made from a representative of the breed, and the gene reintroduced and expressed in the genome of the donor breed. Hence the unique gene is conserved and propagated.

The storage of RNA as cDNA libraries derived from RNA must be an integral part of a conservation programme. RNA allows individual genes to be rapidly isolated, and the gene product expressed. The collection of a representative sample of RNA from an organism is very difficult due to tissue and time specific expression of genes. Hence a broad based collection of RNA could not be considered in the same manner as DNA. Conservation of RNA stocks in the form of cDNA libraries would have to be undertaken on a more selective basis.

The type and amount of stored genetic material should be related to the risk of losing a particular breed and the cost of storing different forms. In general DNA storage is cheap relative to live animal or embryo storage. For breeds at low risk, storage of purified DNA is adequate insurance. However for high risk breeds, DNA, tissue and RNA (in library form) should be preserved for future use. DNA banks should be viewed as genetic information resources for future use.

DNA sequence variation

In the process of domestication, limited population size and an increasing reliance on "superior" animals, genetic variation is reduced. Techniques for the analysis of variability are therefore an essential ingredient for conservation programmes. These techniques can be used to analyze the phylogeny of breed divergence, to follow gene segregation within populations, and ultimately, to associate nucleotide variation with changes in gene function and expression of animal phenotype. The most appropriate techniques for assessing DNA variation in a variety of applications include sequencing, Restriction Fragment Length Polymorphisms and conformational polymorphisms.

Sequencing

DNA sequencing provides the highest level of resolution that can be obtained in genome analysis. Sequence analysis reveals the fundamental structure of genes and allows an understanding of how nucleotide variation can influence gene expression. The concept of total genome sequencing is rapidly gaining acceptance with new automated sequencing technologies beginning to demonstrate the feasibility of the task. The sequencing of full mammalian genomes is understandably a massive undertaking, but not an unrealistic one. It is already practical to use DNA sequencing to analyze nucleotide variation in large animal populations. Using Polymerase Chain Reaction (PCR) and cycle sequencing technologies, highly variable sections of the genome can be rapidly analyzed in a moderate number of individuals.

Restriction Fragment Length Polymorphisms

Simple Length Polymorphism

Nucleotide variation can be highlighted by bacterial restriction enzymes which cut genomic DNA at specific sequences. Variation at the enzyme target site or insertions or deletions of DNA sequences between two enzyme sites produce fragments of variable length. The cut genomic DNA is size sorted by electrophoresis in agarose gels and then transferred to nylon support membranes. The specific DNA fragments of interest can be highlighted on the membranes by hybridization with labelled DNA probes. Unfortunately, simple RFLPs only exploit a fraction of the total variation in DNA sequence because only mutations which change the relative position of restrictive enzyme sites are detected. This is an important consideration in domestic animals since variability is lower than other outbred mammals.

RFLP systems can be made more informative by altering the analysis technique to produce multiple alleles. This can be achieved in two ways. Firstly by using a long DNA probe (e.g. 50 kbp), a haplotype of many restriction fragments may be revealed with the same enzyme. Secondly, the polymerase chain reaction (PCR) can be used to generate a fragment in the region of interest, which is then cut with numerous high cutting frequency restriction enzymes. The resulting multi-fragment pattern can be visualized on a high resolution acrylamide gel. Both procedures do however have practical drawbacks. In haplotyping, the large DNA probe often contains highly repetitive DNA which mask the RFLP signal, and the multicut PCR method requires the nucleotide sequence of the marker region to be known. In many cases, the difficulties of RFLP systems can be overcome by simply using DNA markers that are more polymorphic.

Minisatellites

Another class of RFLPs arises not due to point mutations or chromosomal rearrangements but to variability in the number of repetitive DNA elements. The polymorphism is revealed by restriction enzymes which cut the DNA outside the repetitive sequence.

Minisatellites are fragments of DNA characterized by the tandem repetition of a sequence usually around 25 bp in length. The DNA is visualized by gel electrophoresis, blotting and DNA probing. Variation in the number of repeats can be high, with some loci in humans being heterozygous in 99% of individuals. In cattle the mean heterozygosity of 50 minisatellite loci was found to be 51%. Minisatellite loci exist in high numbers in any genome, and there is a strong sequence similarity between many of these loci. Thus when the genomic DNA is visualized by a minisatellite probe at low DNA hybridization stringencies, many loci become visible simultaneously.

This results in a DNA fingerprint, which permits the absolute identification of animals, and under certain circumstances, provides a means of rapidly screening genomes to find DNA markers that are linked to production genes. When used at high stringency, minisatellite probes reveal only two alleles, but with a high probability that the locus is heterozygous and with different length alleles in each parent in a pedigree. This greatly expands the amount of genotype information available for analysis of genetic linkage between a DNA marker and a production trait. One possible limitation to minisatellite systems is a non-random distribution of genomic loci, with a bias towards chromosome telomeres. There may be some regions of a genome which do not have minisatellite sequences.

Microsatellites

DNA microsatellites are highly variable polyallelic systems composed of DNA repeated in tandem at each locus. The tandem repeats in microsatellites are usually simple dinucleotides (such as $(CA)_n$) with each dinucleotide repeated on average twenty times. The length of each allele is determined by PCR analysis using unique oligonucleotide primers flanking the repeat sequence. The DNA products are visualized on sequencing gels. There are thought to be around 100,000 microsatellite loci in any animal genome, which means that any position on the genome lies within 25–50 kbp of a microsatellite. With such a widespread genome coverage and the ability to run up to five microsatellite loci in a single 'multiplexed' PCR, microsatellite systems have an analytical power approaching the level of minisatellite systems and are more convenient to use.

Conformational polymorphism

Single strand conformational polymorphism (SSCP)

SSCP techniques are a rapid and relatively simple means of detecting most DNA sequence changes. They rely on the concept that the conformation of a DNA strand is altered by a nucleotide change, and this new conformation can be detected as a mobility shift in gel electrophoresis. The method does require either sequence information for PCR primer sites at the site to be analyzed, or a DNA probe that will bind at the site.

DNA variability, conservation and animal improvement

Quantifying genetic variability at the DNA level is an important requirement for rational conservation and improvement programmes. The following sections will discuss in detail how DNA variation can be used to define population structures and how it can be associated with phenotypic variability.

Population structure analysis

The selection of breeds or strains of livestock for conservation or improvement programmes can be hampered by an inadequate description of population structure both within and between populations. Geographic isolation over time has built up a plethora of genetic types but the magnitude of genetic differentiation has rarely been quantified. The situation is further clouded when recent crossbreeding has occurred. A key element of the conservation strategy must be the characterization of breeds and strains to provide an overall picture of genetic diversity. The choice of appropriate populations for conservation or improvement should be based on a combination of phenotypic and genetic data.

General approach

A preliminary classification of livestock diversity, based largely on phenotypic observations has been made. However further refinements are necessary. DNA based measures of variation are potentially very useful in this work. The procedure basically involves four steps:

A. Obtain representative samples from described populations - sample numbers will be determined from breeding structure and planned analysis methods.

B. Measure between and within population genetic variation. A number of alternative systems have been discussed their applicability to population structure analysis.

C. Calculate indices of genetic similarity/dissimilarity between populations. A large number of indices have been proposed, through the most widely used index, probably because of its conceptual appeal, is that of genetic distance. Other measures may be more useful for short term evolution such as the divergence between livestock breeds.

D. Construct phylogenetic trees to describe both the current population structure and the evolutionary history of sub populations.

Clearly the success of each study is very dependent on the effectiveness of the sampling procedure and the extent to which variation in the total genome can be reassessed. A major limitation in the past has been the limited capacity to measure genetic variability at the DNA level. However, this limitation is now removed.

Measurement of genetic variability

Genetic variability can be measured in nuclear DNA or in the maternally inherited mitochondrial DNA. The latter type has the advantage of being unaffected by meiotic recombination. On the other hand, mitochondrial DNA is more subject to genetic bottlenecks. Thus it is advisable to use both sources of genetic information. Where the genetic distance between populations is likely to be relatively small, sensitive measures of variability are required. For this reason, protein polymorphisms or RFLPs are generally not sufficiently variable for efficient use. On the other hand, repetitive sequences such as mini-and micro-satellites, although characterized by hypervariability, will underestimate the rate of genetic divergence because repeat units are both added and subtracted during evolution.

Conventional RFLPs, which reveal less than 20% of total sequence variation, are now being supplemented with conformational polymorphisms such as SSCP, which are of course equally applicable to nuclear and mitochondrial DNA analysis.

However, with the advent of direct sequencing methods, which avoid the need for subcloning steps, the sequence analysis of discrete regions of DNA is now being used for genetic divergence studies. Mitochondrial DNA has been widely used for evolutionary studies because of its rapid evolution. In particular the displacement (D) loop contains several hypervariable (non coding) regions which can be readily sequenced. Such studies have recently been initiated in cattle in an attempt to quantify differences between African, Indian and European cattle breeds. (D. Bradley, personal communication) With automation of sequencing now achieved, it is likely that future studies in other livestock species will also use sequence analysis as the primary method. However phenotype information and, where appropriate protein polymorphism data, should also be considered.

Gene mapping

The future use of animal genetic resources will be based on identification of genes associated with specific phenotypic characteristics. Techniques for rapidly mapping and isolating genes and characterizing them in terms of DNA structure and function are being refined. It is likely that in the near future, breeds and strains of livestock with unique or rare characteristics will be able to be characterized at the molecular level. The advantage of this approach is that utilization of unique or rare alleles will be greatly facilitated through programmes to introduce variants of genes into other populations, or to increase the frequency of such alleles within existing populations.

In the following sections, the current status of gene maps for livestock will be briefly reviewed and strategies for mapping individual genes will be discussed.

Gene maps

Gene maps have three main functions. First, they serve as repositories for gene mapping data ie. the location, order and spacing of genes or genetic markers. Second, maps can be used to facilitate mapping of new genes by providing reference points for searches. Third, by cross-referencing gene mapping information from one mammalian species to another, homologous chromosomal regions can be identified thereby permitting the extrapolation of information on gene location. Thus gene maps are an extremely valuable resource for mapping studies.

Physical maps

Physical gene maps indicate the location of genes on specific chromosomes, chromosomal regions or syntenic groups. The latter comprise groups of genes known to reside on a chromosome of unknown identity. The coordinates and therefore units of a localization will depend on the mapping method used. For example, at present, somatic cell hybrid analysis in cattle can map genes to either the chromosomal or syntenic group level. However, in situ hybridization results in assignment to chromosomal region with reference to a banded karyotype. Recent developments in the use of nonradioactive methods of hybridization to interphase chromosomes have greatly increased mapping resolution. Pulsed field gel electrophoresis is used for fine scale mapping where distances are measured in base pairs of DNA.

A recent summary on the status of mammalian gene maps (Table 1), demonstrates that relatively few of the estimated 50 – 100,000 genes have been localized on mammalian genomes. However, research effect in this area is increasing worldwide, particularly with recent initiatives in human genome mapping.

Table 1. Current status of physical gene maps in various mammalian species

	Haploid Chromosome No.	No. Syntenic Groups	Number of Genes Mapped
Human	23	23	2500
Mouse	20	20	2200
Cattle	30	29	250
Sheep	27	19	50
Pig	19	17	80

As far as livestock are concerned, the cow is the best documented species. However, it must be realized that only around 25% of the mapped genes have been regionally assigned as distinct from localization to only a chromosome or syntenic group. Thus the task ahead for livestock gene mapping is considerable.

On the other hand, there will be considerable spinoffs to livestock from genome research in other species. Much of the basic work on genome organization and function will be carried out in man, mouse and other experimental organisms such as yeast, Drosophila, C. elegans, and E. coli. As will be discussed later, opportunities for making use of this information are considerable.

Genetic maps

Genetic or linkage maps document the order and spacing of genes or genetic markers where distances are measured in recombination units.

The frequency of recombination between homologous chromosomes, a normal event in meiosis, is generally proportional to the distance between two linked loci and can therefore be used as a unit of chromosomal length. The unit, is known as the Morgan (M), and one centimorgan (cM) corresponds to the distance separating two loci exhibiting a 1% recombination rate. For short distances, eg. less than 30cM, the relationship between physical distances and recombination rate is essentially linear. However over longer distances, interference and the occurrence of double crossovers can reduce the concordance.

Measuring recombination rates or linkage relies on being able to distinguish parental and recombinant genotypes. It therefore requires polymorphism to be defined at each locus, and the analysis of segregation from doubly heterozygous individuals. Recently, it has become possible to genotype individual gametes ie. sperm and ova. However, genetic contribution is generally inferred for the genotypes of offspring and linkage studies are carried out within families.

As discussed earlier, there are a wide range of polymorphic markers available. However the most numerous and in many ways the most practical are based on DNA sequence variation. Accordingly, such markers are now being widely studied. Each marker permits the segregation of a discrete chromosomal region to be followed. Pairs of flanking markers provide even greater precision.

It is difficult to assess the current status of genetic maps of livestock for two reasons. First, there is currently a large amount of activity around the world directed at linkage maps in all of the economically important livestock species. Thus even a recently published list is quickly out of date. Second, some research is being carried out in the private sector and for reasons of competitive advantage, is not being published. To take the linkage map of the cow as an example, the most recent published report cites a total of 8 linkage groups comprising 64 markers. However, our own group alone has mapped a further 80 markers in the past two years and we are aware of another group which has mapped more than 100 other markers.

The challenge in the future will be to collate all the linkage information generated within a species into a common framework. In other words, there is a need to avoid the construction of a large number of genetic maps for a single species with little cross-referencing between them. This will arise if different markers are mapped in different sets of families. Although there will probably be some differences in recombination rate between strains and breeds of the same species, their magnitude will be relatively small in most cases.

To this end, the use of common sets of reference families have been proposed. By sharing a limited number of families for use worldwide, the collation of linkage data is greatly simplified. Reference families for cattle are being distributed and such families are being prepared in other livestock species.

A complete linkage map is a powerful tool for gene mapping since it permits systematic and thorough searches of the genome for genes and genetic regions associated with specific traits. An initial goal is a 20cM index marker map ie. where the maximum spacing between polymorphic markers on the chromosome is 20cM. Given that it is not presently possible to choose from where on the genome the markers are isolated, the initial strategy must be to randomly map markers. At some later stage, chromosomal regions which are underpresented with markers can be targeted.

Assuming a total map length of 30M as for humans, and a marker spacing of 20cM, an index maker map of the genome will require around 150 polymorphic markers. In order to achieve this target when markers are isolated at random, in excess of 500 markers will be required for each livestock species. However, 80% genome coverage could be achieved with around half that number. Index maker maps, based on a subset of available markers will be then used in the systematic analysis of the genomes.

Comparative maps

Comparative gene mapping involves the mapping of homologous gene loci in multiple species. The principal aim is to identify the boundaries of genomic conservation between evolutionary divergent species. Although the ultimate goal of comparative mapping is to understand the pathways by which chromosomal evolution has accompanied speciation, it has proved to be a very powerful means of extrapolating mapping data from one species to another based on the establishment of conserved chromosomal segments.

Extensive gene and chromosomal homologies have now been identified between man and mouse and between man, mouse and the cow. Although the boundaries of conserved segments need further definition, it is now possible to both interpolate and extrapolate the position of genes between these three species. Thus as genes are mapped as one species, their likely position in the other species can be predicted. This will be an important source of mapping information in the future since genome research in human and mouse has accelerated rapidly.

Chromosomal homologies between closely related livestock species have been observed at the cytogenetic level. For instance, the banded karyotypes of sheep and cattle have been matched up almost perfectly and homology has been confirmed by in situ localization of a number of genes. Although some minor rearrangements affecting the spacing, and in some cases the order of genes can be expected, it will be possible to exchange information between the cow and sheep gene maps.

Strategies for mapping genes

There are basically two approaches to mapping genes for which the gene product is unknown. The first of these, referred to as the candidate gene approach, relies on some background biochemical knowledge and is therefore limited in its application. The second approach which defines a linked genetic marker as an intermediate step towards cloning the gene is more generally applicable because it requires no knowledge of gene function. The two approaches are not mutually exclusive. Once the search for a gene is narrowed down to a discrete region, other genes may suggest themselves as candidates where previously they were not obviously connected. So in practice, a combination of both approaches is appropriate, especially as mammalian gene maps become denser, providing a larger number of potential candidates.

Candidate genes

The candidate gene approach is an attractive option because it may give a quick answer and involves an element of hypothesis testing. However, the selection of candidates should be based on solid biochemical data or physiological observations. It should be appreciated that an altered level of a particular enzyme or other gene product does not imply an alteration in the structural gene for that product. Gene expression is frequently very complex, involving a number of regulatory genes, in some cases located on distant parts of the genome to the structural gene. Nevertheless, the hypothesis of whether variability at or around the site of a gene exists, can be tested if appropriate reagents and/or sequence information and pedigrees are available. The requirements include multigeneration pedigrees with appropriate genotype and or phenotype data.

The optimum pedigree structures will differ depending on whether simple or polygenic inheritance is expected. Secondly, there is a requirement to measure genetic variability at the candidate gene locus. DNA markers are most frequently used for this purpose. By analyzing for co-segregation at the candidate gene locus and locus of interest, the hypothesis can be tested. Since the candidate gene marker effectively tags a segment of DNA, the involvement of other genes on that segment is tested simultaneously.

There are reports in the literature where candidate gene approaches have been successful. Presumably there are many other unpublished studies which have produced negative results. In cattle, a number of single gene disorders have been mapped and diagnostic marker tests developed via candidate genes. These include Pompe's Disease, and Bovine Leucocyte Antigen Deficiency. The gene for malignant hypothermia in man and pigs was mapped in a similar way. In all cases, detailed biochemical data suggested a strong candidate.

Linked markers

Another approach to mapping genes involves an initial localization to a chromosomal segment via anonymous genetic markers. Detailed analysis of the segment can refine the localization. This approach procedure, part of the so called 'Reverse Genetics' approach to gene analysis, is inherently more laborious, but, if used methodically has a higher probability of success. The approach is equally applicable to simply inherited and polygenic effects although the optimum pedigree structures will vary and there is a limit to the size of gene effects detectable in the polygenic situation. The basic procedure involves genotyping multigeneration families, which have been phenotyped for the trait of interest.

The probability of detecting a linked marker or markers is directly related to the distribution of markers and the number of informative matings for linkage analysis. Ideally, the markers will be chosen from an index marker map to ensure complete screening of the genome with a minimum number of markers. However, such maps are not yet available for livestock.

Assuming there are sufficient informative meioses to be analyzed, linkage between one or more of the markers and the gene or associated phenotypic effect should be found. By localizing the markers, if they have not already been mapped, the chromosomal segment carrying the gene of interest can be defined. This is a very significant step for two reasons.

First, it considerably narrows down the area to be analyzed for closer markers. Second, an approximate localization of a gene allows a re-evaluation of possible candidate genes which have previously been mapped to this region. Homologous regions in other genomes can also be surveyed, thereby expanding the number of potential candidates. Recent reports where the approach of firstly localizing a gene marker followed by successfully selecting from candidate genes in the region include studies on Waardenburg's syndrome and hypertension.

Isolation of a gene by using positional cloning techniques is still not a trivial task, although recent successes include Type 1 - Neurofibromatosis and the testis determining factor. Nevertheless, once a gene has been mapped by flanking markers, it can be efficiently tagged within families, and used in marker based selection programmes.

Analysis of quantitative traits

By and large, the traits related to growth, reproduction, fitness, milk production, parasite and disease resistance and tolerance to climatic variables are characterized by continuous variation. Differences between individuals are of a quantitative rather than qualitative nature. This has led to the assumption that such traits are controlled by a large number of genes, each of small effect . The true genetic basis of quantitative traits has until recently, remained largely unknown, because studies were general based on statistical methods of low power. More recently and with the use of molecular genetic techniques, a more intensive analysis of quantitative traits has begun.

Evidence is accumulating that variability in such traits may be associated with a small a combination of a small number of genes of intermediate to large effect e.g. 0.2 – 1.5 phenotypic standard deviations, and an unknown number of genes of smaller effect. Recent studies on yield traits in maize, water use efficiency in tomatoes, fruit mass, and fruit pH in tomatoes and predisposition to hypertension in rats have strongly suggested a range of gene effects.

The contribution of intermediate - large effect genes to the total genetic variation, will be small if the ir frequency is either low or high. As molecular techniques for genome analysis in livestock are refined, it is becoming feasible to analyze the genetic basis of quantitative traits. It is clear that the utilization of such genes, which may be unique to specific populations, will be facilitated by genetic markers. However the resources required to map such genes are substantial and it will therefore be important to optimize experimental designs in order to maximize the probability of success.

Experimental designs for quantitative trait analysis

Quantitative trait analysis measures the association between specific chromosomal segments tagged by markers and phenotypic effects. The phenotypic effects are assumed to be due to the presence of one gene or several genes on the chromosomal segment. Matings are only informative if one or both of the parents are heterozygous for both the marker and gene. The design of QTL mapping experiments fall into two categories viz analysis of crosses between breeds/lines and analyses of families within populations.

Design considerations have recently been reviewed. In an extension of the crossed line design, M. MacKinnon (unpublished) has evaluated within family analysis of F_1 sires resulting from crosses of divergent breeds.

General conclusions from these studies are:

1. The analysis of either backcross or F2 families is highly efficient where alternative alleles have been fixed or allele frequencies are very different (eg. 0.8 vs 0.2) in the two breeds/lines. However if allele frequency differences are less than 0.5, there is considerable loss of power over some within family designs.
2. F_1 cross sire families are frequently as efficient for quantitative trait analysis as F_2 families, since the availability of polyallelic markers considerably reduce the need to genotype dams. However progeny group sizes must be larger than normal, eg. 100 – 150, for reasonable efficiency. F_1 cross sire families are inefficient at detecting rare alleles in one of the parental breeds and are less sensitive to dominance effects than the F_2 design.
3. The analysis of families within straightbred populations generally has low power because the frequency of sires heterozygous at both marker and quantitative trait locus is normally low. Progeny testing can however significantly improve power.

Overall, the power of mapping experiments can be further improved by selective genotyping, interval mapping and the use of DNA pools. Nevertheless, the required animal and laboratory resources remain substantial. Yet such experiments are likely to be the best approach to analyzing the genetic basis of quantitative traits, and are directly applicable to exotic and rare livestock breeds.

Crosses between resistant and susceptible cattle breeds are being generated in an attempt to understand the inheritance of trypanosomiasis in Africa. Other breeds with unique characteristics or adaptations could be utilized in a similar way.

4

RESULTS OF ANIMAL BREEDING

Domestication has shaped and continues to shape the characteristics of domestic animal species through artificial genetic selection. This has led to considerable differences both between and within domestic animal species, but also to a number of similarities: Domestic species tend to have a reduced brain size, increased reproduction and growth, decreased fearfulness, and increased social motivation compared with their wild counterparts. Domestication started thousands of years ago; however only in the past 50 to 60 years has intensive selection for increased meat and egg production taken place, resulting in large increases in productivity. This intensive selection on increased productivity has contributed to a number of welfare issues, such as cardiovascular problems in broiler chickens. Since the early 1980s, awareness of these welfare issues and research to address them has been increasing.

On the other hand, genetic selection can also be used to alleviate welfare problems in farm animals. This can be done by direct selection against undesired behaviors, such as aggression in pigs or feather pecking in laying hens, but also by more general approaches, aiming to select for animals that are suitable for large-group housing. Genomic tools hold great promise for enabling genetic selection for complex traits, including behavioral traits. A principal aim of new breeding technologies is to advance the rate of genetic progress, and predicted that genomic selection could double the rate of genetic progress in dairy cattle. Genomic tools therefore also enhance the risk of greatly accelerating the rate of any undesirable changes in traits of welfare significance that are correlated to the trait under selection. Approaches where we adapt the animals by genetic selection should always be combined with approaches to optimize the environment of the animals.

Welfare will probably play an important role in future breeding goals for domestic animals. For some species, welfare traits are already part of the breeding index (e.g., lameness in dairy cows and fecal egg count in sheep). This review will focus on the relationship between genetic selection and animal welfare, describing the genetic variation between and within species.

Selective animal breeding already has almost 300 years of history. A lot has been achieved since. Obvious results have been achieved in the field of dog breeding. Selective breeding has produced very tall dogs like the Irish Wolfhound (>71 cm), very heavy dogs, like the Boerboel (50-80 kg), very small dogs like the Chihuahua (20 cm), very fast dogs like the Greyhound (17.5 m/sec), and very many more breeds with different looks and purposes. The size of the genetic improvement from generation to generation depends on the technique used to select animals for breeding. Introduction of new selection techniques made it possible to select the best animals for breeding more accurately and efficiently. Especially the introduction of reproduction techniques like artificial insemination (AI), that made it possible to have (very) large numbers of offspring per father, made it possible to select only the very best males for breeding, without decreasing the population in size.

Techniques with similar effect on number of offspring per parent are not available for the female reproduction, but also in females techniques like embryo transplantation (ET) or ovum pickup have made it possible to produce much larger number of offspring of excellent females than with normal reproduction techniques in species where normally only one or few offspring per year were feasible.

Modern livestock production is characterized by intensification, i.e., a higher number of animals per farm. To achieve successful intensification of livestock production, without negative effects on animals, farmers and farms, certain requirements need to be met. One of these requirements for intensification of livestock production is the capability of the farmer to take care of a larger number of animals. This requires healthy and easy-to-manage animals that need little/less attention time. Resilient animals are animals that need little/less attention time: increasing resilience is therefore desired. Improvement of resilience can be realized by different strategies.

One strategy is to increase resilience by genetic selection in breeding programs. The advantage of genetic selection, in contrast to management improvements, is that it is cumulative and affects all subsequent generations of livestock.

We define resilience as "the capacity of the animal to be minimally affected by disturbances or to rapidly return to the state pertained before exposure to a disturbance". Several definitions of resilience, and resilience-associated concepts have been discussed in literature: robustness, tolerance, resistance, GxE interaction, genetic heterogeneity of environmental variance, plasticity, environmental sensitivity, canalization, (developmental) stability, and residual within-individual phenotypic variation.

EVALUATION OF ANIMALS

Methods of ranking animals for breeding purposes have changed as statistical and genetic knowledge has increased. Along with increases in breeding knowledge, advancements in computing have enabled breeders to quickly and easily process routine breeding evaluations, as well as to develop research needed to rank large populations of animals.

Evaluating and ranking candidates for selection depends on equating their performance record to a statistical model. A performance record (y) can be expressed asy = g + e + e, where g stands for genetic effects, e indicates known (categorized) environmental effects, and e indicates random environmental effects.

The first task in estimating g is to statistically eliminate environmental effects, a process that involves setting up a system of equations to simultaneously solve for all of the genetic effects for the sires and cows. Information from relatives is included in g and increases the accuracy of evaluation of the candidates for selection. All relatives that are available can be incorporated in this type of evaluation. This model is called the animal model.

The animal model is used extensively in evaluating beef and dairy cattle, chickens, and pigs. To apply this model for evaluating large populations requires use of high-speed computers and extensive use of advanced mathematical techniques from numerical analysis. In evaluating the dairy cattle in the United States, a system of equations with more than 25 million variables is needed.

ACCURACY OF SELECTION

In some cases the accuracy of selection for a trait can be measured using a calibrated tool or a scale. Thus, measurements of such traits can be replicated with high reliability. Alternatively, some traits are difficult to measure on an objective scale, in which case a well-designed subjective scoring method can be effective. An excellent example is hip dysplasia, a degenerative disease of the hip joints that is common in many large dog breeds. Apparently, hip dysplasia is not associated with a single allele, making its incidence very difficult to control. However, an index has been developed by radiologists that allows young dogs to be assigned a score indicating their likelihood of developing the disease as they age.

In 1997 American animal geneticist E.A. Leighton reported that, in fewer than five generations of selection in a breeding experiment using these scores, the incidence of canine hip dysplasia in German shepherd dogs measured at 12 to 16 months of age had decreased from the breed average of 55 percent to 24 percent among the experimental population; in Labrador retrievers the incidence dropped from 30 to 10 percent.

Because close relatives share many genes, an examination of the relatives of a candidate for breeding can improve accuracy of selection. The more complete the genealogical record, or pedigree, the more effective the selection process. A pedigree is most useful when the heritability of a trait is relatively low, especially for traits that are expressed later in life or in only one sex.

Reproductive techniques can be used to increase the rate of genetic progress. In particular, for species that are mostly bred by artificial insemination, the best dams can be chosen and induced to superovulate, or release multiple eggs from their ovaries. These eggs are fertilized in the uterus and then flushed out in a nonsurgical procedure that does not impair future conception of the donor female. Using this procedure, valuable females can produce more than one calf per year. Each embryo is implanted in a less-valuable host female to be carried through gestation. The sex of the embryos can be determined in utero at about 50 days of gestation. The normal gestation for Holstein-Friesian cattle is about 280 days, so this early determination of sex saves many days and allows the breeding program to be adjusted. In particular, the donor cow could be collected again, or another superior cow could be bred to produce males. Thus, these reproductive technologies reduce the generation interval and increase selection intensity by getting more than one male calf from superior females. Both superovulation and sex determination are now commonly used procedures. Superovulation is also used when breeders want to increase the number of female calves from a valuable cow.

BREEDING SYSTEMS

Crossbreeding

Crossbreeding involves the mating of animals from two breeds. Normally, breeds are chosen that have complementary traits that will enhance the offsprings' economic value. An example is the crossbreeding of Yorkshire and Duroc breeds of pigs. Yorkshires have acceptable rates of gain in muscle mass and produce large litters, and Durocs are very muscular and have other acceptable traits, so these breeds are complementary. Another example is Angus and Charolais beef cattle. Angus produce high-quality beef and Charolais are especially large, so crossbreeding produces an animal with acceptable quality and size.

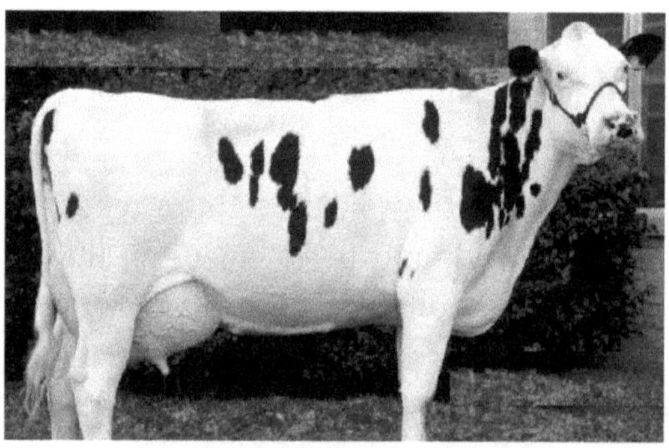

Fig. 1 Holstein-Friesian cow.

The other consideration in crossbreeding is heterosis, or hybrid vigour, which is displayed when the offspring performance exceeds the average performance of the parent breeds. This is a common phenomenon in which increased size, growth rate, and fertility are displayed by crossbred offspring, especially when the breeds are more genetically dissimilar. Such increases generally do not increase in successive generations of crossbred stock, so purebred lines must be retained for crossbreeding and for continual improvement in the parent breeds. In general, there is more heterosis for traits with low heritability. In particular, heterosis is thought to be associated with the collective action of many genes having small effects individually but large effects cumulatively. Because of hybrid vigour, a high proportion of commercial pork and beef come from crossbred animals.

BENEFITS OF IMPROVED LIVESTOCK GENETICS

Farmers breed animals for increased production, disease resistance, successful reproduction, and resilience to climate stresses, most often heat and drought. Highly productive animals use a greater portion of their nutritional intake to produce desired goods such as milk or meat as opposed to simply maintaining their bodies. Increased longevity and reproductive success also means that feed calories are concentrated among most productive, and that a lower number of animals needs to be kept in a herd for replacements.

Animal breeding makes use of the natural variation among animals. It can yield permanent and cumulative improvements in the population because the selected traits are directly transferred from generation to generation.

Genetic recording schemes are already in place in many developed countries. The brief cites research from the United States, where improved dairy cow productivity and associated feed conversion efficiency has decreased methane produced per unit of product by 40%. This indicates the potential for very large reductions in emissions intensity in countries that currently have lower levels of productivity.

The brief identifies rapid pathways for globally improving the genetic performance of ruminants, and associated methane mitigation in tropical, developing countries. Options include genetic improvement programs within a breed, or crossbreeding to transfer traits of interest from one breed to another.

RESULTS OBTAINED IN CATTLE BREEDING

Reproduction is an important consideration in the economics of cattle production. In the absence of regular breeding and calving at the appropriate time, cattle rearing will not be profitable. A healthy calf each year is the usual goal. This is possible only by increasing the reproductive efficiency of the animals.Successful reproduction encompasses the ability to mate, the capacity to conceive and to nourish the embryo and deliver the viable young ones at the end of a normal gestation period. In fact, interruption in this chain of events leads to failure of the cow either to conceive or the embryo to die or to have a premature delivery of the foetus.The reproductive efficiency is a complex phenomenon controlled by both genetic and non-genetic factors, the non- genetic factors being climate, nutrition, and level of management. The reproductive efficiency varies not only between species and breeds but also among the animals within the same breed. Even the best feeding and management can not coax performance beyond the genetic limit of an inferior animal. Improving the genetic merits of livestock populations is important at all levels of management. A sound breeding programme is a necessary part of the total animal production system.

Breeding Efficiency

Factors Affecting Breeding Efficiency

The factors which influence the breeding efficiency of cattle are as follows:

Number of ova

The first limitation on the breeding efficiency of fertility of an animal is the number of functional ova released during each cycle of ovulation. Ovulation is the process of shedding of ovum from the Graffian follicle. In the case of cow, usually a single ovum is capable of undergoing fertilization only for a period of 5-10 hours. Therefore, the time of mating insemination in relation to ovulation is important for effective fertilization.

Percentage of fertilization

The second limitation is fertilization of ova. Failure to be fertilized may result from several causes. The spermatozoa may be few or low in vitality. The service may be either too early or too late. so that the sperms and eggs do not meet at the right moment, to result in fertilization.

Embryonic death

From the time of fertilization till birth, embryonic mortality may occur due to a variety of reasons. Hormone deficiency or imbalance may cause failure of implantation of fertilized ova which die subsequently. Death may occur as a result of lethal genes for which the embryos are homozygous. Other causes may be accidents in development, over-crowding in the uterus, insufficient nutrition or infections in tile uterus.

Age of first pregnancy

Breeding efficiency may be lowered seriously by increasing the age of first breeding. Females bred at a lower age are likely to appear stunted during the first lactation, but their mature size is affected little by their having been bred early.

Frequency of pregnancy

The breeding efficiency can be greatly enhanced by lowering the interval between successive pregnancies. The wise general policy is to breed for the first time at an early age and to rebreed at almost the earliest opportunity after each pregnancy. In this way the lifetime efficiency is increased. Cows can be rebred in 9-12 weeks after parturition.

Longevity

The length of life of the parent is an important part of breeding efficiency, because the return over feed cost is greater in increased length of life. Also, it affects the possibility of improving the breed. The longer the life of the parents, the smaller the percentage of cows needed for replacement every year.

Management Practices to Improve Breeding Efficiency

Some of the management suggestions which will tend to improve breeding efficiency of cattle are listed below.

1. Keep accurate breeding records of dates of heat, service and parturition. Use records in predicting the dates of heat and observe the females carefully for heat.
2. Breed cows during near the end of mid heat or heat period.
3. Have females with abnormal discharges examined and treated by veterinarian.
4. Call a veterinarian to examine females not settled after three services.
5. Get the females checked for pregnancy at 45 days to 60 days after breeding.
6. Buy replacements only from healthy herds and test them before putting them in your herd.
7. Have the females give birth in isolation, preferably in a parturition room and clean up and sterilize the area once parturition is over.
8. Follow a programme of disease prevention, test and vaccination for diseases affecting reproduction and vaccinate the animals against such diseases.
9. Practice a general sanitation programme.
10. Supply adequate nutrition.
11. Employ the correct technique.
12. Provide suitable shelter management.
13. Detect silent or weak heat, by using a teaser bull.

Selection and Culling

Selection and culling are the two sides of the same coin. Selection is the process in which certain individuals in a population are included for becoming the parents of the next generation. Automatically some are excluded for the purpose which are culled. Natural selection has been going on since ages where animals which were stronger, which had better survivability and which were in more unison with the environment around them, found a better chance to reproduce.

Thus certain genes for certain characters got more chance to be selected to form individuals in the subsequent generations. Since domestication of cattle, man has been looking for superior phenotypes in traits useful to him and selecting such animals to form the parental generation. This is man made artificial selection. Now man has progressed one step further in making estimates of genotypes from the study of phenotypes and making use of that information (in artificial) selection.

Selection methods

There is only one way to select and that is to "keep the best and cull the poorest. The various selection methods are techniques for identifying or estimating the genetic values of individual candidates for selection. The procedure discussed here apply to selection for quantitative trails.

Performance testing

Performance test is a measure of the phenotypic value of the individual candidates for selection. Since the phenotypic value is determined by both genetic and environmental influences, the performance test is an estimate, not a measure of the genetic value. The occurrence of this estimate depends upon the heritability of the trait i.e. on the degree to which the genetic value is modified by the environmental influences.

Advantages

- Among simple procedures, the performance test is the most accurate.
- Environmental influences can be minimised by testing candidates for selection in the same pen or in similar environmental conditions.
- The measure is direct, not on a relative basis.
- All candidates for selection can be tested in contrast to progeny testing where only a parent can be tested.
- Generation intervals are usually short.
- Testing can usually be done on the farm under normal management conditions.

Disadvantages

- Accuracy become low when heretability is low.
- Phenotypes are not available for one sexor in sex limited traits such as milk yield.
- Traits which are not expressed until maturity may become expensive or difficult to manage by performance tests since most selection decisions must be made before maturity.

Performance tests should be the backbone of most selection programmes. Although much publicity has been given to other selection methods, it remains a fact that most of the progress in livestock improvement to date has been due to selection on the individual's own phenotype i.e. performance test.

Pedegree selection

A pedegree is a record of an individual's ancestors including its parents. This information is valuable because each individual possesses a sample half of the genes from each parent. If we can precisely know an individual's phenotype, little is gained by considering pedegree in selection. Pedegree considerations are useful when we do not have sufficient accurate records of production of the individual. Also, it is useful in the early selection when the traits in question might not have expressed themselves. It is also useful for selection of males when the traits selected for are expressed only by the female such as milk production in dairy cattle.

Advantages

- It provides information when performance tests are not available for the candidates.
- It provides information to supplement performance test information.
- It allows selection to be completed at a young age. Pedegree records may be used to select animals for performance or progeny testing in multi-stage selection scheme.
- It allows selection of bulls can be selected on the milk records of their female relatives.

Disadvantages

- Accuracy, relative to alternative selection procedures is usually low.
- Too much emphasis on relatives, especially remote relatives, greatly reduces genetic progress.
- Progeny of favoured parents are often environmentally favoured.
- Relatives often make records under quite different environments, thus introducing non random bases into the selection system.

Progeny testing

In this method we evaluate the breeding value by a study of the expression of the trait in its offsprings. Individuality tells us what an animal seems to be, his pedegree tells us what he ought to be, but the performance of his progeny tells us what he is.

Progency testing is, of course, a two-stage selection system because some preliminary selection determines which animals first produce progeny followed by further culling of these which produce poor progeny.

Advantages of progney testing

a. High accuracy when many progeny are obtained.

Disadvantages progney testing

b. Long generation interval.
c. Requires high reproductive rate.
d. Low selection intensity.

Show ring selection

Selection on the basis of show ring performance has had considerable value in the past. Essentially this selection has been directed towards bringing the conformation of the animal to some ideal conformation.

This improvement has been based on two goals:

i. improvement conformation, and
b. correlated response.

Improvement of conformation has economic value because a part of the sale price is determined by the conformation of the individual. The ideal type was chosen so that, in the opinion of the judges, the animal possessing this conformation was most likely to be a profitable producer. In other words, the judges were attempting to stress traits of conformation which are corrected with productive ability.

With the advent of record keeping it was found that direct selection for performance traits resulted in much faster progress than selection through correlated conformation traits. Also, when subjected to intensive study, many of the correlations between performance and show ring were found to be of non-genetic origin.

If the correlations are of genetic origin, direct selection for performance should improve conformation as well as the reverse situation. The show ring has been a good forum for discussion of what constitutes ideal type and good management and has produced dramatic changes in the conformation of some species.

This has resulted primarily from education of the breeders, however, for most animals which are presented in the ring are good and selection differential among these animals is usually so small as to produce little change.

Advantages of show ring selection

1. It enables breeders to exchange ideas and experience.
2. It allows comparisons among superior animals both within and between breeds.
3. It allows new breeders to make contact with established breeders.

Disadvantages of show ring selection

1. Emphasis is usually placed on traits of little economic importance.
2. Clever fitting and showmanship can mask defects of various kinds.
3. Differences between exhibited animals are usually small.
4. Conformation and production traits usually have low genetic correlations.

Choosing Traits for selection

Many factors enter into the choice of traits to be selected for. The following ones are the most important.

1. The goal of the selection programme
2. The habitability of the traits
3. The economic value of improvement in each trait.
4. The range in variation of each trait.
5. Correlation among the traits.
6. The cost of the selection programme.

Selection goals

Often the goal of the selection programme makes the choice of traits quite obvious. The breeder of the race horses must select for speed if he is to be successful and his choice of traits are limited to alternative ways to measure speed. Similarly, the breeder of dairy cattle generally sets out to breed cows with superior milk production characteristics. Thus, his choice of traits is specified by his selection goals.

Heritability

Heritability is defined to be the fraction of the superiority of parents which is, on the average, transmitted to their off-springs. To explain habitability in simpler words: Heritability tells us how much of the observable differences in the animal is caused by genes and how much by environment.

Heritability for the same characteristics may vary from one population to another and also may vary from one characteristic to another even ink the same population. The ability to recognise the breeding values or transmitting abilities of animals is closely associated with heritability. If the heritability is high for a trait, we can proceed straight way to adopt a system of mass selection of superior animals, with little attention to pedegree information, collateral relatives, progeny test or inbreeding and genetic improvement in that trait is low, genetic progress may be disappointing with mass selection and greater attention should be paid to pedegree records, family information and use of progeny tests.

Variability of the trait

Selection operates on the variability in expression of the trait uniform for a trait. there will be little selection response because any selected groups of parents will not be much better than those not selected. Some traits are much more valuable than others. thus the innate variation of the traits should be carefully considered in choosing traits for selection.

Variation can be increased by improving exotic types and sometimes this can result in new combination of genes which are superior to either parent type.

Correlated traits

Sometimes traits tend to be inherited together. These correlations may arise in several ways.

The traits may be of different measures of some underlying trait. For example. weight and height are both measures of body size. thus taller animals are usually heavier and these two traits are said to be correlated.

If the same genes produce response in several traits. those traits will be correlated. This condition is referred to as pleiotrophy.

Correlated responses are common. Selection for increased milk yield produces a correlated decrease in the per cent of fat in the milk of dairy cows. Thus. both direct and correlated responses result from selection and some correlated responses are positive while others negative.

Correlated response may be advantageously used in selection programme. For example feed efficiency is expensive to measure because it requires both weight gain and feed intake on each individual, whereas weight gain requires neither feed weight nor individual feeding.

In summary. definite goals are essential for a successful selection programme. The success in achieving these goals depends on the existence of genetic differences. the degree to which phenotype differences are heritable and the correlated responses in other traits. In comparing the selection programme, the breeder must evaluate the value of the expected response and the cost of the programme relative to the costs and responses of alternative selection programmes.

Systems of Breeding

The ultimate aim of the breeder is to evolve outstanding and improved type of animals which can render better service to man. Selection and system of breeding constitute the only tools available to the breeder for improvement of animals. Since new genes can not be created though they can be recombined into more desirable groupings.

Systems of breeding has been broadly divided as under

1. In breeding -breeding of the related animals.
2. Out breeding -breeding of the unrelated animals.

Inbreeding

Inbreeding is a mating system in which individuals mated are more closely related than the average of the population from which they come. It means the mating of males and females which are related. Animals deemed to be related only when they have one or more ancestors in common on the first 4-6 generations of their pedegree. The intensity of inbreeding depends upon the degree of relationship. Close inbreeding denotes mating of closely related individuals like dam to son (mother x son) or sire to daughter (father x daughter) or full brothers to full sisters.

In breeding makes more pairs of genes in the population homozygous. Wherever there is inbreeding, there will be one or more common ancestors from which, part of the gene samples (gametes) have arisen.

Inbreeding can again be divided into following groups:

Improvement of Dairy Cattle in India

The dairy farming business in many tropical and subtropical countries are characterized by large number of cattle and low yield of milk. For example, India possesses over 230 million heads of cattle and buffaloes, which comes to more than one-fifth of the total world population of cattle and buffaloes. The average annual production of an Indian cow is only 173 kg as against an average yield per milking cow of 3,710 kg in Denmark, 3,250 kg in Switzerland and 3280 kg in the U.S.A.

Twenty six breeds of cattle and seven breeds of buffaloes have been recognised at present in India. However, only a small proportion of the cattle and buffaloes belong to these purebred breeds. The vast majority (more than 75%) are intermixed and do not belong to any specific breed. They are classed as nondescript.

Cattle remain the draught animals in many of these regions. As a result selection over the past many centuries has been to meet the requirements of draught and agriculture. Selection pressure was applied for better capacity and fitness. This has resulted in producing excellent draught animals. Unfortunately, milk production and draught capacity are traits which are genetically negatively correlated. When milk yield capacity goes up, draught capacity goes down and vice versa. As a result attempts to develop and improve some of the dual purpose breeds which are useful for both milk and work, could not progress very far. We could have only a compromise in dual purpose breeds with medium milk production and medium work capacity. If further genetic improvement of either of the two traits is attempted, a set back with respect to the other should be expected.

In India, at present many milch cows yield less than one kg. milk per day. Buffaloes are better milk producers. About 18 -20% of the milch buffaloes yield more than 2 kg per day and only 19% yield less than one kg per day. The reasons for such a low level of production are listed below.

- Acute shortage of feed and fodders.
- Excess cattle numbers.
- Poor genetic potential for milk production.
- The smallness of land holdings and consequently small dairy units make them economically unviable. It also acts against introduction of advanced techniques.
- Adverse climatic conditions of the tropics.
- Poor grazing and environmental factors.
- Inadequate marketing facilities for the products.

The diversity of the breeding stock and the variation available in economic traits of cattle and buffaloes in the country offer greater challenge and scope for their improvement for the animal breeder. At the same time, the task of improving the genetic make up of a large number of extremely diverse, non-descript low producers is a colossal one. Anyone system of breeding can not be applied uniformly to all the animals in all the areas.

Important Reproductive details / Breeding guidelines

Particulars	Indigenous	Exotic / Crosses	Buffaloes
Age at puberty	24 months	12-15 months	24-30 months
Age at first mating	30 months	18-20 months	30-36 months
Optimum weight at first mating	250 kg	180-275 kg	300-350 kg
Oestrus cycle length	17-24 days	21±3	21 days
Duration of oestrus	12-18 hours	12-18 hours	12 -18 hours

Particulars	Indigenous	Exotic / Crosses	Buffaloes
Time of ovulation	12-16 hour after end of estrus		
Optimum time of insemination Mid heat / towards the end of heat			
Gestation period	280-290 days	280 - 290 days	305-318 days
Dry period	80 -90	60 - 70	90 - 120
Calving to first heat	40 days	40 days	40 days
Calving to first service	60 days or less		
Lactation length		305	
Milk yield in litres	1500-2000	3500-5000	1500-3000
Birth weight	20 -25	25-35 305-318 days	30-40

Estrus Period

- Pro estrus: 2 or 3 days
- Estrus: 12 to 18 hours
- Ovulation: 12 to 16 hours after the end of estrus
- Estrous cycle length: 21± 3 days

Puberty

- Puberty is the stage at which animal becomes sexually mature and secondary sex characteristics become conspicuous.
- The term sexual maturity means that the animal is capable of reproduction.
- Puberty is the age at which the first estrus occurs in the heifer and the bull starts giving semen with viable sperms.
- The reproductive organs undergo marked increase in size at the time of puberty.
- Under good feeding a calf attains puberty approximately at 66 per cent of adult body size.

Signs of estrus

- Cow in estrus will be the first cow to rise in the morning.
- The cow become restless does not eat and frequently bellows and seldom ruminates.
- Sudden drop in milk production.
- Searching for male.
- Traits of homosexuality is shown in which the cow will attempt to mount other cows while other females not in estrus tend to mount the estrus cow which she permits.

- The cow is receptive to the act of mating and will stand when the bull mounts her.
- The behaviour of standing quietly while being mounted by the bull or other cow is referred to as the 'standing heat' which is the surest sign of estrus.
- This extends for 14-16 hours and shows other symptom like bellowing, nervousness, anorexia, reduction in milk yield.
- Mucous discharge may be found sticking to the tail.
- In early heat the discharge is watery and copious in mid heat (standing heat) it becomes thick and sticky and in late heat it will be scanty and discoloured.

Bulling

- The best indicator of oestrus is when any cow or heifer repeatedly stands and accepts mounting by one of her herd mates. Unfortunately, they do not do this on demand. Those responsible for oestrus detection must watch for this behaviour and combining what they see with their own previous knowledge/experience, to decide whether to inseminate or not.

Heat detection in buffaloes

- Cows do mount over other cows when they are likely to come in heat and stand for mounting when they are in good heat. This is not seen in buffaloes. Buffaloes neither mount on other buffaloes nor other buffaloes mount on buffaloes in heat. In buffaloes copious ropy hanging discharge is not seen on the contrary it gets suddenly dropped and is not noticed by the owner and the discharge is scanty. Some buffaloes do not bellow and show silent heat, especially high yielding buffaloes.
- The main heat symptoms of buffaloes are as follows. The vulva becomes edematous, swollen. The lower portion of vulva looks oily. The gap is seen between vulvar lips and slight opening is seen. The wrinkles which are present in anoestrus buffalo become shallow or vanish.
- The mucous membrane of vulva becomes reddish, moist and glossy.
- Mucus discharge which is not seen normally can be seen before or after oestrus spontaneously.
- The colour, consistency and fern pattern of mucus help in determination of correct oestrus.
- Engorgement of teats in lactating buffaloes which is due to holding of milk following increased estrogen level in blood is seen when they are in heat.
- Frequent urination. The urine coming in spurting action wetting the part of skin below vulva and above udder (perineum). The drying of the urine leaves white mark on skin.

- Buffaloes in heat remain restless, off feed, raising head in a typical fashion.
- Local non descript buffaloes bellow, become restless and remain off feed. Milk yield is reduced. The bellow is sharp and for longer duration.
- The buffaloes expose their teeth while bellowing which is very characteristic.
- The mucus discharge, in buffaloes is seen in about 49% cases. It is thin on the day of heat, become thick as the time passes and changes the colour from clear to white.
- 60-70 % of the buffalo come in heat from 6 pm to 6 am (after sunset and before sunrise) and this should be borne in mind and attendant should watch the buffaloes in the evening and early morning for expression of heat symptom.
- Teaser bull (Vasectomised bull), can be used for parading in buffalo barn for detection of heat

Other methods to detect estrus

- Crystallization pattern of cervical mucous will show long crystals in a typical fern-like pattern
- There are many estrus-detecting devices available. They are usually attached to the tail or rump of the cow.
- Mounting causes these devices to discharge a coloured fluid which can be observed afterwards even from the distance.
- 'Chin ball mating device' can be used for heat detection. It works on the same principles of a ball point pen and is fixed by means of a halter below the chain of the teaser bull. When the checking animal mount the cow in heat, the dye exuded round a spring-loaded ball of the device marking the back of the cow.
- Russian workers have developed an instrument basically consisting of an ohm meter and electrodes. When applied to the mucous membrane of the vagina, the resistance indicated on the ohm meter shows whether the cow is in heat.
- Pedometer is an instrument used to monitor the movement of animal. The principle is the activity and movement of the cow increases on the day of heat and this can be detected by means of a pedometer tide to the leg of the cow.
- The vaginal temperature can be recorded, which gives an indication about the heat. Generally during estrus, the vaginal temperature increased by about 1°Con the day of heat. Both methods are not very practicable.
- The methods described above had little applicability in developing countries due to technological and economical and managemental reasons. close observation of signs of heat, standing heat remains the most practicable method of heat detection.

- In large farm this can be supplemented with a bull-parade using a teaser bull. A teaser may be a vasectomised bull or bull in which penis has been amputated and the urethra exteriorized.
- An intact bull can also be used by hanging a thick cloth or gunny bag curtain in front of the penis preventing entry of penis and mating.
- Special care should be taken to prevent spread of disease by teasers. Vasectomised bull is more harmful in this regard.

Time of insemination

- Ovulation takes place about 12 hours after the end of estrus. It takes another six hours for it to travel half-way down the oviduct.
- The sperm, even though reach the oviduct within minutes after insemination, must be exposed to the female reproductive tract for about 6 hours to attain the capacity to fertilize.
- This process of preparing the sperm for fertilization is known as capacitation.
- Sperm are viable for 24 hours in the female reproductive tract whereas the ovum remains fertile for only about 10 hours after ovulation.
- This implies that mating or insemination between mid-estrus (middle of standing heat followed by another insemination in about 6 hours after that.
- As a routine practice, if a cow is seen showing signs of early heat in the morning, it may be inseminated in the evening.
- If such signs are first manifested in the evening, the cow may be bred next day morning.
- A cow is expected to show estrus in 30-40 days after calving. Cows that fail to show heat even after 50 days have generally some problem and need examination.
- It may be due to infection or malnutrition and remedial measures may be taken accordingly.
- Insemination should be done only when buffalo is in standing heat. In buffalo to understand standing heat one should know the symptoms of heat.
- Buffaloes normally are not seen standing for mounting by herd mates but standing heat can be known from the changing colour of mucus discharge which is early estrus is clear and watery but in standing heat or mid heat the colour is changed to little buffy with thick consistency.
- In mid heat the oedema of vulva is intense there is little gap in vulvar lips and lower lip looks oily.
- The vulvar mucus membrane is glossy reddish or pink and wet.

Signs of approaching parturition

- Cow will leave the herd and seek isolation.
- Loss of appetite and distress.
- Distention of teat and udder, considerable milk appears in the udder and there may be dripping of milk.
- Relaxation of pelvic ligament one day before calving, the ligament on the sides of the tail head is loosened so that hollows appear on either side of the backbone and the tail head is raised and the quarters are dropped.
- The vulva become enlarged and flabby
- Animal will be restless and will pace about often trying to kick or scratch the flank region.
- The parturition process has three stages a. preparatory stage (uterine contraction and dilatation of cervix) b. active expulsive stage c. expulsion of foetal membrane.
- Cow will deliver the calf within 12 hours after commencement of first stage and lapse in this vaginal examination of assistance by a veterinarian is required.
- Care must be taken to observe expulsion of placenta (after birth). It should be removed immediately so as to avoid cow eating it.

Package of practice to improve reproductive efficiency

- Accurate record kept is very important in ensuring reproductive efficiency of the herd.
- There production detail like date of estrus, date of service and calving should be maintained properly.
- This data should be used to predict the probable date of heat, such animal should be watched carefully in the morning and evening for signs of heat.
- In larger dairy farm teaser bulls can be put in use.
- Complete breeding history, past performance and difficulties of a individual cow should be maintained.
- Irregular estrus and abnormal discharge should be attended immediately.
- The cows with retained placenta should be treated promptly and when such cows are put in breeding next time, the reproductive tract should be examined thoroughly for involution and possibility of infection.
- A manager should examine a cow 24 to 36 hours after service for metestrus bleeding. If it occurs under 24 hours after service, the cows were bred too late.
- If it occurs over 36 hours after service, they were bred too early during estrus. This will help in pinpointing of failure of conception.

- Cow should be examined for pregnancy 45 to 60 days after service so that if they are non-pregnant, steps can be taken to re-breed them at the earliest opportunity.
- If the conception rate under A.I is lower than natural service, time of insemination, insemination technique and quality of semen must be checked.
- Short irregular cycles indicate cystic ovaries, short and long irregular interval point to missed head.
- Silent or quiescent heat : the behavioural manifestation of heat may be very weak or imperceptible in such case. It is very common in buffaloes. But there is a normal ovulation and if inseminated at proper time the animal can conceive.
- Cows go through the normal ovarian changes of the estrus cycle except the behavioral heat and sexual receptivity.
- It is more in summer season than other seasons and more in heifer than adult animals.
- Use of balanced feed, proper summer management, use of teaser bulls can be of use tool in detecting silent heat.
- Anestrus or absence of sexual cycle may be due to under developed genitalia or due to persistent CL. In the former case follicle fail to develop and a heifer will not come to heat at all.
- One of the major causes of under developed genitalia is malnutrition. Besides there can be genetic causes.
- The second probability is the anestrous also may be due to persistent CL, due to certain hormonal disturbances, the C L persist beyond the life expectancy in a normal cycle, thereby preventing further cycling. A common cause for persistent CL is endometritis of the uterus.
- Sometime anestrus is often observed in the early post partum period when the lactation is strong, probably due to the influence of lactation(due to secretion of prolactin) 'e'lactational anoustnum

Care and management of young stock

- Normally newborn animals will be taken care by its mother and required little assistance.
- In case of cattle, sheep and goat immediately after birth the mucus around the nostrils should be whipped out using dry cloth or a hand full of straw can be used for this purpose.
- Calm environment should be provided to the mother and young animals for development of bond.
- The mother should be allowed to lick the newborn; if the dam fails to lick it can be stimulated by sprinkling small quantity of salt or bran over the young one.

- Immediately after birth the naval cord should be ligated with clean sterile cotton thread 1 inch from the body and tincture iodine should be applied to the naval cord.
- With in 1 hour after birth the newborn will able to stand and it should be allowed to drink adequate quantity of colostrum (first milk) which will give immunity to the newborn.
- Young animals should be housed comfortably. Adequate care should be taken to avoid housing young stock with adult stocks.
- In winter condition adequate warmth condition should be provided.
- Adequate bedding materials like straw or hay should be provided to newborn animals.
- For giving extra heat artificial light source can be utilized.
- Proper light, ventilation and hygiene should be maintained to avoid spread of disease.

Care and management of dry animals

- A dry animal means animal, which completes their lactation and drying is essential to give adequate rest to the udder of the animal.
- Dry animals should be separated from other milch animals.
- In case of cow, dry cow can be treated for mastitis to prevent mastitis in next lactation.

Care and management of pregnant animals

- Pregnant animals should be provided with extra ration to meet the requirement of fast growing foetus as well as store energy for future lactation.
- Pregnant animals should be separated in advanced stage from other non pregnant animals.
- They should be housed separately in place called calving pen.
- Adequate bedding materials should be provided in the pregnant animals shed.
- Floor of the pregnant animal shed should be non-slippery.
- Adequate clean fresh drinking water should also be provided in the calving pen.
- In advance stage of pregnancy laxative diet should be provided.

Care and management of bullock

- Bullocks are normally used for agricultural operations and or transport purpose.
- Some bullocks are ferocious and so control them properly with nose rope or nose rings.

- The hooves of the bullocks should be provided with metal shoes to protect the hooves from wear and tear.
- The working hours for bullocks arc recommended as follows :
  - Normal Work - 6 hours of carting or 4 hours of ploughing.
  - Heavy Work - 8 hours of carting or 6 hours of ploughing.
- Sufficient roughages and 1-2 kgs of concentrates may be provided for feeding of bullocks during break period in works, the animal may be left for free grazing.
- The bullocks are housed in separate sheds with sufficient space and protection from hot and cool conditions.
- Free access to drinking water is essential. Regular grooming of animals should be practiced.

Management of Bulls

- The bull is half of the herd. Not only the bulls should be genetically superior quality, but they also have to be in prime breeding condition by proper feeding and management.
- Bulls should be selected based on their pedigree and the bull calves should be separated from breedable cows and heifer by the time of attainment of puberty, which is between 1 ½ to 2 ½ years in zebu and buffalo breeds and still lower in crossbreds.
- The bull calf should be dehorned within a few days of birth by disbudding with chemical or hot iron.
- This practice is considered to make the bull less dangerous.

Restraining of bulls

- The bull should be ringed by the time of about one year of age, by which time he begins to show his strength.
- A smaller ring can be put at this age, and can be replaced with bigger one when he matures.
- Nose rings are made in two semi-circular pieces hinged together and are of aluminum, copper or some alloy which does not rust.
- The free end of the two parts either, dovetails into one another or are in a form of point and socket, secured either by a flush spring or by a screw with counter sunk head, so that the joint is smooth.
- Since the nose is extremely sensitive to touch, ring in the nose enables the attendant to keep the neck extended and the head raised while restringing or parading.

- Nose ring is an essential item in control of bulls. Bull leading poles can be conveniently hitched to the nose ring and this is mostly felt necessary also.
- The bull can be effectively controlled by means of a chain or rope around the horns threaded through the nose ring.

Training of bulls

- The young bulls should be trained for handling and leading.
- It is much easier to maintain control on a mature bull if he was properly trained when young.
- Even when the bull is 4-6 months of old a simple halter may be put over his face and he be accustomed to handling.
- After the nose ring is put he should be led either by chain or pole.
- While leading, the attendant should never walk in front of the bull, but must lead from the side holding the nose always higher than natural level.
- If the nose is allowed to drop, the bull may get inclination to butt.
- While handling and leading, all bulls should be considered as potentially dangerous and no complacency should be shown at any time even in case of old as well acquainted bulls.

Exercise for bulls

- Growing as well as mature bulls should be regularly be exercised. So that they do not put on fat and thus remain in thrifty condition.
- These will also helping keeping their toes well worn. Over grown toes may hinder walking as well as mounting behavior of bulls.

Care of mature bulls

- Breeding bulls should never be allowed to run with the herd. They should be housed in separate paddock, individually.
- This helps in controlling number of services by the bulls for recording breeding data.
- The hair around the prepuce should be trimmed periodically.
- The hair should not be clipped too close which may cause irritation and itching to the prepuce. About 1 cm length may be ideal.

Maintenance of sexual libido of bulls

- There are several factors which can reduce libido in bulls like young or old age, inexperience, tiring exercise, or too frequent usage, semen collection at unusual places in un favourable conditions and using unsuitable fittings, faulty feeding, obesity or run down condition, inherent defects, temporary injury or chronic defect of legs, back and penis. All such problems should be rectified as soon as noticed.

- Some bulls are sensitive to artificial vagina whereas others seem able to withstand considerable rough handling.
- The well known reflexes of mounting the cow, projecting the penis, thrusting and ejaculation can easily be retarded or even inhibited in a bull by unnatural method of handling.
- Majority of the bulls serve well in familiar surrounding and are handled by the same attendant provided these are associated with previous satisfactory experience.
- The sexual reflexes can be inhibited by painful, uncomfortable or even distractive situation.
- In a sensitive bull, inhibition may develop quickly, even when collections are taken carefully.
- The animal should be give rest from collection for as long as possible when inhibition starts developing. This can be overcome by changing the surrounding.
- Overwork is common in young bulls allowed free access to cows and heifers.
- The number of services and not the number of cows served is the important consideration. No bull should be allowed to serve each cow more than twice in a heat period.
- A young bull may be placed with 2 or 3 cow per week and it can be put into service after 2-2 ½ years of age.
- A mature bull may ejaculate many times per week without effect on libido or semen quality.
- The bull with reduced libido should be teased by delaying the service. Bulls become bored in their surrounding, particularly if in small paddock and may lose interest.
- Presence of another bull or change in the surrounding will overcome this problem.
- Summer stress leads to low sexual libido and poor semen quality, especially in purebred exotic and crossbred bulls.
- To overcome such problems during summer, bulls should be housed in cool, well ventilated dry sheds.
- Showering or splashing cold water on bull 2 or 3 times during hot part of the day and protection against direct and reflected radiation were found to be very useful.

Feeding of mature bulls

- A good rule to feed mature bull is to feed daily about 1 kg hay and ½ kg concentrate per 100 kg body weight.
- Thus a 400 kg bull should get 4 kg hay and 2 kg concentrate.
- These amounts should be adjusted according to the body condition of various bulls because there is individual variation in response.
- Excess fatness in mature bull should be avoided at all costs as it reduces libido and may cause severe stress and strain on their feet and legs.
- Excess calcium in bull ration can cause problem particularly in older bulls.
- When legume roughage is fed the concentrate mixture should not contain a calcium supplement.
- Generally bulls do not lose calcium and in time excess calcium may cause vertebra and other bones to fuse together.
- Therefore bulls may need a different concentrate mixture than the milch cows.

RESULTS OBTAINED IN POULTRY BREEDING

Selection methods

The selection and breeding program in poultry has been changing as per the knowledge gained and the needs. In 1940s, the individual poultry flocks were evaluated and after retaining the selected birds, the surplus culled birds were sold as a terminal product. The concept of two-, three-, or four-way crosses in poultry was adapted from maize improvement program in 1980s, which transformed the poultry breeding for production of the high-yielding modern layer and broiler strains. The purebreds were also replaced by commercial hybrids as terminal cross as well the specialized egg and meat type birds replaced dual type birds. The negative correlations in production and reproduction traits necessitated the need of development specialized male and female lines both in layer stocks and broiler stocks. These specialized lines were developed in meat type stocks and egg type stocks.

These specialized male and female lines usually have very different foundation genetic sources. Cornish Game breed was most favored for developing a male line of meat type chicken, whereas developing female lines Plymouth Rock (barred, Columbian, or white) breeds were the most chosen ones for producing commercial broiler across the world. Similarly, for developing brown egg layer male lines, predominantly Rhode Island Red and New Hampshire were used. Plymouth Rock lines were used as female lines. For developing, white shelled egg layers varieties of White Leghorn were used as male and female lines. The modern commercial lines across the world are now a composite of the founding breeds having minor contributions from other suitable breeds.

The present poultry breeding, therefore, involves both pure-line selection (PLS) and crossbreeding program. The selection in poultry is therefore combined crossbred and purebred selection (CCPS). Purebred performance and crossbred performance (rpc) are treated as genetically correlated traits assuming the infinitesimal model. Depending on genetic parameters like heritability estimates and correlations, the method such as phenotypic selection primarily followed for improving body weights, whereas for egg production, the index selection (Osborne index) was employed in PLS.

The number of traits is now included in selection program, the modern programs, therefore, rely on breeding value estimation with animal model best linear unbiased predictor (BLUP).

Pure-line breeding for development of specialized lines:

Specialized sire and dam lines were developed through unique selection program based on different set of traits for sire and dam lines. The dam lines are selected for their reproductive performances, e.g., egg production, egg size, egg weight, shell quality, age at sexual maturity, and hatchability besides juvenile growth. The sire lines are primarily selected for improving the rate of growth, body confirmation, feed conversion ratio, and carcass quality and fertility.

Therefore, with the involvement of these specialized lines in the development of commercial broiler stocks thrive toward lowering the cost of production. Crossing of these genetically diverse lines results in gene recombination producing a heterotic effect in progeny for different economic traits. Therefore, intense selection within pure-lines and crossing those genetically diverse lines is the most characteristic feature in broiler breeding program. While practicing the artificial selection, care is taken to minimize the inbreeding, and its related consequences in the population.

A control population with the same increment in inbreeding as the selected population may be maintained for comparison and evaluation of the selected population.

1. Layers: for layer, the objectives primarily is "To obtain maximum number of sale-able eggs per hen housed at low feed cost per egg or per kg egg mass and the eggs should have optimal internal and external qualities. Stock should have low mortality and high adaptability to different environments." Layer breeders apply selection to improve over 30 traits important for commercial egg production. Breeders today select for (or at least monitor) the age at sexual maturity, the rate of lay, livability, egg weight, body weight, feed conversion, shell color, shell strength, albumen height, egg inclusions (blood and meat spots), and temperament. The selection strategies to improve egg production include part-time egg production records, persistency of lay, clutch length, FCR/Residual feed consumption (RFC), skeletal problems (majorly osteomalacia and osteoporosis).
2. Broilers: for broilers, selection strategies concentrate on rapid growth and carcass traits. The most practiced strategy for broiler PLS is "selection at commercial weight," which employs selection at a weight that matches the market weight and

the age at selection becomes progressively earlier as growth potential increases. The other two strategies are the selection at a commercial age and multi-stage selection. Different breeding and selection technologies at different period of time were employed for the genetic improvement of poultry. Breast muscle weight, meat quality, and FCR are major traits; in addition to these, thrust is also being given on skeletal abnormalities, metabolic disorders and welfare. The selection basing on breast area measured through length and width of the breast using a pachymeter along with body weight resulted in a genetic gain of 277% per generation while keeping feed conversion and fertility in the actual levels. The nondestructive means like needle catheters, ultrasonic apparatus etc. were found more accurate for measuring the thickness of the breast muscle. The other non-invasive methods like computed tomography scan (CT scan), magnetic resonance imaging (MRI), and echography are more accurate for measuring the muscle thickness and dimensions of internal organs etc., but these methods are far more expensive. Therefore, among the various non-invasive means, ultrasound offers a viable and advanced solution for breast muscle analysis. In developing or maintaining a strain of broilers, geneticists must consider a balance of characteristics related to growth versus reproduction

Breeder Management

- The layer breeder management is more or less similar to the management of commercial layers.
- Since the parent stocks are costly and their hatching eggs and pullet chicks fetch higher income, more care has to be taken on parent stock, to generate more profits.
- Moreover, in parent stock management, the management of male breeding stock and the hatchery are additional activities, to be carried out more carefully.

Rearing systems and space requirements

- The layer parent stock can be reared successfully on deep litter, slats, slat cum litter or in breeder cages.
- The floor space requirements will be 1860 cm^2 in deep litter, 1400 cm^2 on slat/wire floor and 450 cm^2 in cages for females and 700 cm2 in breeder cages for male breeders.

Males and Artificial Insemination

- Day old male parent chicks are supplied dubbed and detoed. Males are reared separately from 0-21 weeks of age.
- Start with 12% males in case of natural mating and 8% in case of artificial insemination.

- At the beginning of the breeding season (22 weeks), introduce 8 males per 100 females.
- Replace weak, lame and sick males promptly. In case of A.I. maintain at least 5% males which can yield about 0.5 ml neat semen per ejaculate with not less than 60% motility.
- Inseminate females once in 5 days, with 0.03 - 0.05 ml of neat semen; within 30 minutes after collection.

Debeaking

- Both males and females are debeaked at 10-14 days of age and again at 12-14 weeks of age.
- For females, leave 2mm beak from the nostrils, whereas for males, cut half of the beak between nostrils and tip of the beak.
- Both upper and lower beaks are cut off straight. Give vitamin K in water 1 day before debeaking and electrolytes for 2 or 3 days from the day of debeaking.

Vaccination programme and health care

- It is more or less similar to the programme followed for commercial layers.
- The programme varies from place to place and time to time, depending on the prevalence of diseases in the area.
- The only difference will be, killed vaccines are given, for diseases like N.D., I.B.D., I.B., REO and M.G., before the onset of egg production.
- Sometimes, N.D., I.B.D. and I.B. killed vaccines are repeated at 45 weeks of age in problematic areas, to increase the maternal acquired immunity in the chicks. Fowl cholera vaccine has to be given at about 10 weeks of age in endemic areas.
- Moreover, the flock has to be tested for Mycoplasma and Salmonella at around 16 weeks of age, to eliminate the positive reactors.
- Deworming will be done every month or once in 6 weeks in deep litter system and once in two months in case of cage and slat reared breeders.
- LaSota vaccination will be invariably followed after deworming.

Feeding

- The feeds given to layer parents will be more or less similar to that of commercial layers in respect of major nutrients.
- But the breeder feeds, especially the breeder hen feed is enriched with all micronutrients like trace minerals and vitamins in order to obtain high rates of fertility and hatchability besides peak egg production.

- Moreover, the breeder feeds must be practically free from all mycotoxins, because mycotoxins will not only affect the egg production and health status of the birds but also fertility and hatchability.

Sex separate feeding

- The breeder males must be fed with a low protein diet having 13-14% protein only because high protein diet will affect sperm quality as well as semen volume.
- Therefore, sex separate feeding of breeder hens and cocks will be followed.
- The females will be fed a 18% protein and 3.0 to 3.5% calcium feed while the cocks with 13-14% protein and 1-1.5% calcium feed with higher levels (40mg/kg) of vitamin E; on other aspects, both the feeds are comparable.
- The male and female feeds are offered in separate feed hoppers in slat and deep litter system. In cage system, sex separate feeding can be followed with 100% accuracy since they are reared in different cages.

Uniformity

- Flock uniformity is a major goal to be achieved in breeding flock management for peak egg production, less number of culls and more uniform sized chicks.
- From 4 weeks of age, group the chicks according to body weight.
- The weak chicks should be taken extra care for attaining uniformity.
- At any stage, the flock must be having at least 80% uniformity.

Hatching egg collection and care

- In slat or deep litter system, keep nest boxes at the rate of one hole for 4 to 5 hens at 18-20 weeks of age. Close the nest holes during night time, to discourage broodiness and soiling of nest material.
- Introduce males around 22 weeks of age at 8 cocks/ 100 hens or as per the recommendation of the principal breeder.
- Collect hatching eggs when they reach at least 48-50g weight or from 25 weeks of age whichever is later.
- Collect eggs at hourly interval during forenoon and once in 2 hours in the afternoon in deep litter and wire floor sheds. In cages collect eggs 2 or 3 times a day.
- Separate clean, soiled dirty, broken, misshapen and abnormal eggs soon after collection.
- Save clean eggs with sound shell, shape and size for hatching; without any cleaning.
- Dry clean soiled eggs with the help of a sand paper, dry cloth or cotton and also save them for hatching.

- Do not practices wet cleaning of eggs. Discard other eggs which can be sold for table purpose.
- Fumigate hatching eggs with formaldehyde gas at 3 X concentration and store in an egg store room, until 6 hours before setting.
- Do not store hatching eggs for more than a week. In case of cage system, netlon or rubber mat is placed over the cage floor to prevent hair cracks (checks) in hatching eggs. Otherwise, plastic coated steel mesh is used as cage bottom.

Hatchery operation and sanitation

- The eggs are set according to the demand or order for pullet chicks.
- Depending upon the size of the hatchery, the eggs are set 1 to 6 times a week. Set 250 eggs for every 100 pullet chicks required.
- The remaining hatching eggs may be either sold as hatching eggs for other needy hatcheries or sold for table purpose.
- The cockerel chicks produced may be either sold for specialized cockerel market or destroyed and recycled in feed as "male chick meal", replacing fish meal.
- Discard weak female chicks also, weighing less than 32 grams.
- Unlike the old design, the modern hatcheries locate the tray cleaning room etc., atleast 30 m away from the main hatchery, on sanitation grounds.

Production targets and standards

- The recommended body weights, feed consumption, egg production and mortality are reported in table.
- But these values vary marginally from strain to strain. The breeder must aim at achieving these targets for optimal profits.

Nutrient requirements layer breeder of different age groups

	Age (in weeks)				
	Chick (0-8)	**Grower (9-15)**	**Pre-layer (16-18)**	**Layer Phase-1 19-34)**	**Layer Phase-2 (35-72)**
Protein (%)	20.00	17.00	17.00	19.00	17.50
M.E. (Kcal/kg)	2750	2550	2550	2550	2500
Linolenic acid (%)	1.40	0.10	1.20	1.40	1.20
Lysine (%)	1.10	0.80	0.80	0.88	0.75
Methionine (%)	0.50	0.40	0.45	0.50	0.40
Methionine + Cystine (%)	0.75	0.60	0.65	0.73	0.62
Calcium (%)	1.10	1.10	2.50	3.80	4.00
Available Phosphorus	0.45	0.45	0.45	0.45	0.42

Sodium (%)	0.20	0.18	0.20	0.20	0.20
Vitamin A (IU/kg)	20,000	16,000	20,000	20,000	20,000

	Age (in weeks)				
	Chick (0-8)	**Grower (9-15)**	**Pre-layer (16-18)**	**Layer Phase-1 (19-34)**	**Layer Phase-2 (35-72)**
Vitamin D (IU/kg)	4,000	3,200	4,000	4,000	4,000
Vitamin E (mg/kg)	60	40	60	60	60
Vitamin K (mg/kg)	4.00	3.20	4.00	4.00	4.00
Riboflavin (mg/kg)	20	50	20	20	20

Production standards for breeding stock	
Trait	**Standards**
No. of sire/ 100 dams in deep litter or slats	10
No. of sire/ 100 dams in cages	3
Feed/ bird upto start of egg production (kg)	6.0
Feed/ hen/ day during laying period (g)	110
Feed/ cock/ day during breeding period (g)	100-105
Period of hatching egg production (week)	24-72
Total no. of hatching egg/ hen (dam)	260
Total no. of straight run (unsexed) chicks/ day	230
Total no. of pullet chick/ dam	110
Total no. of saleable chicks/ dam	105 (female)
Average body weight of day old chicks (g)	35
Average body weight of male at maturing age (kg)	1.6
Average body weight of female at maturity age	1.25
Average body weight of male at culling age	2.0
Average body weight of female at culling age	1.5
Average mortality during growing period	5%
Average mortality during laying period	8%

Parent stock performance potential		
Traits	**Male**	**Female**
Body weight (g) at 4 week of age	300	250
Body weight (g) at 8 week of age	725	580
Body weight (g) at 12 week of age	1100	850
Body weight (g) at 16 week of age	1350	1100
Body weight (g) at 20 week of age	1550	1300
Body weight (g) at 40 week of age	2000	1600
Body weight (g) at 72 week of age	2300	1700

Traits	Male	Female
Flock uniformity	>80%	>80%
Feed intake (kg) 0-8 weeks	3.0	2.5
Feed intake (kg) 9-20 weeks	4.5	4.0
Feed intake (kg) 0-20 weeks	7.5	6.5
Feed intake (kg) 20-72 weeks	38.0	40.0
Layer feed/ hatching egg (g)	145	
Total feed/ hatching egg (g)	188	
Mean livability (%) 0-20 weeks	94	
Mean livability (%) 21-72 weeks	92	
Mean mortality (%) 0-72 weeks	14%	
Hen housed egg number		
(20-72 weeks of age)	280	
% Total hatchability	90	
Saleable pullet chicks/ hen housed	110	

Fertility Disorders In Breeders

- There are a variety of possible causes for fertility disorders, such as improper mating ratios and male body weight control.
- The fertility disorders is divided into four egg laying sections - early, peak, mid-lay, and late period.

Early egg lay hatches (26-28 weeks)

- Insufficient number of active males. Four to five active males per 100 females at beginning of mating period are recommended.
- **Physiological Castration** - Some normal appearing males at housing may have been "physiologically castrated" temporarily (or permanently) due to a very stressful event.
- **Rough appearing and/or non-uniform males at housing.** Flock may have an excess of culls, "crow-heads", and small males. Some males may be permanently damaged.
- **Male Aggression:** Frightened females will remain on the slats or hide in the nests, resulting in reduced mating activity. No more than 4-5 active males per 100 females are recommended at the beginning of mating period.
- Eggs set before flock is 25 - 25½ weeks old. Expected range of hatchability for eggs set between 24-25 weeks of flock age may be only 65-73% with a fertility Tange of 83-88% - when there are no other complicating factors.

Peak egg lay hatches (29-39 weeks)

- Some possible causes for reduced fertility during this period are:
    - Insufficient Active Males or Male Aggression: The effects of either problem that occurred during the early mating period will generally (but not always) carry through the peak hatchability period.
    - Reduced Male Feed Consumption: This causes some males to "cull out" while other normal looking males stop semen production due to body weight loss. This can occur when no adjustment has been made in feed allotment for the males when they can no longer "steal" from the female feeders. The average male body weight may actually increase somewhat afterwards due to no energy being spent on sexual activity by these non-productive males - and, thus, goes toward growth.
    - Insufficient Water Consumption
    - Disease or Leg Problems.
    - Crowding (floor space): High bird density in the hen house can affect male mating activity - as well as egg production. A minimum of 1.80 ft2/hen (no more than 6 hens/m2) is suggested in slat floor houses.
    - Male Feeder Space: Decreased hatch sometimes noticed with 12-13 males per pan feeder versus recommended 9-10 males. Some males may not be able to consume sufficient feed, especially later on with more "timid" spike males.

Mid-egg lay hatches (40-50 weeks)

- Reduced Male Feed Consumption.
- Insufficient Water Consumption.
- Disease or Leg Problems.
- Crowding (floor space).
- Male Feeder Space.
- Insufficient Active Males - Usually need to "spike" with 2-3% younger males (2-3 males per 100 females) to achieve 8-1/2 - 9-1/2% total males in the flock. Possible causes of insufficient males during this period are:
    - Overweight males - reduced mating ability.
    - Bad feet/legs - often weight related.
    - Ratio reduction - due to male mortality and normal culling.
- **Male Aggression** - The aggressive behavior is often established during the early mating period. One can usually find frightened hens, many with cut backs and flanks, remaining on the slats or hiding in the nests.

- Excessive Feather Loss - Hens with tender backs avoid the males by staying on the slats or hiding in nests. This can be caused by a combination of factors such as low feed consumption, borderline or low energy and/or protein (amino acids) in the diet, cold weather (increased energy requirements), etc.
- Hot Weather - Both fertility and egg production can suffer.

Late egg lay hatches (50-65 weeks)

- Due to age-related reduced mating activity, semen quantity and quality, etc. a minimum of 9 - 9-1/2% total males should be maintained to have 7-8% active males during this final mating period. Some possible causes of reduced fertility are:
    - Generally the same causes mentioned during the 40-50 week period carry through this period.
    - Overweight Hens - Female effect in fertility. This can especially be a problem in hot/humid weather.
    - Overweight Males - Although mentioned in previous sections, this cannot be over emphasized. The average male weight should not exceed 10 lbs (4.54 kg) - 9.71 lbs to 9.81 lbs (4.40 to 4.45 kg) is better! Individual males weighing more than 11-1/2 lbs (5.2 kg) will probably not be active at this age.

Selection and Culling of Breeder Flocks

- Culling refers to the identification and removal of the non-laying or low producing hens and poor or infertile males from a breeder flock.
- Unless the birds are diseased, they are suitable for marketing or home cooking.
- Usually males are selected based on its vigor and spermatozoa concentration.
- In case of natural mating, the mating ability of the males is important, in addition to its semen quality.
- In case of females, their egg production qualities are to be taken into account.
- Removing the inferior birds reduces the cost of producing eggs, reduces the incidence of disease, and increases the available space for more productive hens.
- Hens eat feed whether or not they are laying. Removing the cull birds will make more feed and space for more productive birds.
- Two types of culling are usually used to remove the inferior birds:
    - Sight culling at the time of housing and
    - Culling by individual inspection, which evaluates the bird's ability to lay or her past productive performance.

Artificial Insemination

- Artificial Insemination (AI) is an important tool to improve the reproductive performance of birds especially broiler breeders and turkey where fertility is low due to heavy body weight.
- Eventhough AI is well developed technique in cattle, is not so well developed in poultry because no standard technique is available to store poultry semen for a long period.
- The techniques available at present permits to collect semen and use it for insemination immediately with or without dilution using semen diluents at 1 : 2 ratio. Semen collected from one cock is sufficient for inseminating 5 to 10 hens depending upon the semen volume and sperm concentration.
- At farms, where AI is practiced the males are kept separately in individual cages where sufficient space is available for movement of the birds.
- There should be a particular team of workers to associate collection and insemination of semen.
- Frequent changes of personnel in the team may affect the normal behaviour of birds.
- Rough handling should be avoided, if not it may develop fear reaction, which affects the semen volume during ejaculation.

CHARACTERISTICS OF POULTRY SEMEN

- Usually cock start producing semen from the age of 16 weeks but the fertilizing capacity of the semen is low.
- So the cocks from 22 or 24 weeks of age are used for semen collection.
- The natural colour of poultry semen is white or pearly white.
- Heavy breed male can produce 0.75 to 1 ml semen and light breed male can produce 0.4 to 0.6 ml of semen.
- A male can be used thrice in a week for semen collection with a gap of one day.
- Although every day semen collection will not change the fertilizing capacity but the volume of semen will be low.
- Semen consists of spermatozoa and seminal plasma.
- Fowl semen is generally highly concentrated (3 to 8 billion spermatozoa per ml for broiler fowl).
- This is due to the presence of limited amount of seminal plasma since the accessory reproductive organs are absent in avian species.
- The seminal plasma is derived from the testes and excurrent ducts.

- At the time of ejaculation a lymph-like fluid (also known as transparent fluid) of cloacal origin may be added to the semen in varying amounts.
- The addition of transparent fluid to semen at the time of ejaculation act as an activating medium for the previously non-motile spermatozoa, thus ensuring their transport from the site of deposition to the sites of sperm storage tubules in the utero-vaginal junction of the hen's oviduct.

Equipments needed for A.I

- Small glass funnel with stem plugged with wax.
- Inseminating syringe
- Wide mouthed glass vial.
- Small pyrex semen cup
- Large flask to hold water at 180 C to 200 C range for short time holding of semen.

Steps in A.I

- AI in poultry is a three-step procedure involving semen collection, semen dilution and insemination.
- The second step may be omitted if 'neat' semen (undiluted) is to be used for inseminations within 30 minutes after collection.

Semen collection

- The first step in AI program is manual collection (milking) of the semen.
- For semen collection, a team of two members are generally involved, one for restraining the male and the other for collecting semen.
- The bird is held in a horizontal position by a person at a height convenient to the operator who is attempting to collect the semen.
- To collect semen the operator should place the thumb and index finger of the left hand on either side of the cloaca and massage gently.
- By his right hand the operator should hold a collecting funnel and with the thumb and index finger massage the soft part of abdomen below the pelvic bones.
- Massage should be rapid and continuous until the cock protrudes the papilla from the cloaca.
- Once the papilla is fully protruded, the previously positioned thumb and index finger of the left hand are used to squeeze out the semen in to the collecting funnel.
- Avoid contamination of semen with faeces and feather.

Semen evaluation at the time of collection

- Normal colour of the semen in pearly white or cream coloured.
- Yellow semen and semen contaminated with blood, urates, faeces or other debris should be avoided.
- Do not allow semen to contact water.
- If debris or contaminants are observed in pooled semen, carefully aspirate contaminates from the sample before mixing with additional diluent with the semen
- Place the diluted semen in a cooler or refrigerator (3 to 12 oC) to cool down.

Insemination

- All equipment used for insemination should be thoroughly cleaned and dry before Use.
- Insemination must be carried out when majority of the birds completed laying since a hard shelled egg in the lower end of the oviduct obstructs insemination and lowers fertility.
- In practice, inseminating chicken after 3 pm obtained better results.
- In turkey flocks much better results are obtained if insemination is done after 5 pm.
- It is difficult to inseminate non-laying hens.
- Usually insemination is done when the flock reaches 25% egg production.
- Hens are inseminated twice during first week. Then at weekly intervals.

Procedure

- Bird is held by the legs with the left hand down and tail tucked back and against the operator chest.
- The thumb of the right hand is placed against the upper lip of the vent then with a rounding motion press the abdomen muscle.
- Do not squeeze with fingers but apply pressure evenly with the palm of the hand.
- When the oviduct is everted, the second operator inserts the syringe into oviduct as far as it is going inside without exerting pressure.
- The insemination apparatus is introduced into the vagina about 1 inch and semen is deposited at the junction of vagina and uterus.

Dose and frequency of insemination

- Chicken : 0.05 ml, once in a week
- Turkey : 0.025 ml once in every 2 weeks

- Ducks : 0.03 ml once in every 5 days
- Goose : 0.05 ml for every 7 days.
- It has been observed that the males produce more semen of good quality during morning and females produce more fertile eggs when inseminated around 9 p.m.

Semen volume and sperm concentration in different species of poultry

Species	Volume (ml)	Sperm concentration (million per ml)	Need of sperm concentration
perinsemination (million)			
Broiler type chicken	0.7	3500	150 to 200
Layer type chicken	0.5	4000	150 to 200
Tom	0.25	9000	300
Gander	0.6	2500	250
Drake	0.3	4000	300

RESULTS OBTAINED IN HORSE BREEDING

There are approximately 60 million horses in the world, most of them living in America, Asia and some European countries. Currently China has the largest herd (around 8 million), followed by the United States (7 million), Mexico (a little more than 6 million) and Brazil (a little less than 6 million). Together, these four countries have close to 45% of the world's equine population.

The world's export trade of live horses is concentrated in Europe and America, together representing 84% (58% and 26% respectively) of 2.1 billion dollars moved around yearly. According to this source, the United States were the main exporter (148,472 animals, representing 48.8% of the world trade), raising around 474 million, in average $ 3,200 per animal.

Similar to the exportation, the world trade of live horses in relation to imports is highly supported by Europe (49.8% of the world trade), followed by Asia (26%) and Mexico (82,854), Canada (63,240) and Italy (46,333) are the main importers in number of animals, although the highest global expenditure in this aspect occurred in the United Kingdom (U.S. $ 498 million), UAE ($ 236 million) and Ireland (U.S. $ 233 million), representing together 46% of annual turnover

Horse breeding

The expression "improvement of equine species," dates back to the French articles about horses and donkeys in the"Histoire Naturelle" by Buffon in 1753. Despite the strong creationist dogmas of that time, these articles anticipated evolutionist ideas, while they described the concept of race degeneration due to the influence of location or climate. Adopted by the French Veterinary schools, it was believed that in order to return to an ideal type of creation, it would be necessary to mate mares and stallions with opposite types, to compensate traits that differed from the ideal. This meant basically to look for stallions on distant lands or regions.

Only decades later, after Darwin's evolution theory introduced the concept of selection is that the improvement of native populations emerged to counterbalance the situation, and effectively replace the desire to keep local types. Later, and gradually, the management of purebred animals predominated over crossbreeding, ending in the Thoroughbred Studbook's creation (first worldwide). It was a very important step for the use of animal production techniques in the 19th century. According to the author, these techniques required precise identification procedures records of races held at different times and places in order to relate them to the same horse. The Stud Book, from the animal lineage certification, not only made it possible to relate the own horse performance information, but also their relatives. This fact prepared the way for the pedigree selection and progeny tests.

In addition, until the beginning of last century, horses were the focuses of experimental tests of inheritage theories. In this sense, historically the main concepts introduced by the horses, especially by the Thoroughbred breed, were: performance selection in a purebred, introducing of a precise method for identifying an animal and its relatives, thinking about the male and female roles in the herd and the widespread use of planned matings.

Currently, although research in several countries are published every year in the literature involving some kinds of horse breeding study, few of them have ongoing consistent selection program. It means, in a way that most of research results in this area don't generate practical application and therefore it adds little to the species' development.

In most cases, this fact occurs because the breeders don't show interest in using the research results and not because of the research quality. The studies, depending on the availability and quality of information, usually do not consider the breeders' interests. Thus, in most countries there is wide gap between research institutes / universities and breeder associations. This gap is particularly due to the fact that more than in other species, horse breeders consider other breeders as potential competitors and give little importance to joint actions needed in breeding programs.

On the other hand, closer relation in Japan, Canada and some European countries, have allowed major advances in horse breeding. In Germany, for example, a country that stands out for jumping and dressage competitions and export of horses, the opinion, awareness and cooperation among breeders gave associations set guidelines that would meet not only their needs, and those of the research institutes / universities, but also the interest of the country. So the Breeders' Associations, supported by these institutions, publishes annually a Sire Handbook containing productive traits considered of general interest.

Horse Breeding Basics

A healthy stallion is necessary to have a successful horse breeding program. Having a working knowledge of stallion management is also essential. The following article discusses stallion management practices.

Role of the Stallion in Reproduction

The stallion must deliver healthy spermatozoa (which contain his genetic contribution) into the vagina of the mare at time of service. He should have enough libido (sex drive) to tease and service frequently and be able to sustain production of healthy spermatozoa throughout the breeding season (Table).

Quantitative Data on Semen and Spermatozoa

Volume per ejaculate	25 to 150mL
Sperm per cubic millimeter	60,000
Total sperm in ejaculate	6,000,000,000

The male reproductive system consists of two testes, three accessory sex glands and a series of tubules through which spermatozoa are transported to the female reproductive tract.

Spermatozoa are produced in small coiled seminiferous tubules in the testes that can be extended 400 to 500 feet in length. Since these developing cells cannot live at body temperature, heat regulation of the testes is critical. Scrotal muscles contract and expand as temperatures change in the normal process of temperature regulation. "Ridgling" or cryptorchid horses are sterile in the testis maintained in the body cavity, but are fertile in the suspended testis. Since this condition is hereditary, it should not be propagated, as castration of a cryptorchid horse is usually a serious operation.

The accessory sex glands are the seminal vesicles, prostate and bulbourethral gland. These furnish alkaline fluid secretions that neutralize the urethra, through which spermatozoa are transported from the epididymis to the end of the male genitalia glans penis.

The sperm life in the mare's tract is from 24 to 48 hours. Only in highly irregular or exceptional cases does it exceed this time span. Sperm has been found in the Fallopian tube 15 to 18 minutes after coitus, but the normal time to travel from the site of deposit to the Fallopian tube is five to eight hours. The average egg life is also only five to eight hours.

Because of a long estrous cycle and short life span of the spermatozoa and egg, it is not uncommon to have a lower than 50 percent conception rate.

Care and use of a healthy stallion

Breeding rates

Yearlings should not be used for breeding. Two-year-olds may settle 10 mares; 3-year-olds, 30; and mature stallions, 50 mares when hand-mated. About half this number can be pasture-mated. A short breeding season will reduce the number, and sexual individuality of the stallion will greatly affect his siring ability.

Feeding and management

The breeding stallion should be fed like a horse at hard work. An estimate is 1½ pounds of grain and 1 pound of hay per 100 pounds body weight. If he is worked under saddle, more feed will be required. Because of diverted interests, a ration high in palatability may be necessary for some stallions to get adequate intake.

- Regular exercise usually results in increased vigor (libido) and fertility.
- Regular grazing of good grass, even for short periods of time, is recommended.
- For safety's sake, fences should be strong and tall when stallions are grazed loose; and mares should not be in adjoining pastures unless extremely tall fences are used.

Methods of mating

Pasture mating, hand mating and artificial insemination are the three methods used, with variations of each. Breed registry regulations vary regarding the use of artificial insemination.

Information on constructing a breeding stall is given in Figure 2. Information on constructing a teasing stall is given in Figure 3.

Pasture mating reduces labor, affords convenience to the owner, "catches" shy breeding mares, and creates an opportunity for a high settling percentage. It has the disadvantage of reducing the number of mares a stallion can serve and obscures breeding dates. Some risk to the stallion exists.

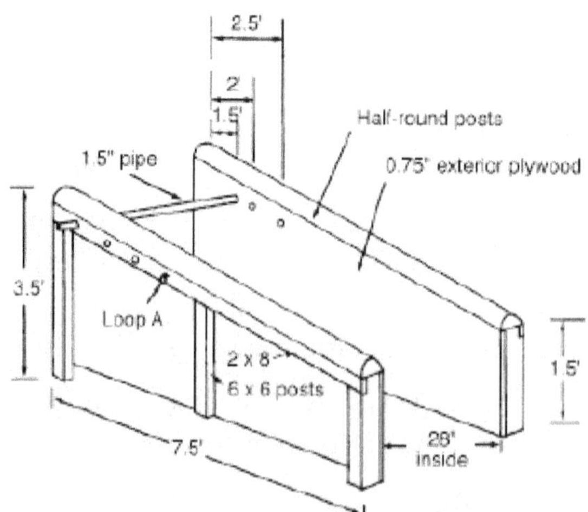

Fig. 2: Breeding stall. A 3/4-inch rope is attached to loop A, brought behind the mare above the hocks, and wrapped twice around the end of the pipe at the mare's right shoulder. The end of the rope is securely held by an attendant who can release it if necessary in an emergency.

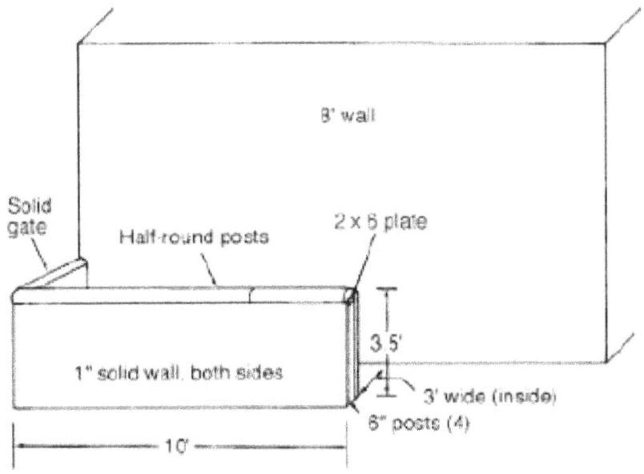

Figure 4: Teasing stall. If stall is positioned against a building, be sure the roof overhang cannot be reached by a rearing horse. A colt pen 20-30 feet in front of the mare is very desirable. It should be easy to see through but should be constructed of mesh wire small enough that a colt's feet do not go through.

Stallions should be hand-mated a few times as 2-year-olds, then turned in a large pasture with a few older mares when they are to be used in a pasture breeding program. Even so, they are likely to carry some scars from their experience. For this reason, pasture mating is seldom used with breeds whose owners discriminate against blemishes, whereas it is extensively practiced with stock horses in the range country.

A combination of hand mating followed by pasture mating will extend the number of mares bred and increase settling percentage.

Hand mating is practiced under a wide variety of conditions, ranging from rather casual selection of mares and sanitation conditions to those that are highly supervised with a veterinarian in attendance.

Stallions used with hand mating should be adept at teasing mares. This may be done at a teasing pole, over a stall door, or any other sturdy fixture that does not injure the horses or attendants.

Signs of heat are frequent urination, vaginal discharge and intensified interest in the stallion. As ovulation approaches, hormones released by the ripening follicle cause an intensification of these signs. The character of vaginal discharge may change from limited amounts of stringy consistency to profuse amounts of liquid consistency.

After the mare has been teased and found in heat, she may be hobbled or placed in a breeding stock. Hobbles have the advantage of convenience and safety to the mare but may entail some risk to the operator. Stallions also have been known to become entangled in them.

The mare's hindquarters may be washed in mild soap and rinsed, and her tail bandaged with a roller bandage. The stallion is allowed to mount quietly from directly behind the mare when ready. A stallion should not be permitted to be rough in the process of breeding. Front shoes should be removed before the breeding season.

- How to increase your percent foal crop
- Breed only healthy animals.
- Breed as often in the heat cycle as possible.
- Pasture breed when practical.
- Don't breed at foal heat.
- Have mares in good condition, but not fat when bred.
- Know the characteristics of each mare's heat cycle.
- Tease mares regularly after breeding.
- Have mares pregnancy-checked by a competent veterinarian.

Some advantages and difficulties in horse breeding

Comparing to other farm animal species, there are some advantages and difficulties specifically related to researches on horse breeding, when quantitative genetics principles are used.

The advantages are fundamentally the amount of performance information and pedigree extension.

- **The depth of the genealogy in most breeds is high:** Traditionally, horse breeders associations consider the "pedigree" as a key factor to select their animals, so that in most of them, herd control is efficient. This fact goes back to the world's first Stud Book opening in 1791 (General Stud Book) for Thoroughbred animals. It was the basis for the other StudBooks, not only for horses, but also for all other domestic species.

  Most of the breeds that were studied based on breeding, it is possible to track the animal's genealogy back to the fourth or fifth generation (depending on when the breeders' association's started), so that genetic evaluations in this aspect are efficient.
- **Economic important traits can generally be measured in both genders:** In most of the breeds, especially the ones for some kinds of performance, the possibility of measuring both genders generates a greater information and knowledge volume about the behavior of traits in the population, what enables more efficient genetic evaluations. Racing, jumping, dressage, barrel, performances meets three classical disciplines: dressage, cross country and jumping. It is a form held in three days.

  On the other hand, even in breeds (or strains within a breed) where the breeding economic interest is the production of animals only for the conformation, not for performance, both genders can be evaluated.
- **Economic important traits can usually be measured repeatedly in short time periods:** In horses it is possible to get repeated performance in relatively short

time periods in a large portion of the population, while that doesn't happen with some domestic species, where economic important traits aren't repeated in the animal life (weight at weaning, weight at the year), or require a relatively long time to repeat (milk production, weight of the fleece).

On the other hand, certain difficulties related to equine species and others due to various issues have been some of the major problems when research on horse breeding is done.

Inherent to the species

Low reproductive rates

Since the early ancestors emerged from 55 to 60 million years ago, horses are adapting in order to develop a reproduction model that ensures survivability in the wild, adopting different reproductive strategies to ensure that their progeny are born in the appropriate time of year. However, domestication has strongly influenced reproductive performance, with selection pressure on fertility being either small or null, and mating usually dictated by the functional performance of the animals.

Thus, considering that reproductive traits usually have low heritability estimate, and have been selected on horses by an indirect way, genetic alterations in order to enhance characteristics of this nature are evidently neither fast nor simple, especially in a species with a long generation interval such as the equine's.

Hence, horses have low reproductive performance when compared to other farm animal species. The birth rate ranges from 59% to 74% the higher percentages being usually found in tests involving a small number of mares. Table below illustrates the result of 42,750 matings done with 7278 Thoroughbred mares.

Occurrences after mating

Occurrence	No. of observations and %
Male	29.35%)
Female	12,927 (30.23%)
Abortion	603 (1.41%)
Empty	3878 (9.07%)
Without information	9864 (7.23%)
Stillborn	866 (2.02%)
Not mated	1945 (4.54%)
Mated with another breed	135 (0.31%)

It was observed that birthrates for males and females were 49.26% and 50.74%, respectively, whereas abortion and stillborn foals were 1.41% and 2.02%, respectively. It was also recorded that 9.07% of coverings were classified as empty, whereas 23.7% of matings did not show any latter records to track success.

This relatively low fertility is described in different races, countries and purposes, and may be related to hormonal dysfunction, genital infections in mares, parasitic infestations and inadequate handling practices before the breeding season.

These factors are even more imposing in the case of animals used in sports, since they have very different handling from those that are exclusively used in breeding.

Furthermore, maintenance of older mares and stallions due to their progeny's superior sporting performance can decrease the rate of conception in the herd, as the rate decreases progressively with increasing age.

In the southern hemisphere, an interval of 12 months between July 1st and June 31st. In northern hemisphere countries, begins on January 1st and ends in December 31st also contributes to the decrease in reproductive rates. This is because, in certain competitions, animals are usually grouped according to, among other parameters (awards, past performance, gender, etc.), the horse's age defined by the racing year.

Thus, breeders try to get the products born closer to the beginning of the equestrian year (July 1st - southern hemisphere or January 1st - northern hemisphere) in order to seize a competitive advantage (better developed, mature and trained horses) in relation to the animals born later that year.

Number of observations (N), conception rates and apparent fertility according to the parturition order of Thoroughbred mares.

Parturition Order	N	Conception rate (%)	Apparent fertility rate (%)
1	5.531	75	71
2	4.534	73	68
3	3.655	71	68
4	2.794	69	67
5	2.155	67	65
6	1.560	64	61
7	1.070	62	59
8	777	59	56
9	513	56	54
10	329	54	52
11	171	48	47
12	92	48	46
>13	79	41	38

With that objective, the breeding season, that usually lasts for 4 to 5 months, usually starts in August 15th in the southern hemisphere (or February 15th in the northern hemisphere). However, the percentage of mares that naturally ovulate in this period is quite low, since mares are seasonal poliestric, with the onset of the natural breeding season in spring, associated with increases in photoperiod, temperature and food availability.

In this sense, researchers found in Thoroughbred horses raised in Ireland (Northern Hemisphere), that the change of the beginning of the breeding season from February 15th to April 15th (hence delaying the beginning of the racing year by the same amount - January 1 to March 1), would better accommodate the natural reproductive cycle of females and could potentially increase the pregnancy rate by approximately 10%.

Similar gains were likely to occur in countries in the southern hemisphere if the beginning of the breeding season changed from August 15th to October 15th, consecutively postponing the beginning of the racing year from July 1st to September 1st. Following this guidance, Australia postponed the beginning of the national racing year to August 1st (breeding season between September and December), mitigating the problem, although considers the best breeding season in that country to be between November and February.

High generation and parturition intervals

Generation interval represents the time needed to replace the next generation, and the shorter it is, the greater the expected annual gene change rate. Thus, considering that in horses this interval varies from 8 to 12 years, overall genetic changes due to selection tend to be slower when compared to cattle (4-6 years), sheep (3-5 years) pigs (1.5 to 2 years) and birds (1 to 1.5 years). Sportive breeds, in which reproductive technologies are not permitted, typically show higher ranges as the superior performance animals, especially females, usually start into reproduction after the end of their competitive life.

The generation intervals of some equine breeds are described in the Table.

Generation intervals from a few equine breeds

Breed	Generation Interval (years)
Andalusian	10.1
Thoroughbred	7.10
Icelandic Toeler	9.7
Friesian	9.6
Hanoverian	8.4
Mangalarga	9.5
Arabian	9.7
Lusitano	10.5
Mangalarga Marchador	8.9

The parturition interval is the amount of time between two consecutive parturitions, including the time from the parturition until the appearance of the first heat, from the first heat to the conception and finally the duration of pregnancy. It is an important component when estimating the herds' reproductive efficiency, with great influence on the economic return and breeding, due to its effects on the generation interval and selection intensity to be applied.

Among the domestic species, the mare has the capacity to provide fertile estrus a few days after birth, the so called foal heat. The main advantage of this phenomenon seems to be the maintenance of a 12 months foaling interval. According to these authors, due to the enrollment of horses in sport activities, there is great pressure in order to have as many pregnant mares as possible in the breeding season. In this sense, efforts are made to cover mares in the foal heat.

Considering the average pregnancy lasting around 11 months and the possibility of new pregnancy in the close postpartum days, a 12 months foaling interval would be obtained. Thus, most breeders seek to take the opportunity of the foal heat, being aware that during this heat mares ovulate quickly, conception rates are lower and early embryonic mortality rate is higher.

There is a great variation among the equine foaling intervals, depending on the breed and breeding purposes, although most studies point values greater than 365 days (Table).

Foaling intervals in some equine breeds

Breed	Foaling interval (days)
Halflinger	468
Thoroughbred	490
Marwari	535
Kathiawari	567
Mangalarga Marchador	548
Arabian	387

Relatively long gestation period and low number of offspring per parturition

Although the duration of a pregnancy isn't directly associated with a breeding farm's production costs, its study may be extremely important in the preparation of breeding plans.

The gestation period can be defined as the time between fertilization of egg and the fetus' delivery. The average duration of a mare's pregnancy is typically 340 days, ranging from 300 to 400 days. This wide time range until the birth of the foals indicates that mares may be highly susceptible to both internal and external factors afecting the duration of the pregnancy. The ages of mare and stallion, year and month of birth, breeding season, foal sex, breed and nutritional status are factors that should be considered in the study of the pregnancy's duration.

Studies focusing the stallion used on coverings also deserve special attention when studying the pregnancy period in mares. The pregnancy's duration for females mated with specific stallions may be a criterion when choosing the stallion. This is because when a mare is bred late in a breeding season, yet the owner wants to mate her during this season, choosing a stallion associated with shorter pregnancy durations may be profitable.

Working with horses in the northern hemisphere observed that the mating season was the most important factor affecting the duration of pregnancy in mares. According to these authors, the pregnancies that derived from mating during the period from December to May were 10.4 days longer than those derived from mating from June to November.

Studying Arab mares in Egypt, observed that pregnancies with longer durations were the ones that ended in the winter, suggesting that the mares seem to be able to adapt the length of the gestation so the births happen in spring, which may be important for the survival of the species in the wild.

Gestation periods in some equine breeds

Breed	Gestation period (days)
Carthusian	332
Thoroughbred/Quarter Horse	341
Andalusian	336
Standardbred	349
Mangalarga Marchador	327
Arabian	334
Criollo	335
Freiberger	336

Regardless of the discrepancy between studies and breeds, mares have a relatively long gestation period compared to other domestic species such as cattle (270-290 days), goats (145-151 days), sheep (144-152 days), pigs (112-115 days) and buffalo (298-317 days). Furthermore, as a uniparous species, twins (or multiple) are rare in mares, incidence varying from 0.5 to 1.6% of parturitions, so that the annual availability of animals for selection is comparatively small.

Other aspects

Use of reproductive technologies

Although reproductive technologies (artificial insemination and embryo transfer) make possible different practical advantages such as lower disease and injury transmission, long-term storage of genetic material, easier transportation, earlier onset of reproduction in females and, in the case of embryo transfer, reproduction during the sports career, in the context of animal breeding they are usually considered additional tools to optimize breeding programs.

The commercial impact of these techniques in horses varies greatly. For example, in Thoroughbred horses meant for racing, the use of artificial insemination

"The fecundation of mares can only be made by direct sexual contact, not admitting artificial insemination, but may exceptionally be authorized by the Brazilian Stud Book, by virtue of proven physical impairment of the player, the use of immediate reinforcement with fresh semen collected during the coverage. This procedure, when authorized, will be held only by a veterinarian authorized in advance by the Brazilian Stud Book " is officially banned worldwide, while in several sportive breeds, especially in Europe, the percentage of inseminated animals exceeds 80% (French Saddle Horse - 84%, Hanoverian - 91% Holsteiner - 95%, Belgian and Dutch Warmblood - over 95%).

On the other hand, according to the International Embryo Transfer Society (IETS) the higher number of embryo transfers occur in the United States, Argentina and Brazil, in order of importance, countries which together represent over 90% of the activities in this area worldwide. In 2005, 5,700 embryos were transferred in Brazil, none frozen, while across Europe only 711 transfers were done in horses.

In this context, it is observed that, although several countries present a prominent role in the worldwide scenario with respect to the use of these reproductive biotechniques, especially embryo transfer, there are few studies about their impact (generation interval, accuracy, selective intensity, inbreeding) on horses breeding programs. Research in this subject would be important to understand the direction that has been given to these tools in different countries and monitor their actual benefit for the horse population.

Knowledge of interesting traits' economic values

A fundamental requirement for any breeding scheme aiming the improvement of quantitative traits is the establishment of the breeding objectives, involving the relative values of genetic change for all desirable features included in the breeding program. Typically, these values are expressed in monetary terms as weights to be applied to each feature of economic importance.

However, few scientific studies have been performed in order to obtain economic weights for traits involved in horse selection programs, were a combination of empirical experience, some biological factors and intuition of designers prevail. There are a few reasons for that.

It's often very difficult to determine, in horses, the value of one unit of expression for a given trait in relation to the animal's total value. Economically quantifying units for traits such as speed, dressage, jumping, etc., is far more complex than attributing values to liters of milk, kilos of meat or wool.

The long period of time between mating and expressig the traits of interest in the progeny, besides the difficulties in determining an appropriate function for profitability, provide part of this deficiency. Moreover, according to recent authors, another problem arises from the fact that not always the relative economic weights are linear in a breeding program. Thus, the amount of increase in the genotype for certain character can be strongly dependent on the values of other genetic traits. For example, in horses with outstanding ability to jump, the additional genetic values affecting their training capability is almost neglected, whereas in animals with a low ability to jump, a genotype corresponding to training characteristics can greatly increase its value.

Diversity of goals within certain breeds

There are equine breeds that are commonly selected by breeder in only one direction, as is the case of the Thoroughbred, where the objective is basically to obtain animals with superior performance in races. In Quarter horses, in addition to races, performance in work tests and conformation may also be targets of breeders since the race is subdivided amongst these strains.

Moreover, in breeds in which animals are involved in a wide variety of uses (work on farms, horseback riding, trekking, exhibitions, equine therapy, equestrian tourism, unskilled riding sports, etc.) breeders seek very different traits, depending on the purpose of raising the animal, hindering the implementation of breeding programs that cover all segments. Brazilian breeds such as the Mangalarga and the Mangalarga Marchador fall into this category.

In these cases, studies involving quantitative and molecular aspects of traits that can meet the desire for the greater proportion of breeders can result in meaningful contributions to selection of reproductive, behavioral, immunological and other traits.

5

NEGATIVE EFFECTS OF ANIMAL BREEDING

Animal breeding has increased production rates in livestock species bred for economic purposes. Traits such as meat, milk and eggs production, carcass composition and food conversion are directly related to the economic efficiency of the production systems and they consequently receive special attention in breeding programs.

High accuracy of genetic values associated with genetic variability of the populations and moderate to high heritability of the productive traits, have allowed the success of breeding programs. However, together with the desirable effects of selection for high production and economic efficiency, negative effects have become more evident. These effects are generally associated to behavioural, physiological and immunological traits, because selection for high production efficiency may result in a correlational response in other traits, because the traits involved may be genetically correlated.

It is not all positive that has come out of animal breeding practices. There are examples where selective breeding has been taken too far. There are also examples where selective breeding has not only improved certain performances, but simultaneously and unintendedly also deteriorated other performances that were not under selection: the so-called negative correlated responses. Both types of negative responses to selective breeding are difficult to predict and are usually only noticed afterwards. This is the case because it takes a while to realise that the negative effects are structural and not coincidence, and that they occur at increasing frequency throughout the population. Even then it sometimes takes stepping back to realise the negative consequences.

SIDE EFFECTS OF ANIMAL BREEDING IN DAIRY CATTLE

In most of the dairy cattle breeding programs, selection is directed at milk production. Such high-yield production comes at the cost of shortening of life expectancy, increase in animal mortality, reduced fertility, and compromised health.

Digestion

In order to establish and to maintain a high-yield production, cattle have to be fed with a diet richer (than their normal grass diet) in easily digestible nutrients with a lower content of effective fibres. However, this new feed composition has exposed animals to digestive disorders. Their physiology is not well adapted to this new diet, and they were not co-selected for physiological traits.

Among main digestive disorders is the metabolic acidosis, which is caused by the increased intake of grain or other highly fermentable fodder. Clinical signs of the disorder are appetite loss, depression and potentially death.

In addition, it may cause laminitis. This hoof disease develops due to fibre-digesting bacteria which function only in a very stable pH environment and do not adapt well to fluctuation in acidity (caused by the fermentation of low-fibre but starch-rich diet). The resulting endotoxins and exotoxins may then be absorbed into the bloodstream.

The endotoxaemia results in impaired circulation, in particular in the feet, which in turn results in laminitis. Thus, lack of quality and quantity of fibres, respectively, are important parts of the etiopathogeny of laminitis.

Reproduction

An antagonistic relationship between high milk production and some fertility traits has been observed, because high-yield cows allocate their energy into the trait they were selected for, thus decreasing their body fat supply, which in turn has a negative impact on the animal's reproductive performance. Loss of body condition in the beginning of lactation is high in high-yield cows, creating a greater negative energy balance in these animals, which is associated with metabolic disorders and reduced fertility, such as more days open, days to first service, reduced conception at first service, longer intervals between parturitions and a greater number of services per conception/parturition.

The reproductive traits are also strongly influenced by environmental factors in dairy cattle. In addition, there is also a correlation between the negative energy balance and the return of luteal activity.

The negative energy balance has genetic causes and may be included in the genetic evaluations, but it also can be mended with management and nutritional arrangements.

The quality of embryos and oocytes is reduced in these selected animals. Therefore the selection for reproductive traits in dairy cattle as well as management and nutritional adjustments may be an important tool to profile these trades-offs.

Besides, for many years it has been highly commented among dairy cow breeders and milk producers that a superior dairy composition, associated with a high angularity of the cow's phenotype, is associated with greater milk production. However, greater angularities implies worse body condition and lead to compromised fertility. Moreover, heifers sired by bulls selected for better angularity have a greater incidence rate of metabolic disorders as well as of foot and leg diseases.

Foot and leg

The progress made in dairy cattle in the selection of genes for productively desirable traits was not accompanied at the same speed by improvements in foot and leg stability. These traits, besides not having been of initial concern and thus largely ignored, are traits of low heritability, and are strongly vulnerable to environmental effects. Therefore, many generations have to pass until satisfactory breeding results will be obtained (Ferreira et al., 2005). Low impact absorption capability, excessive wearing of hoof and great pressure to the joints due to weight - associated to animals selected for high production - are the main factors which cause hoof problems in cattle.

Diseases Susceptibility

High-yield cows of high genetic merit display a greater incidence rate for disorders of skin, of skeleton formation, as well as infections of the mammary glandule and adjacent tissues edema and mastitis. A QTL (quantitative trait loci) affecting both milk production and mastitis is reported, and class I bovine lymphocyte antigen complex alleles were associated with mastitis, milk and fat production.

Bovine class I MHC (major histo compatibility complex) alleles were also associated with fat production, indicating an association between immunological responses and fat contents in milk. Brown Swiss cows carrying the Weaver gene, which causes gradually the loss of their control on hind limbs, have a greater milk yield. In cattle, selection for high milk production appears to be associated with a reduced heat tolerance.

SIDE EFFECTS OF ANIMAL BREEDING IN SWINE

In swine production, selection is usually directed towards high growth rate, minimum backfat thickness, high rate of lean meat deposition and low feed conversion. Selection for high growth rates is associated with physiological and anatomical dysfunctions.

Reproduction

Selection for sexual precocity in gilts must be prudent because of the economic limitations the animals might present, especially concerning a low conception rate and the number of piglets per litter, which has been observed mainly in genotypes selected for low backfat thickness and high meat yield . The problem seems to be related to the fact that sows are still not fully grown and therefore experience physical stress during the first lactation which may lead to low ovulation and fertilization rates during the next oestrus. Sows with a high percentage of carcass lean meat have a delayed puberty, a less intense and shorter pro-oestrus, and a vulva less red and swollen, despite of the environmental effects which have a great impact on reproductive traits.

Selection against feed conversion may also affect significantly the reproductive performance, especially in litter size and weight, and growth rate is inversely correlated with the ability to exhibit a standing reflex, oestrus duration and age of onset of puberty.

Moreover, favourable alleles of estrogen receptor gene for litter size were associated with a decrease of average daily feed intake in pigs.

Males with a higher growth rate are less able to mate a sow in oestrus than males with an intermediate growth rate, and the sperm quality is inferior in males with a bigger growth rate, pointing that those males do not present physiological maturity for precocious reproduction.

Unfavourable side effects for reproduction may occur as a result of the direct selection for high growth rates. However, fertility in swine has increased enormously during the last decades, showing, for example, growing litter size and more litters per year, which is due to direct selection for this kind of trait applied during the last years. This situation indicates the importance of considering both performance and fertility selection objectives in the selection process.

Litter development

Selection for large litter size is directly related to the weight reduction at birth, thus increasing variability in piglets' weight, number of weak piglets and risk of mortality, therefore delaying the development of the animals. Piglet weight is positively related to backfat thickness and a strong correlation between the size of placenta and foetus weight was found, as well as between placenta blood flow and foetus weight, showing that piglets of larger litters are lighter because uterus blood flow decreases with the increase of the number of foetuses. Searching for individuals who display/ exhibit compensatory growth during their productive life may be an alternative to counteract the low weight at birth.

Skeletal formation

Animals selected for high growth rate and lean meat deposition tend to have bone weakness in limbs, and the length of productive life of an animal is intensely influenced by reproductive disorders and also by bone weakness, since there is a genetic association found between length of productive life and leg soundness score.

The occurrence of osteochondral lesions were associated with high food conversion rate, low daily weight gain, besides low initial meat pH and high paleness, both associated with poor meat processing and sensorial attributes. Continuous selection for large amounts of muscle meat deposition and high growth rate can intensify this problem.

Carcass and meat quality

Growth rate and daily feed intake are positively and genetically associated in swine. However, daily feed intake is directly correlated to fat deposition and carcass meat yield, selection for growth rate without intake limitation results in increase of appetite, fat deposition and in reduction of carcass meat deposition. A QTL affecting both growth and backfat thickness is reported.

An alternative to high feed intake is the selection for residual feed intake (RFI), which is the difference between observed feed intake and expected feed intake, whereby the latter is based on metabolic body weight and growth; its negative values indicate a higher efficiency in the conversion of the food intake into weight, reducing waste of intake and consequently the fat deposition. Selection for muscle deposition increase might be associated with the arising of the PSE (pale, soft, exudative) phenomenon in meat, which is caused by recessive homozygosis for the Halothane gene.

Breeds with muscular hypertrophy tend to develop this condition (Seller, 1998) because the genes involved in both aspects are located in the same linkage group. Recessive homozygote pigs show better feed efficiency, and greater carcass yield and carcass lean content. A QTL affecting lean meat quantity and meat paleness is also reported.

The PSE phenomenon is triggered by animal stress before slaughter, and this situation can be increased due to the lower ability to stand environmental stress evidenced in selected pigs (Rauw et al., 1998). Therefore, management procedures to avoid stress conditions before slaughter could prevent PSE phenomenon.

Diseases Susceptibility

Swine with greater growth rate exhibit high incidences of gastric, cardiac, renal and pulmonary problems such as pneumonia and pleuritis. These factors may bring the necessity of a limited selection emphasis for high daily growth, resulting in reduction of animal productive performance, increase in mortality and production costs and impairing animal welfare.

SIDE EFFECTS OF ANIMAL BREEDING IN POULTRY

Selection in poultry is focused on fast growth, food efficiency and high carcass yield. Nearly 85 to 90% of existing growth speed and body weight increase has resulted from animal breeding for weight increase at a young age. However, growth rate increase in broiler has caused several metabolic disorders.

Reproduction

Rapid growth selection turns into responses correlated negatively with reproductive traits such as an increase in numbers of defective eggs and infertility. Both might be attributed to neuralendocrine unbalance, disruption of gametogenesis synchrony, disorders in ovulation, oviposition and libido. Selection for muscle weight increase might generate problems related to natural mating, because natural mating becomes unfeasible due to male sizes, therefore provoking injuries to dorsum lumbar region in females. Nevertheless, artificial insemination has allowed carrying on with body weight selection.

Excessive body weight also seems to be associated with fertility decrease in broiler via reduced semen quality. Concentration, volume and sperm mobility reduction and an increase of death or abnormal sperm cells are reported. High body weight selection is also associated with an enlarged number of eggs; however, it is related to a high incidence of defective eggs as well (extra calcification, two yolks) which is caused by a lack of syntony during ovulation. There is also a reduction in eclosion and a high frequency of chromosome abnormalities in embryos. Regarding to laying hens, selection for body weight decrease might result in a population of reduced size which has their reproduction capacity impaired.

Skeleton formation

There is an important association between leg problems and the selection for growth in broiler carcass traits. For modern broiler lines tissue growth rate is extremely high, which starts in a very early phase post hatching on an immature skeleton. In this context, broiler often suffer from tibial dyschondroplasia, an abnormality of growth plate cartilage featured by the presence of non-vascularised, nonmineralised tissue under the epiphyseal plate (growth plate) occurring in the proximal end of the long bones.

The manifestation of tibial dyschondroplasia is thought to be the result of a very fast growth in the early phases of development whereby the development of the bones does not keep up with the rapid weight gain of the muscle mass. Therefore, the animal is unable to support its own weight, thus causing a decrease in performance as well as the discard of the animal. Tibial dyschondroplasia has a genetic component, although it is mainly caused by environmental effects such as nutrition, housing and husbandr.

Cardio respiratory system and metabolic rate

Ascites syndrome is characterized by the extravasation of liquid from the liver to the abdomen cavity due to the increased pulmonary arterial pressure and the fatigue of the cardiac muscle. This extravasation of fluids occurs when there is a lack of oxygen which results in systemic hypoxia and an increase of cardiac debt. In order to cut the oxygen debt, broiler compensate with a high cardiac frequency, causing increased blood flow and pulmonary hypertension. Although this syndrome is multifactorial and influenced by the environment a genetic predisposition for it has also been observed.

Owing to genetic selection for muscle development and food conversion, the cardio-respiratory capacity is insufficient due to the out-of balance relation between heart/lung size and broiler weight. The high demand for oxygen in broilers selected for rapid growth, necessary to sustain the high metabolic rate, makes oxygen a limiting factor, predisposing broilers to heart failure.

Moreover, a genetic tendency to a reduction of the absolute and relative heart size in a male chicken line breed was found, due to indirect selection for economic traits. The selection of animals for blood parameters, such as cardiac and haematocrit rate may help to avoid ascites.

The intense pressure for body weight selection has altered growth standards. Today broilers reach their slaughter weight at a younger age and have a higher content of body fat, as well as higher insulin and glucagon concentrations in the plasma. Associated to that, an increase in the food passage rate in addition to high enzymatic activity in the intestine has been observed.

Carcass and meat quality

Selection for body weight increase has also altered endocrine and neural control mechanisms which affect feed consumption, therefore causing obesity in broilers. However, the main effects of these disorders remain unknown in broilers because they are slaughtered at young age. In these poultry breeds voluntary consumption is beyond metabolic demands, only limited by the maximum capacity of the digestive system.

This is largely due to a failure of the hypothalamus to regulate appetite. Other side-effects are the tendency for an increased abdominal fat deposition and an enlarged intestine. As described for swine, the selection for RFI could be used in order to avoid the excessive fat deposition in broiler.

The number of fibres is relative and changes during animal growth and development; broilers selected for rapid growth have a higher number of fibres than broilers with normal growth rates, moreover, the muscular fibres diameter increases according to the age and genetic potential for breast meat production.

However, selection for high breast weight seems to decrease the number of muscular fibres but to increase the diameter and area of these fibres and thus may reduce meat quality because of water loss and increased shear force of meat, a measure for meat tenderness.

Therefore, the selection for a large number of fibres with small diameters and fibres areas may improve meat quality by reducing water loss by exudation, defrosting, and cooking, as well as by increased tenderness, which are important traits for the industrial meat quality. A balance between histological traits, body and breast weight and meat quality is demanded, and it can be established by the selection index.

The pectoral myopathy incidence, an ischemic necrosis that develops in the deep pectoral muscle, has also been associated with rapid growth and muscle increase in poultry, and there is a positive correlation between age and rapid growth on one hand and the occurrence of degenerated breast muscles on the other. Selection for rapid growth has produced muscles that grow more than the vital system can stand, causing injuries to the muscle and carcass discard.

Stress and Disease Susceptibility

Metabolic properties of muscles are related to the animal's capacity to cope with environmental stress. Muscles with a low proportion of glycolytic fibres (white fibres), a high blood capillary supply, high oxidative capacity and small fibres are more efficient to maintain their energy reserves, and therefore are more able to stand the environmental stress.

It has been suggested that commercial broilers are more susceptible to stress because they have a high proportion of glycolytic (rapidly contracting) fibres and only a low proportion of oxidative (slowly contracting) muscle fibres. Glycolytic fibres have high growth potential, suggesting that the increase in the proportion of glycolytic fibres is associated with the selection for a high growth rate.

Additionally, high growth rate broilers display a reduced immune response when challenged by several microorganisms. The animals show a low resistance to sanitary challenges, they exhibit low antibody responses and high mortality rates.

In layer hens, this impaired immune response is reported for individuals with low RFI. Genetic selection for immunological traits may be used in these situations, but correct management against stress and biosecurity procedures should co-operate in order to prevent disease occurrences.

THE NEGATIVE EFFECTS OF DOG BREEDING

By disregarding the health and working ability of their dogs, irresponsible breeders directly contribute to some of the worst problems that come with dog breeding. This includes contributing to overpopulation and exacerbating problems within the breed. At the same time, responsible breeders are working to combat these issues.

Worsening Dog Overpopulation

According to the ASPCA, 6.5 million of our pets enter animal shelters in the USA every year – a sobering statistic for any dog breeder. Irresponsible breeding contributes to dog overpopulation in a number of ways. By breeding without regard for temperament or characteristics, many backyard breeders have contributed to this tragic issue.

Dogs with poor temperament are often bred by backyard breeders. This produces puppies with behavioral problems who are quickly surrendered to shelters or abandoned as owners struggle to cope. In the same vein, irresponsible breeders who fail to socialize their puppies, ignore their critical development periods, and remove them from their dam too early are dooming puppies to the same fate.

A responsible dog breeder will make sure that there is a market for their puppies before they are bred. For some, this might involve creating a waiting list for puppies before they are even born to ensure that there is interest. They will also ensure that their puppies come from parents with excellent temperaments to avoid behavioral problems for their future owners.

Lastly, a responsible breeder will always meet with the prospective buyer. This is to ensure that the buyer is knowledgeable and prepared for their new puppy. Some breeders will even take their puppies back if the owner is unable to care for them. However, until these practices become the standard for all dog breeders, the problem of overpopulation will sadly continue.

Breed-Specific Exaggerations

Many of the dog breeds we have today are the result of hundreds of years of artificial selection for certain characteristics. Among the most infamous examples are the English Bulldog, known for its stout body and flat face, and the German Shepherd, now with its sloping back and wider chest.

So, for both of these breeds, painful arthritis and difficulty walking are now commonplace. Irresponsible dog breeders, or those ignorant to the health conditions that accompany these breed changes, will not strive to improve their breed. Instead, they allow for, or even select for, these unhealthy traits.

Fortunately, many responsible breeders with a passion for their breed are now actively working to reverse these problems by selecting dogs who show less dramatic traits. For some, this involves outcrossing programs. Some breeders go a step further and cross-breed to introduce new genetic material to the breed. However, until prospective puppy buyers and the majority of dog breeders become aware of the health problems that come with these traits, they are likely to persevere in these breeds. As such, it is important that responsible breeders continue to educate others through their work.

Puppy Mills

While there is demand for puppies and a lack of law enforcement, puppy mills thrive. According to the Humane Society, there are at least 10,000 puppy mills in the USA alone. Fewer than 3,000 of these are regulated, and many more are likely hidden. Sadly, puppy mills produce a staggering 2 million puppies every year.

Also, considering that over 1 million dogs are euthanized in shelters every year, this is a very sobering statistic. Until the public is better educated on puppy mills, these highly unethical puppy mills will prosper. As a prospective puppy buyer, you must always see your puppy in person, meet their dam, and check the breeder's credentials. Or, better yet, seek a puppy from a shelter if you're looking for a new furry friend to bring home.

Inbreeding & Small Gene Pools

Due to unethical breeding practices, the gene pool of several breeds has become alarmingly small! Perhaps the most infamous example of this is seen in the Pug. In the UK, 10,000 Pugs are so inbred that their gene pool is the equivalent of just 50 individuals. To combat this problem, some breeders are now looking to out-cross their Pugs to totally unrelated Pugs. To do this effectively, the two dogs must share no common ancestors in a four-generation pedigree.

Some breeders are going a step further and crossing the Pug to other small breeds, such as the Parson Russell Terrier or Jack Russell Terrier, in an attempt to lessen the brachycephalic features of the breed. The resulting mix is known as the "Retro Pug." Many Retro Pug breeders aim to keep the breed at around 80 to 90% Pug. Cross-breeding in this way also introduces new genetic material to the bloodline. However, some breeders reject the idea of bringing new breeds into the picture. They worry that the breed will take on new diseases and change in temperament.

Culling Practices

Culling can mean two things: removing a dog from a breeding program or euthanizing them. While euthanasia for cosmetic reasons is uncommon today, past breeders engaged in the culling of puppies in a few breeds. One notable example is the white German Shepherd. White German Shepherds fell from grace in 1959. At this time, they were labeled as "albino." Some countries then refused to register them altogether or made them an automatic disqualification. This mutation was rumored to be responsible for blindness as well as deafness.

Today, culling like this is not common practice. Instead, puppies with severe deformities and health problems are usually the only candidates for a cull. That's not to say that cosmetic culling doesn't happen, however. Because of this, it's especially important to avoid breeders who breed for color alone. Be wary of breeders who only offer "rare" puppies.

An ethical breeder will sell puppies with undesirable coloration for a lower price. They may also ask the buyer to sign a contract to say that they will not breed from the dog later on. These practices help to ensure that the breed continues to thrive. If you buy a puppy with undesirable coloration, make sure to check the breed standard before entering shows. Your puppy may have an automatic disqualification due to their coat color.

FINAL CONSIDERATIONS

In many cases selection for high productive efficiency in livestock species are accompanied by undesirable side effects for some physiological and reproductive traits, impairing animal welfare, health and productivity, and consequently increasing production costs. Animal breeding has made animals more sensitive to these problems, changing their body composition and production capacity, causing a great impact on their homeostasis.

The undesired side effects differ in their impact in different species, breeds, lines and populations, because the selective pressure applied varies among them and thus also the impact of genetic changes due to the breeding. Most frequently undesirable effects can be found in species with reduced generation gap, as broilers, or in precocious breeds, since these effects rapidly arise in these cases and consequently can be more evident.

In several species it is possible to observe that the undesirable effects are due to their multifactorial nature. Then, the identification and the control of environmental factors concerning these undesirable traits become essential to minimise them, although several studies have proved genetic correlation between productive traits and undesirable effects. On the other hand, if at favourable management and environmental conditions the undesirable effects may not become so evident, and the control of environmental conditions may be expensive.

Therefore, it is necessary to redefine animal breeding strategies within a wider perspective of traits as well as further studies on physiological processes under genetic selection performance. Understanding genetic selection for economic traits upon physiological mechanisms might offer an important tool to understand and prevent unfavourable side effects of animal breeding. In this manner, the selection objectives need to be reevaluated and redefined in breeding programs. The Behavioural, physiological and immunological traits should be included as selection objectives in the selection process and/or the selection intensity for economically interested traits must be adjusted according to the dimensioning of their unfavourable correlational responses. It could be done even with withdraw of the genetic gains for economical traits decreases; nevertheless it would reduce productivity losses, discards of animals and environmental control costs.

Breeding technologies could also contribute for the optimization of the genetic gains and for the success of animal breeding programs. Reproduction techniques and DNA technologies may be helpful to correct some undesirable effects, e.g. sperm preparation techniques, sexed semen, embryo transfer and in vitro fertilization may increase the fertility indexes, and DNA analysis could be used to identify the loci involved in the trade-offs of indirect selection for behavioural, physiological and immunological traits.

6

BASICS OF ANIMAL BREEDING

ANIMAL BREEDING PROGRAM

Animal breeding is based on the fact that traits of parents are reflected more or less in their offspring. This is caused by the fact that traits are more or less heritable and that 50 % of the DNA, comprising the heritable ability for the traits of an animal, is passed from a parent to its offspring. In animal breeding potential parents are selected for certain traits and the best ones are indeed used as parents. In this way the next generation will be genetically improved for the desired traits. For the long term the subsequent breeding activities are carried out in a breeding program illustrated in the scheme below:

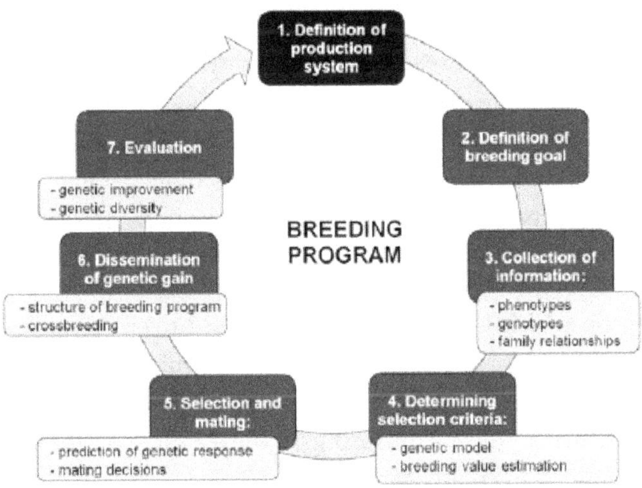

Diagram of breeding program

In animal breeding potential parents are selected for certain traits and only the best ones are used as parents. In this way the next generation will be genetically improved for the desired traits. Over a long period of time breeding activities are carried out step by step following a breeding program.

The starting point for an animal breeder is always a clear definition of the breeding goal. That means breeders need to identify the traits which should be improved in a certain population. Information on performance of animals and their genetic relationships has to be collected and those showing the best genetic potential have to be identified.

Next, the necessary proportion of the population which needs to be included in the breeding program in order to achieve a certain genetic gain in the next generation is determined. Animals are selected and mated. The final step is to map the resulting offspring against the originally defined breeding goals.

Each generation which is bred follows this circle of steps. Thus, each time an adjustment to the parameters can be made to a certain extent. However, the overall breeding goal should not be changed in every generation because one single generation will not allow for much genetic improvement. Breeding is more about the cumulative success of multiple generations. Goals can be modified, responding to changes in the markets or to adjust the actual breeding program to counteract an unwanted genetic change in the population. Adaptations have to be made timely to avoid cumulative effects of an undesired response to selection. Almost every chapter will focus on a specific step of the breeding program. The main goal of the respective step will be explained as well as challenges and ways how to master them.

SET UP OF A BREEDING PROGRAM

Production system

First step in the setup is a description of the production system (1). This includes the analysis of the way in which animals are kept and which purpose they will serve. For a small dog only kept as a companion animal in a comfortable house behaviour and health are important. For heath sheep kept in rough conditions the whole year, fitness traits and grazing behaviour are more relevant. In the broilers industry with its intensive systems and high production costs, daily growth rates are of highest importance.

Breeding goal

Second, the question which traits should be improved over the next generations has to be answered. What will be the goal(s) of breeding? This issue is highly related to the reasons for which animals are kept. This process requires a thorough study and a long term perspective because animal breeding is only effective when a breeding goal is consequently maintained for many generations.

Examples of breeding goals are defined improvements in traits of production, product quality, health and welfare traits, conformation traits, sport performance, fertility etc.

Collection of information

In a third step all information relevant for the defined breeding goal has to be collected such as traits of animals (called phenotypes) that can help to establish the value of an animal with respect to the breeding goal. If performance in jumping is a breeding goal trait in horses, data on jumping are collected. If fertility of pigs is in the breeding goal, litter traits are recorded. Other relevant information is the pedigree of the animals.

Animal breeding is all about passing genetic abilities from one generation to the next. When breeders want to trace or influence this process of passing heritable traits, it is crucial to registrate the parent-offspring relationships, i.e. pedigrees of animals have to be kept. Today DNA-analysis are also possible and already practiced in animal breeding. They can be used to trace or influence the process of passing genetic abilities for traits.

Breeding value estimation and selection criteria

Fourth, knowing the breeding goal and after recording relevant traits of potential parents, the population of animals is divided into two groups: Animals with the potential to be used in breeding as future parents and animals which will be excluded from reproduction. Based on a genetic model i.e. a statistical model including pedigree information, a breeding value for a trait is estimated. Because today DNA information of animals is available, this information can also be used to estimate breeding values. The estimated breeding value indicates the value of a specific animal with respect to the breeding goal: the lowest values will have a negative effect on the breeding goal traits, the highest values will improve them.

Selection and mating

Fifth, given the estimated breeding values of sires and dams, the actual selection of parents has to take place. Parents with a higher than average estimated breeding value will improve the breeding goal traits in the next generation. When for example a group of dairy sires with the highest breeding value for milk yield is selected as sires for the next generations, their daughters will produce more milk than the present generation of dairy cows. Proper selection of parents leads to a positive selection response in the next generations. Selection creates progress in breeding goal traits. After the selection of the parents another choice has to be made: Which sire should be mated to which dam? The choice can be made on the basis of the pedigree information available or on the traits of the sires and the dams.

Dissemination of genetic gain

In many breeding schemes the number of animals from which traits are recorded is rather small compared to the population of animals used for human purposes. The dissemination of the selection response depends on the structure of the breeding programs.

In commercial pig and poultry programs selection takes place in the top of the breeding program and via a few "multiplying generations" the selection response obtained in the top is disseminated to the animals producing meat or eggs. In cattle breeding artificial reproduction techniques, in particular AI techniques, given the opportunity to produce high numbers of offspring, thus disseminating the genes of the superior animals widely.

Selection of a small number of animals may have a large impact on the traits of a population. Within commercial breeding schemes e.g. for poultry and pigs specialized lines are crossed. These lines are selected for specific traits and crossed in the multiplying phases. Crossbred progeny is obtained with the breeding goal traits by combining the traits of each of the lines.

Evaluation of results

The breeding program should be evaluated regularly. The first question which has to be answered is if breeding goals have been reached. Is the new generation of animals better with respect to the breeding goal traits? Are there any unwanted effects of selection? E.g. has a better growth of meat producing animals been achieved on the cost of more leg problems compared to the parent generation? The second question is: what has happened with the relatedness among animals of the new generation. Are they more related to each other than their parents, due to the fact that selection has only been made only a few heavily related animals as parents for this generation? Has the genetic diversity of the population decreased? Following these evaluations the breeding circle starts again with a critical review of changes in the production system. Questions to be answered are: do market requirements change, e.g. for pork of a different quality? Do production circumstances change, e.g. are milk production quota for dairy farms expected to be abolished in the next future?

GENETIC BASIS OF ANIMAL BREEDING

DNA is the carrier of genetic information passed on to the next generation. Breeders want to transfer the best genetic material available from the present to the next generation of animals. This genetic material is stored in the chromosomes, in the nucleus of each cell inside those animals which may be selected as parents for the next generation. The process takes place when chromosomes containing the genes are transferred via sperm cells and oocytes. The combination of a sperm cell and an oocyte into a zygote is the starting point of a new animal with a unique genetic composition. In the transfer of chromosomes from parents to offspring the meiosis plays an important role. It ensures that the transfer follows to some extent the laws, recognized by Mendel, and is also driven by random processes. The laws connect genetically relatives, e.g. parents and their offspring. The parents each share for 50% the same chromosomes, the same DNA and thus the same genetic value with their offspring.

Therefore phenotypic traits of parents, can be found in the phenotypic traits of their offspring, based on the genes they got from their parents. The conclusion of this is, that offspring and parents share a part of their DNA, they have a genetic relationship. This relationship is higher in generally related animals.

Structure and composition of chromosomes

Chromosomes are units of DNA. Body cells of mammals and birds have a nucleus where pairs of chromosomes (units of DNA) are found (Table 1).

Table 1. Number of chromosome pairs for different species

Species	Number of chromosome pairs
Man	23
Cattle	30
Horse	32
Pig	19
Sheep	27
Goat	30
Rabbit	22
Chicken	39
Duck	40

Each species has a specific number of chromosomes as illustrated in the table above. The different number of chromosomes impedes the production of crosses between species. When a zygote forms out of a sperm and an oocyte their single chromosomes are regrouped into pairs. This process fails if the number of chromosomes from the paired species is not equal i.e. when sperm cells and oocytes originate from different species with different number of chromosomes.

Chromosomes are double-stranded helices, consisting of two long biopolymers made of simpler units called nucleotides. Each nucleotide is composed of a nucleobase (guanine, adenine, thymine, and cytosine), recorded by using the letters G, A, T, and C, as well as a backbone made of alternating sugars (deoxyribose) and phosphate groups (related to phosphoric acid). The nucleobases (G, A, T, C) are attached to the sugars. Within a species and also within a breed the nucleotides and nucleobases are placed in a fixed sequence.

The transfer from chromosomes and genes from parent to offspring

To understand the genetic relationships among related animals it is necessary to know what happens during the creation of sperm cells, oocytes and zygotes as the start of a new animal. In mammals and birds all body cells of an individual are diploid: All chromosomes (Fig. 2) in the nucleus of a cell are present in twofold, grouped in pairs.

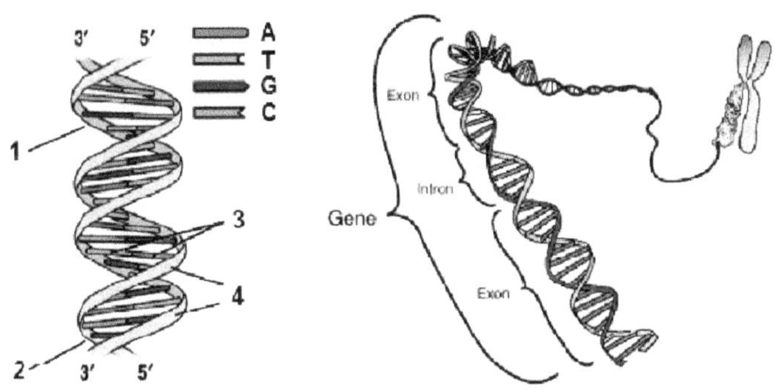

Figure 2. DNA structure (left), chromosome shape and gene (right).

Left: Major chain (1), minor chain (2), nitrogenous bases (A - adenine, T - threonine, G - guanine and C - cytosine) that form base pairs (3) on the phosphate-deoxyribose skeleton (4). DNA has 5% of regions that encode different characters. The remaining 95% of regions are assumed to have no role in encoding processes or characters. Right: a gene, related to the double helical structure of DNA and a chromosome. The chromosome has the shape of the letter "X" because it is in division. Introns are regions often found in eukaryotic cells that are removed through the sizing process (after DNA is transcribed into RNA). Exons are the only regions that encode protein synthesis. Image modified after "DNA structure and sequencing:

The expression of genes, of their alleles, in the phenotype

In all body cells the chromosomes are present in duplo: one originates from the sire and one from the dam. Therefore also all genes are present in duplo. These genes might be identical: the allele originating from the sire is identical to the one from the dam. In this case an animal is homozygous for that gene. It implies that progeny of this animal always get that allele from this parent. However, the alleles originating from sire and dam can be different which makes the animal heterozygous for that gene. Progeny of this animal might get one of the two different alleles of its parent.

For a certain gene three different genotypes can be distinguished,e.g: EE, Ee or ee. These combinations of alleles may cause different phenotypes. Suppose E is responsible for the production of the protein eumelanin in skin cells of dogs that gives a black pigmentation of the skin and e is responsible for the production of phaeomelanin in skin cells of dogs that gives a red pigmentation. It is obvious that EE animals will be black and ee animals will be red. But what will be the colour of Ee dogs? They are also black!. This phenomenon is called dominance: The expression of the e-allele in heterozygous is not expressed in their phenotype. The allele E is dominant over e or, from a point of view from allele e: It is recessive to allele E.

In cases where a gene is involved in the expression of a quantitative trait e.g. body weight of a mature goat the alleles might have a different expression leading to small differences in mature body weight. The following two examples explain this in more detail:

1. GG animals weigh 40 kg, Gg animals 38 kg and gg animals 36 kg. The body weight of the heterozygous animal is exactly the average of the two homozygous animals. The two alleles have an additive effect. This is called co-dominance.
2. GG animals weigh 40 kg, Gg animals 42 kg and gg animals 36 kg. The body weight of the heterozygous animal is higher than the average of the two homozygous animals and even higher than the value of the highest homozygous parent. This is called overdominance.

In addition to the effects of different alleles of a gene at a single locus, alleles of different genes at different loci might influence each other. That might be expressed in the phenotype of the trait they influence. There are two possibilities. 1): The effects of different alleles at different loci are additive: the effect is the sum of the effect of the individual alleles. 2): When these effects are non-additive, this is called epistasis.

Plumage pattern in chicken is amongst other genes, determined by interacting alleles of two different loci: the E-locus and the S-locus. The E-locus has two alleles E and e+. The S-locus: S and s.E is dominant over e+ and causes a uniform black plumage. In the e+e+ animals the black colour is restricted to restricted parts of the plumage. In the non-black parts of the plumage the SS or Ss animals have at these places the silver colour, while the ss animals have there the golden colour. Thus the golden or silver colour is only expressed in the e+e+ animals: black at the E-locus is dominant over golden and silver determined by the alleles at the S-locus.

Differences among related offspring

In sperm cells and oocytes the chromosomes are no longer present in twofold, grouped in pairs. In these cells all chromosomes exist in singularity. In the testis and in the ovary the pairs of chromosomes split in singular chromosomes and each chromosome goes by chance to a sperm cell or an oocyte. This process is called meiosis and is illustrated below with three chromosome pairs of a male (Fig 3):

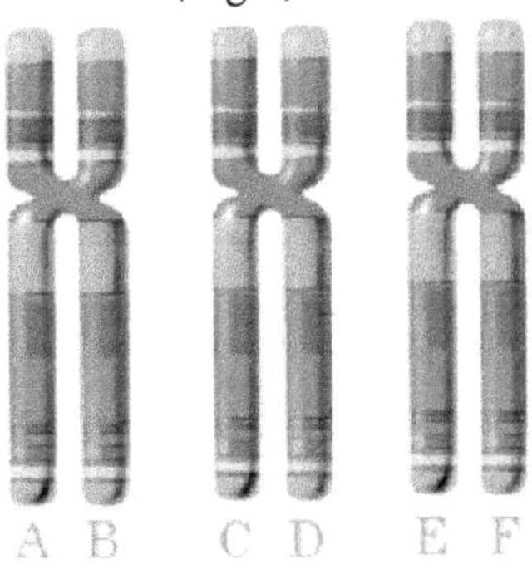

Figure 2.2. Combinations of chromosomes

Chromosome pair 1 consists of chromosome A and B, pair 2 of C and D and pair 3 of E and F. In the meiosis the pairs the chromosome pairs split and go by chance to a sperm cell. In this way sperm cells are created with 8 (23) different combinations of chromosomes: ACE, ACF, BCE, BCF, ADE, ADF, BDF and BDF. When a species has n chromosomes the parents create 2n different sperm cells or oocytes.

Relationship between relatives with share similar DNA

Due to the processes during meiosis phase a sperm cell and an oocyte contain 50 % of the DNA of the parent (a natural law in the transmission from DNA of parents to offspring) and express a unique combination of chromosomes of the parent (random process in the transmission of DNA between generations). After fertilization of an oocyte with a sperm cell the nucleus of the zygote contains again chromosomes in twofold, grouped in pairs.

This implies that each animal receives half of its chromosomes, half of it genetic value from its sire and half of its dam. Thus the genetic relationship between an animal and each of its parents is 0.5.

This is called the additive genetic relationship. But each sperm cell and each oocyte from a parent contains a unique combination of the chromosomes of that parent. This is the reason why the offspring, while having the same combination of a sire and a dam (full sibs), still show differences in traits.

The additive genetic relationship of full brothers and full sisters (full sibs) is 0.5, because on average they share 50 % of the DNA of their parents (Table 2).

Relationship	Percentage of similar DNA they share
Parent-son or daughter	50
Grandparent-grandchild	25
Great-grandparents- great-grandchild	12.5
Full brother(s) – full sister(s)	50
Half-brother(s) – half-sister(s)	25

Thus relatives share similar DNA. The average percentage which they share is obvious, but without further knowledge of their DNA (genotypes) or their phenotypes, it is not clear which part of the DNA, which alleles they share.

Production systems in animal husbandry

Animal husbandry represents for the economy of any country, the branch that ensures long term survival, including prosperity, food requirements of the population, superior capitalization of feed resources, rational use of work force, efficient use of nutrients from manure and many other factors. Over time, animal husbandry has been the most dynamic sector, being the branch in which the processes of concentration and specialization of production materialized the earliest. Modern industrial technologies have been introduced.

The resources which are related to this branch of agriculture belong to different categories of entrepreneurs: family farms, agricultural companies of different kinds, etc. Regardless of ownership and level of organization of the processes, the main production systems in animal husbandry can be considered the following:

- The system of production (S.P.) of milk from cattle
- S. P. beef cattle,
- S. P. of wool, S.P. of meat and S.P of skins in sheep;
- S. P. pork;
- S. P. of eggs and S.P. poultry meat;
- S. P. honey and bee by-products;

- S. P. fish in fish farms and recirculating water systems;
- S. P. of donuts from silk butterflies;
- S. P. productions from thoroughbred horses;
- S. P. from breeding animals
- S. P. ecological, etc.

The various production systems listed above include different approaches to breeding and exploitation of species i.e. breeds from which productions can be obtained.

Characteristics that are subject of animal breeding

Each production is the result of a set of complex characteristics, which themselves are based on a group of simpler characteristics. These being determined by a number of genes. In farm animals, regardless of the species, the characteristics which are subject to improvement can be classified into four broad categories:

Production traits or characteristics:

- milk production;
- meat production;
- wool production;
- speed of movement or milking;

Reproduction characteristics:

- fecundity;
- birth;
- prolificacy;
- the influencing characters of fertility

Resistance characteristics/ traits to:

- hereditary diseases
- diseases caused by environmental factors
- diseases caused by pathogens

Conformational characteristics:

- aesthetic characteristics (recreational animals)
- external characteristics turned into production (skin of fur animals or Karakul lambs)
- external characteristics positively correlated with some production (carcass characteristics)

The improvement of these characteristics from one generation to another depends on the genetic basis that determines their phenotypic value. Obviously, breeders want to transfer the best genetic material from the best animals to the next generation.

KEY ISSUES IN BASICS OF ANIMAL BREEDING

1. A breeding program is characterized by a series of subsequent activities: defining the breeding goal, registration of phenotypes, genotypes and pedigrees, estimation of breeding values for selection traits with a genetic model, selection of parents for the next generation based on estimated breeding values, mating of parents and dissemination of genetic superiority towards the production animals and evaluation of the program with respect to the genetic diversity maintained and realized selection response.
2. Animals can be raised and exploited in different production systems, breeding and exploitation systems, according to the requirements of different technologies. Since all components are dynamic, systems must allow for viable production (economically efficient, environmentally sustainable and socially accepted);
3. Body cells of mammals and birds have a nucleus where pairs of chromosomes are found. The different number of chromosomes among species impedes the production of crosses between species. Chromosomes are strings of DNA, Deoxyribo Nucleic Acid, which is a macromolecule in the form of a doublestranded helix that carry the genetic information in all cells of higher organisms.
4. A gene is the hereditary unit, a region of DNA on a chromosome containing genetic information which is transcribed into RNA. RNA is translated into a polypeptide chain with a physiological function. A gene can mutate to various forms, called alleles.
5. In all body cells the chromosomes are present in duplo: one originate from the sire and one from the dam. Therefore all genes are present in duplo. These genes might be identical: the allele originating from the sire is identical to the one from the dam. Then an animal is homozygous for that gene. The alleles originating from sire and dam can also be different. In this case an animal is heterozygous for that gene.
6. Alleles can be dominant or recessive (interaction between two alleles at a locus). The effects can be additive: Co-dominance (the value of the heterozygous lies exactly between the two homozygous genotype) or over-dominant (the heterozygote has a genotypic value more extreme than parents).
7. Alleles of a gene can also interact with alleles of another gene: Epistasis.
8. Due to the processes during meiosis a sperm cell and an oocyte contain 50 % of the parent DNA. After fertilization of an oocyte with a sperm cell the nucleus of the zygote contains again chromosomes in twofold grouped in pairs. This implies that each animal receives half of its chromosomes, half of it genetic value, from its sire and the other half from its dam. Thus the genetic relationship between an animal and each of its parents is 0.5. This is called the additive genetic relationship.

7

CHALLENGES FOR ANIMAL BREEDING

Modern selection approaches are expected to bring about the cumulative and permanent improvement of animal performance and profitability of animal production. Breeding values of traits along with trait economic values (EVs) are utilised for economic selection purposes with many species all over the world. Currently, some challenges related to trait EVs in animal breeding should be considered. First, the selection response based on the higher accuracy of genomic selection may be reduced due to improper weighting of the trait breeding values of selection candidates. A comprehensive approach applied in bioeconomic models allows suitable trait EV calculations.

Further challenges comprise the new breeding objectives associated with climate change, environmental mitigation and animal adaptability. The estimation of EVs for traits influencing greenhouse gas (GHG) emissions has been mostly based on including the value of CO_2 emission equivalent in the trait EVs, on calculating EVs for feed efficiency traits and on methane yield as a direct trait of GHG emission.

Genetic improvement of production, functional, feed efficiency and methane traits through the application of multi-trait selection indices was found to be crucial for mitigation of emissions and farm profitability. Defining the non-market values of traits connected with climate protection could be a useful solution for including these traits in an economic breeding objective. While GHG emissions mostly change the costs per unit of production, animal adaptability in its complexity influences animal performance.

Clear definitions of disease, fertility, mortality and other breeding objective traits allow the proper calculation of trait EVs, and an accurate estimation of trait genetic parameters could lead to sufficient economic selection response. This complex approach could be beneficial for more effective utilisation of inputs and overall economic and environmental sustainability of animal production.

Demand for animal protein is set to increase dramatically over the next few decades. This represents a significant challenge in terms of increasing productivity against a backdrop of reducing resources including land and water. It will require the application of many different technologies including genetic improvement. Whilst the largest cost of production is associated with feed, another significant element is the impact of disease. The cost of disease may be underestimated due to its multifactorial nature and the relative success, at least in the developed world. Researchers state that the role of genetics in improving animal health will become increasingly important as focus increases on tackling antimicrobial drug resistance.

Technological innovations have been drivers of social and economic change. They have played a pivotal role in enhancing the quality of life and the safety of animals and humans. In the last four decades there has been an unprecedented surge in the development of biotechnology in animal production and health, with gene-based biotechnologies becoming most prominent in the last decade. While the vast majority of these technologies has been developed and utilized in developed countries, they have the potential to alleviate poverty and hunger, reduce the threats of diseases and ensure environmental sustainability in developing countries. Some of the technologies have a long history of successful use, others have been used with varied success, and many more are at different stages of development and commercialization.

In selective breeding, the potential of individuals to transmit good genes to the next generation is estimated (i.e. their breeding value is calculated). With genomic selection it is possible to estimate an animal's breeding value quite accurately without the need for own performance or performance of large number of offspring. Modern breeds of livestock differ markedly from their ancestors as a result of breeding strategies.

For example, milk production per cow has increased among Holstein dairy cattle. Similarly, breeding programs have resulted in lean, fast-growing pigs. Chickens from modern breeds each produce more than 250 eggs per year, approximately double that produced in 1950, again mainly due to genetic selection. Currently countries that are following genomic selection are United States of America, Canada, New Zealand, Netherlands, Australia, Denmark, Sweden and Brazil. Benefits of genomic selections have well been demonstrated in developed countries that include reduced generation interval accuracies of above 70% have been reported for young genomic proven bulls, higher rates of genetic gains.

Genomic systems in developed countries are characterized with large reference populations, collaboration among countries, well defined phenotypes but mostly within pure breeds.

THE BREEDING GOAL

The first step is always the definition of a breeding goal. After that, a breeding scheme has to be set up which ensures genetic progress in line with the goal. The main components of structured breeding programs with the relevant traits are collection of performance data,

data analysis to identify superior animals and the use of superior animals to produce the next generation.

In most cases, when describing animal breeding, reference is made to a breeding program that aims to improve certain traits. However, sometimes the purpose of breeding is not to make genetic improvements to the population, but to preserve the genetic diversity of a given population.

This second type of breeding objective is often found in small populations that are not raised (only) for animal production (zoological populations, local breeds). Even when the goal of breeding is genetic improvement of the population, genetic diversity is still an issue.

From a descriptive point of view, the improvement objective (H) has six essential characteristics. Basically, the objective of improvement is characterized by the fact that:

i. aims at the challenges of the future
ii. includes all the desired features in the improvement objective
iii. contains breeding values grouped in "genotypic aggregations"
iv. allows the weighting of the characters subject to improvement v) includes all the desired features in a single criterion (index)
v. may include not only economic values, but also non-economic aspects

CHALLENGES

Although the constraints that breeds of small census size are faced with are not insurmountable, they are not trivial either. A first major challenge is simply a strong inertia built up by a typical small breed's history; small breeds are usually not small by accident. Some breeds are small because they were developed and adapted to a given region and isolated by geographical constraints from expansion into wider markets.

Others are small because of either deliberate policies to remain exclusive or a lack of effort or success in promotion and marketing. Others have never been as productive as the best breeds and were thus not competitive enough economically to appeal to a wide number of breeders. Small breeds suffer because they cannot take advantage of economies of scale in breeding and marketing programs. Larger breeds have a greater opportunity to increase selection response, because a larger number of individuals allows for greater selection differentials, especially when artificial insemination and other reproductive biotechnologies can increase the number of offspring per individual.

Breeding companies also have more interest in larger breeds because the potential market is greater and because the truly superior animals are more extreme and thus more valuable. This vicious cycle basically condemns breeds to remain small under "standard" conditions. However, this reality does not preclude that particular interventions can be undertaken to overcome these obstacles.

Challenges for animal breeding

The major challenge for food production in agriculture is the continuous growth of the human population towards 9 billion in 2050.

Challenges for human society needs

Livestock systems play an important role in agriculture by producing high quality food. In developing countries animals provide not only meat, milk and eggs, but also fibre, fertiliser for crops, manure for fuel and draught power. For these countries productivity and fitness traits are the major challenges of animal breeding.

They make food production and food supply to consumers efficient. In developed countries who run intensive animal production systems, health and welfare traits became a new challenge for animal breeders. Breeding business is influenced by a wide range of factors. Needs and priorities of several interest groups have to be balanced: Animal owners, consumers of animal products, the food industry, and increasingly the general public.

It is a continuous process where future developments have to be anticipated and planning has to be done carefully to establish effective breeding programs.

Challenges for breeding depending on the production system

In addition to food production, animals fulfil a variety of functions for mankind: They provide labour, are held as companion animals, participate in leisure activities, cultural events and have also a role in nature management. The use of animals and user requirements determine to a great extend the breeding goal and the breeding programs.

If breeding programs have another focus than food production some additional traits become important in addition to those which are obvious for any selective breeding goal traits as: health and welfare of the animals, adaptation to feed of lower quality and extreme climates to be capable to produce and reproduce.

Before defining the breeding goal many questions regarding the production system have to be answered. For what reason are animals kept? What are the distribution channels? What are important aspects of feeding and management? Are the breeders organized? Is there already a breeding program in place? What traits can be recorded? Is artificial reproduction applicable? Hence, these aspects of production systems determine the possibilities for breeding programs and for the selection of breeding goal traits.

Challenges for animal breeding by size of populations

Small populations limit breeding opportunities for food limited. In such populations nearly all animals, at least the females, have to be used as parents for the next generation to get enough offspring. This gives no opportunity to select for traits related to food production. In small populations, the main concern is to maintain the population by conserving the genetic diversity and to manage inbreeding. This is important because inbreeding causes lower fitness levels and increases the incidence of recessive genetic defects.

In populations where almost all males and females have to produce offspring, selection for breeding goal traits cannot be made. The first step in initiating a breeding program is the choice of the most appropriate breed, considering the given environment or production system. The adaptive performance of a breed is also an important decision factor. There are numerous examples of animals of high productive breeds (e.g. Holstein Friesian dairy cow) which have been imported into tropical countries without success. The animals are not adapted to the high temperature, they hardly reproduce and heat stress impedes high production levels. In addition many tropical diseases lead to high mortality.

In all food production systems adaptation of animals to the conditions of the system is important. When this is ignored, fitness levels of the animals will be reduced. Adaptive fitness is characterized by survival, health and reproduction related traits. In warmer regions and tropical areas, pathogens and epidemic diseases are widespread, climatic conditions are stressful, feed and water are scarce. Under those conditions, locally adapted autochthonous breeds have a far greater level of resistance. Their evolutionary roots fit better into the environment compared to imported breeds.

The categories of breeding goal

Breeding goal traits can be quantitative. Milk, meat or egg production, body measurements or performance expressions are examples of quantitative traits. They are measured in units: in kg or simply in numbers: kg of milk, grams of growth and number of eggs.

Breeding goals can also be qualitative e.g. the quality of a product or an important trait in the breed standard. Product traits, scores for body traits, disease incidences or performance impressions are examples of qualitative traits. They are measured in classes: e.g. a 1 (good), 2 (moderate) or 3 (bad) for meat quality or simply 0 (not present in the animal) or 1 (present).

Some breeding goals traits cannot be measured at the time when it is relevant. In meat production, for example, meat quality is an important breeding goal trait. However, carcass composition of a young calf, piglet or lamb cannot be measured at the moment it is considered to use the animal for breeding. It can only be measured after slaughter and then breeding with that animal is impossible. Indicator traits, obtained by scanning live animals for body composition before making breeding decisions can help to predict carcass composition.

Some breeding goals traits cannot be measured at the time when it is relevant. In meat production, for example, meat quality is an important breeding goal trait. However, carcass composition of a young calf, piglet or lamb cannot be measured at the moment it is considered to use the animal for breeding. It can only be measured after slaughter and then breeding with that animal is impossible. Indicator traits, obtained by scanning live animals for body composition before making breeding decisions can help to predict carcass composition.

In females age at puberty, interval between litters, number of offspring raised per year are examples of underlying traits. In jumping horses the conformation of the horses and gait are very important breeding goal traits. For working dogs, trainability is an important trait in addition to health, behaviour and conformation. The latter three traits are of high relevance in all species used for companion purposes.

Weighing of traits in the breeding goal

Breeding goals can be simple or complex. In commercial breeding programs many traits are recorded and have an influence on the profit made by production of animals. In extensive production conditions or in hobby breeding only a few important traits are recorded and more simple breeding goals which consist only of a few traits are used.

To be able to rank the individuals which are candidates for the breeding goal traits the values for the respective traits have to be consolidated into one single selection criterion. The value of this criterion can be obtained by summation of the breeding value for each trait multiplied by a weighing factor expressing the relevance of that trait in the breeding goal. The relevance might be based on the relative economic value of the trait. The formula used is shown below.

$$H = v_1A_1+v_2A_2+ \qquad (1)$$

where:

H - the objective of the breeding, which usually includes several characters depending on their importance and heritability; v1 = (economic) value of character 1, A1 = breeding value for objective 1, v2 = (economic) value of objective 2, A2 = breeding value of objective 2… and so on..

The traits included in the breeding target can be expressed in weighted terms, depending on the economic value or the genetic progress desired for each trait. These characteristics may be limited to the wishes of breeders' associations, the demands of producers and processors or may be extended to the requirements of consumers or the expectations of society.

The more characters (n) are introduced in the breeding objective, the less progress from one generation to another will be and will represent 1/"n compared to the value of the genetic progress that would have been obtained if the breeding objective had been aimed at improving a single character.

Economically efficiency in the breeding goal

Sustainable production systems need long-term and equitable solutions, emphasize resource efficiency, profitability, productivity, product quality, environmental soundness, biodiversity, social viability and ethical aspects. The focus should be on long-term biologically, ecologically, and sociologically sound breeding goals. The economic value of an animal is based on many traits having different effects: production, quality (composition) of the product, disease problems, fertility, and ease of handling and management.

Breeding goals need to weight market and non-market values which can be done by various procedures. In these procedures animals are seen as an integrated part of a production system (at farm level?). Economic values and frequencies of expression of the genetic gain obtained are most often used criteria. The methodology to weigh the traits with respect to resource efficiency and economy is well developed

The composition of traits affects the structure of a breeding program. The breeding goal traits determine from which animals traits have to measured: from parents of the selection candidates, the candidates themselves, their sibs or their progeny? When sib or progeny records are required, it is necessary to breed sufficient numbers of offspring to obtain accurate information for the breeding value of the candidate.

Progeny of selected animals produce at various times. Therefore it is necessary to relate future income into the present costs of selection.

Improving milk yield in dairy cattle has a favourable impact on greenhouse gas emissions as fewer cows and followers are required to achieve the same production level at a farm. Improving the average lifespan of dairy cows by one year has a large favourable impact on greenhouse gas emissions. The expected annual milk yield per cow increased when selection index weights were shifted from current economic weights to environmental weights.

The Need for Selection Programs in Small Breeds

As explained, the inferior economic performance of a breed leads to decreased interest among farmers and eventually extinction. Therefore, some approach to selection is needed to increase economic performance: more output, less costs. In principle, all livestock breeds should be able to benefit from the advances in animal breeding and improvement. Obviously, differences exist across world regions and among breeds. For each breed, a critical first step is to undertake a SWOT (strengths, weaknesses, opportunities and threats) or similar analysis to identify logical breeding objectives and strategies to achieve those objectives. Some local breeds already have sufficiently high production to achieve profitability, but low performance with regard to secondary characters, such as with the udder conformation in the Reggiana cattle from Italy. Other breeds may obtain greater benefits by improving output while maintaining their characteristic secondary traits, such as adaptation to the environment.

For example, the Valdostana cattle are uniquely adapted to their mountainous production environment, but have relatively low milk yield. A well-designed selection program may seek to improve milk yield, but do this gradually to avoid creating energy demands that cannot be met by mountain pastures. At the same time, selection must avoid increasing body size and maintain leg conformation because these cows must go up to mountain pastures and negotiate steep slopes, meaning their center of gravity must remain low. In less economically developed countries, the importation of exotic breeds is often still proposed as a quick solution, but without adaptation failure is likely to occur, especially during years when climatic extremes occur. On the other hand, the time and capital invested in selection within breed will eventually lead to adapted and profitable populations.

GENETIC VARIATION WITHIN BREEDS

In conservation genetics, maintenance of both within-breed and across-breed genetic diversity are primary aims, as they play different but critical roles in sustaining animal production. Selection can negatively affect both these components, and breeding programs should cautiously monitor genetic variation. Within a breed, the level and rate of inbreeding, which is negatively correlated with effective population size, is generally used as parameter of within breed variation.

Index selection based on information from relatives leads to the reduction of effective population size and increases the probability of co-selecting close relatives. This is particularly true for traits with low heritability. In designing selection programs for small populations, a main challenge is to maximize genetic gain at an acceptable inbreeding rate. Inbreeding rate per generation should be below 1.0%, which may preclude selection when the population size is particularly small.

However, as the population size increases, selection intensity can be increased, resulting in a continuum of situations with respect to selection differential. Different strategies are available to achieve genetic response with control of inbreeding, ranging from the earlier methods using sub-optimal criteria of selection, to considering genetic relationships among selected animals, to the most-sophisticated selection with optimal contributions.

Various studies have compared OC selection retrospectively with the observed values after truncation selection. Potential for up to 30% more genetic gain at a given inbreeding rate was revealed in Meatlinc sheep and Aberdeen Angus populations. Researchers observed 13% more genetic gain from OC selection compared to the actual breeding program for German Holstein bulls, under the same average relationship constraint. These studies determined that a lack of inbreeding control had resulted in unbalanced use of ancestors in these populations and underline the benefits of OC selection. This is particularly true in local breeds with limited population size, where inbreeding rates are expected to be high using conventional selection.

When acceptable rates of inbreeding are not known a priori, it is possible to generate a response surface of inbreeding versus genetic gain to facilitate the choice of the inbreeding level to be adopted.

Genetic Variation among Breeds

The genetic diversity of a livestock species is generally addressed by keeping a sufficient number of breeds. However, species-wide diversity must also be considered during selection within a breed. In general, FAO (2013) suggests that selection should conserve breeds as genetically and cultural distinct genetic resources. Selection for increased output while ignoring traits correlated to traits of conservation interest such as adaptation, specific genetic variants, and quality of products, can reduce breed distinctiveness and between-breed variation. Identification of selection traits in local breeds should be accurate and based upon knowledge of the trait biology. Advances in genomics and bioinformatics have allowed the identification of genomic similarities/differences among livestock breeds.

Some of these genomic signatures may contribute to explain the phenotypic uniqueness of breeds and facilitate prioritization and the use of genomic breeding tools to preserve these important traits. A further option is the landscape genomics approach, whereby the association between alleles and geographic locations and/or climatic variables is targeted and assumed to be suggestive of signatures of adaptation, giving information on the environmental forces acting on the genome.

Economic Sustainability

Genetic improvement programs require significant investments. Although well-designed genetic improvement can be expected to eventually provide positive returns on investments, in local breeds the costs will often be relatively high on a per-animal basis. The breeding strategy and system that maximize genetic response may not be optimal from an economic standpoint. Recording of performance and pedigrees may not be economically sustainable, even if restricted to a portion of the population (e.g., the nucleus).

Lack of infrastructure in marginal areas where local breeds are often found may impair the introduction of genetic improvement programs, and the development of the infrastructure may be costly. When considering artificial insemination, the production of few semen doses per donor, as expected in small populations, can substantially increase per-dose semen costs relative to large populations.

Therefore, a cost–benefit analyses should be conducted before implementing selection in local breeds to determine the optimal approach. In genetic improvement programs, economic returns should be evaluated in the long term, given generation intervals and genetic cumulative effects. Additionally, organizational and infrastructural shortcomings are often associated to local breeds: these could be circumvented by taking advantage of existing organizations and infrastructures developed by larger breeding organizations: examples are the genetic evaluation for Meuse–Rhine–Yssel cattle carried out by CRV[1] in the Netherlands, and regional breeds cattle data managed by ICBF[2] in Ireland.

BEEF CATTLE

South America is a major beef cattle producer, with approximately 25% of the worldwide cattle population. The cattle industry is based on a plethora of systems varying from small-holder farmers with low-productivity levels, basic management issues (e.g., nutritional, disease control) and minimal use of technology, to very large producers with intensive adoption of precision livestock technologies. These production systems include divergent genetic resources, with a predominance of Zebu cattle (Bos taurus indicus) in tropical regions (e.g., Brazil, Paraguay, Colombia, Venezuela, Peru, and Bolivia) and Taurine breeds or crosses in sub-tropical regions (e.g., South of Brazil, Uruguay, Argentina, and Chile). The three main beef cattle producers in South America are Brazil, Argentina, and Uruguay. Beef cattle production is pasture-based, with certain regions also finishing animals in feedlots. Nellore (Zebu cattle) is the main beef breed raised in South America.

The main current breeding goals, according to its relative importance on economic indexes, are: growth (particularly growth rate and cow maturity weight) and reproduction. New initiatives are evaluating the inclusion of feed efficiency and meat/carcass quality (ultrasound-based carcass measurements) as index components. In order to meet such goals, there are around 10 Nellore breeding programs currently established in Brazil, evaluating over 0.5 million cows per year. There are breeding program initiatives for other breeds as well (e.g., Angus, Montana Tropical Composite, Braford, and Hereford). The data collection system in most breeding programs is mainly performed by technicians that periodically visit herds spread out across the country (mainly to evaluate animals by visual scoring), in addition to data transfer uploaded into independent databases (owned by each breeding program).

Undergoing research in the area of beef cattle phenomics

As previously mentioned, improved feed efficiency is a key breeding goal. However, the cost and difficulty to quantify individual feed intake, especially in pasture-based systems, have limited the inclusion of this trait in breeding programs. Over the past decade, various research groups in South America have concentrated efforts on identifying the best indicator variables of feed efficiency, unveiling the genetic relationship with traits already evaluated, and investigating the feasibility of developing a training population for genomic selection. Recent studies have shown that a 35-d test with automatic tools for weight collection can attain sufficient phenotyping precision for traits considered in the Brazilian genetic evaluation of Nellore cattle.

Automated feeding systems have been implemented mainly in feedlots or research farms. For instance, data from experimental farms have been used to derive feed efficiency-related traits, such as RFI, feed conversion ratio, average daily gain, and dry-matter intake. Furthermore, these systems are usually coupled with other innovative tools (e.g., sensors and scan cameras) to measure (or predict) additional variables to be potentially included in breeding programs. These traits include in vivo carcass yield, body condition score, meat quality, and behavioral traits (e.g., feeding behavior, temperament, and social dominance).

Over the past years, various studies have focused on identifying more specialized phenotypes related to reproductive traits. For instance, the number of antral follicles influences heifer pregnancy rate and the success of reproductive technologies (ovum pick-up, in vitro fertilization), which are widely used in Brazil.

Testicular hypoplasia, a disorder attributed to incomplete development of the germinal epithelium of the seminiferous tubules has also been studied, which enabled the identification of important genomic regions affecting this reproductive disorder.

Animal resilience and adaptation is paramount in South American livestock production systems. For instance, tick infestation causes large economic losses and welfare issues, especially in Taurine populations. Therefore, infrared thermo-imaging was investigated as a potential tool to quantify (count) the number of ticks in the body surface of Brangus cattle.

However, the results were not satisfactory as the suggested approach only captured a small contrast between ticks and the animal hair coat. Alternative adaptation traits include scoring (subjective) protocols for traits such as prepuce (navel) length, hair length, ocular pigmentation, and tick resistance (based on tick count in one side of the animal body). These indicator traits were shown to be heritable and can be implemented in genomic selection schemes.

Zebu breeds are known for having lower meat quality (marbling and tenderness) compared to Taurine animals. However, there is enough genetic variability to enable selective breeding. As meat quality traits are usually difficult to measure (slaughter of potential selection candidates), genomic selection will play an important role. Furthermore, near-infrared reflectance spectroscopy (NIRS) has been investigated as a non-destructive alternative to predict meat quality traits in Nellore cattle. NIRS was shown to be useful to predict tenderness and meat color, but not indicated for subjective traits such as marbling. The genomic background of meat fatty acid profiling has also been investigated as an additional breeding goal in Nellore. Better assessments of carcass yield and meat quality traits are still needed. Another potential alternative could be through collaborations with commercial slaughterhouses.

However, there is limited interest from the beef industry on sharing and using such data for breeding purposes. In this context, image analysis and visual computing could be promising tools to predict carcass yield in different ages. Sensors (e.g., Microsoft Kinect—MK) can be applied for this purpose. MK can minimize imaging interferences due to the ambient light through deep mapping image technology. Subsequently, these image sections from the width of chest, thorax, and abdomen; body length; and, dorsal height can be used to predict carcass yield in cattle.

A common challenge associated with pasture-based production systems is the long period of food scarcity caused by the seasonal patterns of rainfall, and high temperature and humidity. In this context, genetic selection for improved animal resilience and adaptation in such environments is gaining importance. Another major issue is GxE, especially because of the outdoor production systems (pasture- or feedlot-based).

Additionally, the feasibility of using datasets recorded in a particular environment to improve the genomic predictive performance and subsequent selection of breeding bulls in untested environments has become an important topic of research. For instance, one could be interested in using proven bulls from Argentina to breed (through artificial insemination—AI) with cows raised in harsh environmental conditions in Brazil. Environmental covariables can be used to predict the performance of individuals in untested locations.

This can be achieved through the use of geographical information systems (GIS) as environmental index in GxE models. In our conceptualization of GxE based on environmental index obtained from GIS, a particular geographical area is considered as a geoprocessing environment corresponding to a grid of pixels, and for any single environmental variable, a value can be assigned to each pixel. The value distribution of a particular environmental variable in this set of pixels is termed "envirotype" for each geographical area.

OPPORTUNITIES IN BEEF CATTLE PHENOMICS

There are several challenges for wider adoption of phenotyping tools in beef cattle, but at the same time, modern technologies are becoming more accessible and producers more interested in their adoption. For instance, researchers suggested a more aggressive strategy including the concentration of pregnancies early in the breeding season to improve reproductive efficiency. These authors and other research groups recommended the use of AI in all females at the beginning of the breeding season, and an early identification of non-pregnant cows, using color Doppler ultrasonography with subsequent AI.

The DNA pooling technique is another technology that could be used to build a training population for genomic selection and to identify genomic regions affecting fertility traits in beef cattle. This strategy requires the identification of animals with divergent phenotypes (e.g. females pregnant at the first compared to those nonpregnant after three rounds of AI) and the genotyping of pooled biological samples of females clustered in the same phenotypic group, instead of genotyping each single female. The DNA pooling strategy could be also applied for other purposes, such as in feedlot systems (phenotype extremes defined based on high or low growth rate).

Furthermore, Brazilian start-up companies have recently been granted funding for the development of 3D cameras to predict cattle live weight, and to install automated scales and image analysis in feedlot operations to determine the optimal slaughter time.

This could be used to identify the selection candidates (e.g., sires) more related to each DNA pool, assuming that all selection candidates are individually genotyped.

A common challenge associated with pasture-based production systems is the long period of food scarcity caused by the seasonal patterns of rainfall, and high temperature and humidity. In this context, genetic selection for improved animal resilience and adaptation in such environments is gaining importance. Another major issue is GxE, especially because of the outdoor production systems (pasture- or feedlot-based). Additionally, the feasibility of using datasets recorded in a particular environment to improve the genomic predictive performance and subsequent selection of breeding bulls in untested environments has become an important topic of research.

For instance, one could be interested in using proven bulls from Argentina to breed (through artificial insemination—AI) with cows raised in harsh environmental conditions in Brazil. Environmental covariables can be used to predict the performance of individuals in untested locations. This can be achieved through the use of geographical information systems (GIS) as environmental index in GxE models. In our conceptualization of GxE based on environmental index obtained from GIS, a particular geographical area is considered as a geoprocessing environment corresponding to a grid of pixels, and for any single environmental variable, a value can be assigned to each pixel. The value distribution of a particular environmental variable in this set of pixels is termed "envirotype" for each geographical area.

Challenges and opportunities in beef cattle phenomics

There are several challenges for wider adoption of phenotyping tools in beef cattle, but at the same time, modern technologies are becoming more accessible and producers more interested in their adoption. For instance, Baruselli et al. (2017a) suggested a more aggressive strategy including the concentration of pregnancies early in the breeding season to improve reproductive efficiency. These authors and other research groups (e.g. Pugliesi et al., 2019) recommended the use of AI in all females at the beginning of the breeding season, and an early identification of non-pregnant cows, using color Doppler ultrasonography with subsequent AI.

The DNA pooling technique is another technology that could be used to build a training population for genomic selection and to identify genomic regions affecting fertility traits in beef cattle. This strategy requires the identification of animals with divergent phenotypes (e.g. females pregnant at the first compared to those nonpregnant after three rounds of AI) and the genotyping of pooled biological samples of females clustered in the same phenotypic group, instead of genotyping each single female. The DNA pooling strategy could be also applied for other purposes, such as in feedlot systems (phenotype extremes defined based on high or low growth rate).

Furthermore, Brazilian start-up companies have recently been granted funding for the development of 3D cameras to predict cattle live weight, and to install automated scales and image analysis in feedlot operations to determine the optimal slaughter time. This could be used to identify the selection candidates (e.g., sires) more related to each DNA pool, assuming that all selection candidates are individually genotyped. Through this approach, phenotypes from commercial farms (or slaughter plants) could contribute to improve the performance of genomic evaluation for certain traits.

Dairy Species

Dairy cattle are the main milk producing species in South America, but sheep, goats, and buffaloes are also raised for similar purposes. Milk production in South American countries are mainly characterized by pasture-based production systems. However, an intensification trend has been observed after the inclusion of several large dairy operations, characterized by advances in nutrition and management practices. Girolando, a composite dairy breed developed in Brazil by crossing Holstein and Gyr cattle, is the main genetic resource used for milk production in the tropical regions of Brazil.

Dairy goats (especially Alpine and Saanen breeds) have, to a lesser extent, economic importance in certain regions of South America, including the Northeast and Southeast of Brazil.

Buffaloes are also raised for milk production (and cheese-making), especially in the Southeast and North of Brazil, Bolivia and Colombia. There are some dairy sheep producers, mainly in Argentina, Uruguay, Chile, and Brazil. However, these are usually small-holder farmers with no routine recording of phenotypes, with exception of a few research flocks.

Over the past decades, selection for improved milk production (total yield) was the main breeding goal, as the large majority of producers were paid only based on milk volume. Genetic improvement for additional traits was also achieved by importing semen from bulls (or other dairy species males) selected for additional traits including milk composition, conformation, health, and reproductive ability. In the past two decades, the breeding goals in South America have been refined to include other traits. Currently, the main trait categories are as follows: milk production and composition (especially fat and protein), udder health (based on somatic cell count), fertility and reproduction (e.g. age at first parity and interval between parities), workability (especially milking temperament in dairy cattle populations with genetic contribution from Zebu breeds), and conformation traits. For instance, the Brazilian Girolando and Gyr national breeding programs currently report breeding values for milking ease and temperament, 305-d milk yield and composition (fat, protein, and total solids), age at first calving and conformation. Adaptation and environmental resilience are also key breeding goals in dairy species raised in the tropical regions. The main indicator traits are heat tolerance, survival, and resistance to endo- and ectoparasites. However, genetic selection for these traits is still incipient.

Even though the breeding goals for dairy goats are similar to those described above, phenotypic selection for morphological traits was heavily weighted as there were no production or reproduction records and pedigree information. In Brazil, milk recording in dairy goats started only in 2005. In addition to milk yield, other breeding goals include lactation length and reproductive traits (e.g., kidding interval and age at first kidding).

The high adaptability of buffaloes to tropical regions has contributed to the population expansion in South America, especially in the Amazon region and Southern Brazil (>3 million animals). There are also some incipient breeding programs for buffaloes and the main breeding focus is milk yield, lactation persistency and milk composition.

RESEARCH CHALLENGES AND OPPORTUNITIES IN DAIRY CATTLE PHENOMICS

The dairy industry payment system is an important challenge for dairy improvement. For instance, mastitis (clinical and subclinical) is a great welfare and economic issue in South America as producers are usually paid only based on total milk yield and penalized based on microbiological aspects of the milk. This has started to change in some regions, but still needs more research and investment. The usefulness of mid-infrared (MIR) analysis has been investigated as a phenotyping tool. For instance, researchers predicted milk components in Brazilian Holstein based on MIR and validated the results through gas chromatography.

Matrix-assisted laser desorption/ionization time-of-flight mass spectrometry (MALDI-TOF) has been offered as a service by some laboratories and also at the research level as an alternative method for bacteria identification. On-farm culture systems, aiming to fast identify milk pathogens, have been implemented on several herds across South America.

Systems for monitoring individual feeding and drinking behavior have been recently tested in dairy cattle.

The frequency and duration of each visit can be captured (feed and water), as well as feed and water intake. Correlations between the true data (obtained via video observation and manual weights) and predicted parameters were extremely high (0.917 for duration of feed visit, and >0.963 for all others). Computer vision is an expanding area in precision livestock, which enables identification of individual animals and posterior assigning of phenotypic records (e.g., eating time) to each individual (Fig. 1).

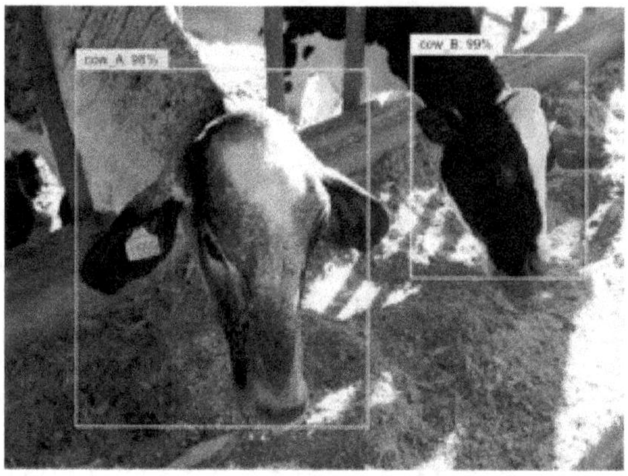

Fig. 1 An example of computer vision use (pilot project) in which two cows were video identified with high similarity after an automated search in the image database. After identifying the animals, the data collected can be linked to their individual IDs.

There are several challenges involving dairy production in South America. First, there is a lack of centralized institutions integrating on-farm data collection, laboratory analysis of milk samples, and technical assistance to producers. Second, similarly to other regions around the world, the low profit margin and unstable milk prices make it difficult for producers to commit to investments in data recording. In most large dairy operations, protein and fat are usually controlled at the bulk tank level and not individually per cow. Somatic cell score, as part of a management protocol, is generally evaluated once a month in most herds. The lack of adequate payment and incentive to producers with regards to milk composition does not incentivize phenotyping and selection for such traits. However, there are some cases of success regarding data collection and genetic evaluations.

KEY ISSUES IN REASONS TO KEEP ANIMALS DETERMINE THE BREEDING GOAL

1. Breeding challenges have a large impact on the breeding goal. They are determined by the needs and priorities of animal owners, consumers of animal products, the food industry, and increasingly by the general public. Finding the right balance between the different demands is a continuous process, and requires anticipation at future conditions and careful planning to establish effective breeding programs.
2. A breeding goal is the specification of the traits to be improved including the emphasis given to each trait. It points out the direction in which the population should be developed. Most breeding goals are only reached after several generations of selection. This requires persistency of the breeders involved.
3. In small populations nearly all males and females have to produce offspring. Selection for breeding goal traits is hardly possible.
4. In addition to selective breeding for the obvious breeding goal traits also some additional traits play an important role in breeding programs: Health and wel-

fare of the animals, and adaptation to feed of lower quality and extreme climates to be capable to produce and reproduce.

5. The selection of the most appropriate breed to be uses in a given environment or production system should be the first step when initiating a breeding program. Also due attention to the adaptive performance of a breed should be given, otherwise the fitness of the animals will be reduced. Adaptive fitness is characterized by survival, health and reproduction related traits.
6. In commercial breeding programs for dairy cattle, pigs and poultry sophisticated breeding programs with complex breeding goals are in place. For other species breeding programs are less complicated, the number of breeding goal traits is limited. Breeding goal traits are heritable traits which can be easily and accurately measured.
7. To be able to rank the individuals which are candidates for the breeding goal traits the values for the respective traits have to be consolidated into one single selection criterion. The value of this criterion can be obtained by summing up the breeding value for each trait multiplied by a weighing factor based on the relevance of that trait in the breeding goal. The relevance might be based on the relative economic value of the trait.

8

GENETIC MODELS

Livestock breeding has shifted during the past decade toward genomic selection. For the estimation of breeding values in purebred breeding schemes, genomic best linear unbiased prediction has become the method of choice. Systematic crossbreeding with the aim to utilize heterosis and breed complementary effects is widely used in livestock breeding, especially in pig and poultry breeding. The goal is to improve the performance of the crossbred animals. Due to genotype-by-environment interactions, imperfect linkage disequilibrium, and the existence of dominance and imprinting, purebred and crossbred performances are not perfectly correlated.

Hence, more complex genomic models are required for crossbred populations. This study reviews and compares such models. Compared to purebred genomic models, the reviewed models were of much higher complexity due to the inclusion of dominance effects, breed-specific effects, imprinting effects, and the joint evaluation of purebred and crossbred performance data. With the model assessment work conducted until now, it is not possible to come to a clear recommendation as to which existing method is most suitable for a specific breeding program and a specific genetic trait architecture.

Since it is expected that a superior method includes all the different genetic effects in a single model, a dominance model with imprinting and breed-specific SNP effects is proposed.

Further progress could be made by assuming realistic covariance structures between the genetic effects of the different breeding lines, and by using larger marker panels and mixture distributions for the SNP effects.

Genetic resources are genetic material of actual or potential value, whether embodied in live animals or in material such as cryopreserved semen or embryos. Animals here include all animal species that are used, or may be used, for food and agriculture, and the populations within each of them, in other words all species of livestock, including both mammalian and avian species.

Livestock species populations generally include a number of subpopulations referred to as breeds. According to the definition used by FAO, a breed is "either a subspecific group of domestic livestock with definable and identifiable external characteristics that enable it to be separated by visual appraisal from other similarly defined groups within the same species, or a group for which geographical and/or cultural separation from phenotypically similar groups has led to acceptance of its separate identity."

Animal genetic resources provide crucial options for the sustainable development of the livestock sector, whether in terms of increasing food production, mitigating and adapting to climate change or promoting the supply of a broad range of ecosystem services.

Erosion of the world's animal genetic resources has accelerated in recent decades as a consequence of the rapid changes affecting livestock production systems.

BENEFITS FROM AND THREATS TO ANIMAL GENETIC RESOURCES

Benefits

Livestock populations, or animal genetic resources for food and agriculture (AnGR), provide crucial options for the sustainable development of livestock production. Diverse animal genetic resources provide the capacity to adapt and resilience in the face of climate change, emerging diseases, pressures on feed and water supplies and shifting market demands. However, these resources are often poorly managed and under threat. Efforts to manage them sustainably need to be stepped up urgently.

Threats

The proportion of the world's livestock breeds classified as being at risk of extinction increased from 15 percent to 17 percent between 2005 and 2016. A further 58 percent of breeds are classified as being of unknown risk status because no recent population data have been reported. The number of breeds at risk is therefore likely to be underestimated.

Monitoring of population trends is a prerequisite for prompt and effective action to protect breeds from extinction. Erosion of within-breed diversity can be a problem even in breeds whose total population size remains large. Action to prevent the loss of livestock diversity will be more effective if the factors that drive genetic erosion and extinction risk are well understood.

While there is broad agreement among stakeholders regarding the range of factors that can be considered potential threats to animal genetic resources, the magnitude of these threats and the ways in which they combine to affect particular breeds in particular circumstances are often unclear.

GENOMIC MODELS

Genomic models for crossbred data are extensions of purebred models. The extensions were made in several directions. Most genomic models for the analysis of crossbred data are developed for two-way crosses. A two-way cross XX is created from a sire line AA and a dam line BB, which are usually not inbred. The pure lines have breeding values aAaA and aBaB for PP, and breeding values cAcA and cBcB for CP. Typically, some animals are genotyped, whereas others are not. The goal is to obtain accurate predictions of the breeding values for CP by utilizing phenotypic information from genotyped and ungenotyped purebred and crossbred animals.

The SNP alleles are usually assumed to be biallelic, so they may be coded as alleles 1 and 2. Most authors use centered allele content matrices as proposed by VanRaden. The centering does not affect the predictions, but affects the model-based reliabilities. We denote with

$Z_G^A = G^A - 2P^A$

the centered allele content matrix for the genotyped animals from line A, whereby the allele content G_{im}^AÎ{0,1,2} of animal i from line A is the number of copies of allele 2, animal i has at SNP m, and P_{im}^A is the frequency of allele 2 of SNP m in line A. Moreover, we denote with

$Z_X^A = G_X^A X- P^A$

the centered allele origin matrix for alleles from cross XX that originate from line AA. That is, $G_{Xim}^A \in \{0,1\}$ is the number of copies of allele 2, crossbred animal i has obtained from sire line A at SNP m. These matrices are needed to define genetic values of purebred and crossbred animals. The vector with breeding values for CP for animals from line AA has the representation

$$c^A=Z^A_G a^A, \tag{1}$$

where a^A is the vector with allele substitution effects for CP. The vector with breeding values for PP has the representation

$$a^A=Z^A_G a^{\sim A} \tag{2}$$

where $a^{\sim A}$ is the vector with allele substitution effects for PP. The equations for aBaB and c^B are similarly.

Most genomic models for two-way crosses utilize, that the vector a_X with additive genetic values of the crossbred animals can be decomposed into a contribution c_X^A that comes from sire line A, and a contribution c_X^B that comes from dam line B. That is,

$$a_X=c_X^A+c_X^B \tag{3}$$

where

$$c_X^A=Z_X^A a^A, \text{ and } c_X^B=Z_X^B a^B. \tag{4}$$

The contribution c_X^A from line A can be further decomposed into a contribution that comes from the breeding values cAcA for CP, and into a vector m_X^A that contains the Mendelian sampling terms of the transmitted gametes. That is,

$c_X^A=0.5\ Z_X^A c^A+m_X^A$, (5)

where matrix Z_X^A assigns animals from line A to their crossbred offspring.

Different models have been developed for predicting CP, which can broadly be classified into additive models and dominance models. While some models predict the breeding values for CP directly with Equation (5), others predict the vector ±AáA with allele substitution effects for CP. In the latter case, the estimated breeding values c_A for CP in line A are obtained by substituting a^A with the prediction $a^{\hat{}A}$ in Equation (1).

Additive Models

Different additive models have been proposed in the literature. Some models assume that the crossbred animals are genotyped, whereas others do not. The general additive model for a two-way cross is a trivariate model that has two equations for the parental lines, and one equation for the cross. It has the general representation

$$y_A=X_A b_A+Z_A u_A+a_A+E_A$$

$$y_B=X_B b_B+Z_B u_B+a_B+E_B$$

$$y_X=X_X b_X+Z_X u_X+\ldots+E_X,$$

where y_A, y_B, y_X are vectors with phenotypic records of the respective subpopulation, b_A,b_B,b_X are vectors of fixed effects with design matrices X_A,X_B,X_X, and u_A,u_B,u_X are vectors of non-genetic random effects with design matrices Z_A,Z_B,Z_X. Finally, a_A,a_B are the breeding values for P, and E_A,E_B,E_X are the residual terms. The term "..." in the third equation depends on the respective model.

The first two model equations are needed because PP and CP are genetically correlated, so phenotypic records of purebred animals increase the reliabilities of the breeding values for CP.

The Parental Additive Model

The parental additive model is based on Equations (2), (3), and (5), and is suitable when the crossbred animals are not genotyped. The model assumes that the Mendelian sampling terms are part of the residuals, so the model equations become

$$y_A=X_A b_A+Z_A u_A+a_A+E_A$$

$$y_B=X_B b_B+Z_B u_B+a_B+E_B$$

$$y_X=X_X b_X+Z_X u_X+0.5\ Z_{XA} c_A+0.5\ Z_{XB} c_B+E_X,$$

where $a_A=Z_G^A a^{\check{}A}$, $a_B=Z_G^B a^{\check{}}B$, $c_A=Z_G^A a_A$, and $c_B= Z_G^A a_A$.

The BSAM and ASGM Model

The model with breed-specific allele effects (BSAM) and the model with breed-independent allele effects, which is also called the across-breed SNP genotype model (ASGM) are based on Equations (2–4), and require that the crossbred animals are genotyped. While the ASGM model predicts one effect per SNP, the BSAM model predicts one effect for the paternal allele, and one for the maternal allele of the crossbred animals. Origin-specific allele effects may occur e.g., due to a different LD pattern between the marker and the QTL, different gene frequencies at the QTL, imprinting effects, or the epistatic effects may be different in the pure breeds. This results in different effects of the marker alleles and thus affects the estimated breeding values.

The first two equations of the BSAM and ASGM model are as above, whereas the third model equation becomes for the BSAM

$y_X=X_Xb_X+Z_Xu_X+Z_X^Aa_A+Z^{XB}a_B+E_X$.

An equivalent representation for the ASGM model is

$y_X=X_Xb_X+Z_Xu_X+a_X+E_X$.

Researchers predicted CP of the parental lines from genotyped crossbred animals with BSAM and ASGM, whereby the breed-specific allele substitution effects of the BSAM model were a priori independent. The allele substitution effects were estimated with BayesB, which is a method that assumes that many of them are actually zero. An oligogene trait was simulated with breed-independent QTL effects. Although the SNP effects are expected to be breed-specific due to differences in LD between markers and QTL, the authors found that the BSAM model outperformed ASGM only if the number of markers was low, the number of records for training was high, and if the parental breeds were distantly related.

Researchers used the BSAM model with normally distributed SNP effects to predict breeding values for CP from crossbred data, and compared the results with conventional GBLUP. The model provided similar prediction accuracies as conventional GBLUP for the traits litter size and gestation length in pigs. It may be not superior to GBLUP because the allele substitution effects of the different breeds were implicitly assumed to be uncorrelated, which is an assumption that is not likely to be fulfilled.

Researchers extended the BSAM and ASGM model toward a three-way cross and distinguished SNP that showed a strong trait association from all remaining SNP. For the trait associated SNP breed-specific effects were estimated, whereas for the remaining SNP one effect was estimated, regardless of the allele origin. This model was compared with the BSAM model and with the ASGM model for the trait daily gain by assuming normally distributed SNP effects. Purebred as well as crossbred data was used for training. The results showed a superiority of their method only if the estimated genetic correlations between PP and CP for the trait associated SNPs and the remaining SNPs were unequal.

Researchers derived equations for predicting the reliability of genomic breeding values for CP for BSAM and ASGM models and assumed normally distributed SNP effects. The authors found that BSAM outperformed ASGM for a specific parental line, if the effective number of chromosome segments in the crossbred reference animals that originate from the parental line is less than half the effective number of all chromosome segments that are independently segregating.

Model Evaluation

Researchers compared a Bayesian dominance model with the corresponding BSAM model and the corresponding ASGM model. A BayesCp type method was used to estimate the marker effects, so the prior assumption was that the SNP effects are either zero, or come from a normal distribution. The comparison was done for a simulated two-way crossbreeding program. A number of 20 generations of selection was simulated with the aim to improve CP in both parental lines. The marker effects were estimated only once in generation one from crossbred animals and used in all subsequent generations. The simulated traits showed a different degree of dominance variance, ranging from "large" to "realistic," or null. The dominance model was superior to the BSAM model and to the ASGM model. This superiority depended on the fraction of dominance and thus heterosis in the data, but even for situations where no dominance was simulated, the accuracy of the dominance model was similar to the additive model, indicating the robustness of the model. It can tentatively be concluded, that the use of a dominance model is in general advisable, even if dominance is not an important source of trait variability.

Researchers used a dominance model with line-dependent effects for a two-way cross and the parental breeds. The SNP effects were normally distributed, and the additive and dominance effects of the three different populations were correlated. The authors found that the increased predictive ability of the dominance model arose solely from capturing inbreeding depression. This suggests that dominance effects of individual QTL have not been captured. The reason may be that a 60K SNP panel is not sufficient for achieving high LD between markers and QTL, and that the normality assumption is unlikely to be fulfilled.

Researchers compared a Bayesian dominance model with the corresponding Bayesian ASGM model at the example of litter size in a two-way pig cross, whereby BayesC of researchers as used for prediction. Training was on the parental lines. The prediction accuracies for PP and CP obtained with the dominance model were both higher than those for PP obtained with the ASGM model.

Phenotype in a model

Anything which has happened during the life history of an animal may have an influence on the current phenotype. For example, if the height of an animal is measured, then this measure would be its phenotype. Genetics play a role here because the final height is determined by genes. If genes determine that a specific animal will stay small it will never exceed this genetically set boundary, no matter how much food it eats. However, bad nutrition, disease, cold climate, disease of the mother during pregnancy are factors which will hinder the organism to even reach the genetically determined boundary. Compared to an animal with same genetic makeup which has best growing circumstances this disadvantaged animal will stay smaller. The environmental influences are not always easy to pinpoint because they start very early (oocyte and sperm experience environmental influences as well), and because it is not always clear which factors do have influence and which not.

In general, the following basic model can be considered:

Phenotype = Genotype + Environment

or $P = G + E$

The symbols P, G and E are important to remember. They are very commonly used to describe phenotype, genotype, or 'environment'.

MONOGENIC GENETIC VARIATION

Genetic differences between animals are a result of differences in their DNA. If a trait is determined by only a single gene, like for example in the case of cattle having horns or not, the phenotype depends on the combination of alleles for that single gene. Having horns only occurs in case of homozygosity for the recessive allele h. Being polled (having no horns) is a dominant trait, so both Hh and HH animals are polled, and only hh cattle have horns. Especially in dairy cattle the calves are de-horned when they are still very young. In Holstein-Friesian cattle some animals are naturally polled because they carry the H-allele.

Some aspects of coat colour are also determined by only a single gene with two alleles. But this might result in more phenotypic variation compared to the previous example of horned or polled cattle. In chestnut horses, individuals with no dilution factor (DD) are chestnut (brown coat and brown mane and tail). If they have a single dilution allele (Dd) they will be palomino (lighter manes and tail, slightly lighter coat), and with a double dilution allele (dd) they will be cremello (almost white in coat and mane and tail, and also lighter eyes). This dilution gene therefore results in three different phenotypes (Fig. 1), whereas the polled gene only produces two. It may look as if monogenic traits are never influenced by environmental factors, meaning $P = G$. This is not always the case.

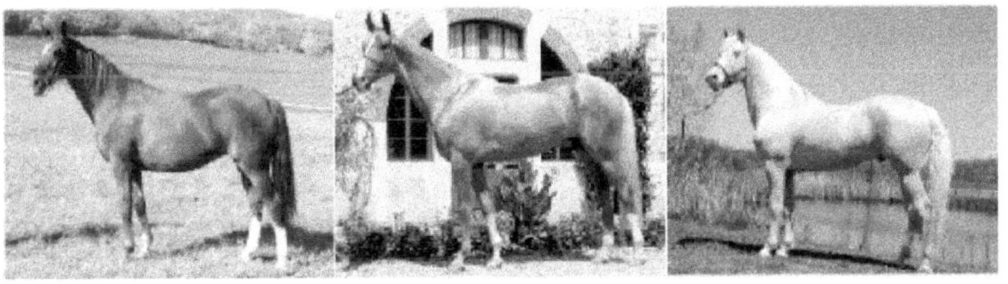

Fig. 1. Coat colour in horse: chestnut (left), palomino (middle) and cremello (right).

Polygenic genetic variation

Many traits are determined by more than a single gene. Figure 2 shows an example of three genes that together determine skin colour. With only three genes 64 different genotypes can be formed! However, due to epistasis, these 64 genotypes result in not more than 6 different phenotypes: The expression of genes depends on the combination of alleles and the 64 genotypes result in only 6 different grades of expression. Plotting the frequency at which these genotypes occur per phenotype leads to a bell-shape curve.

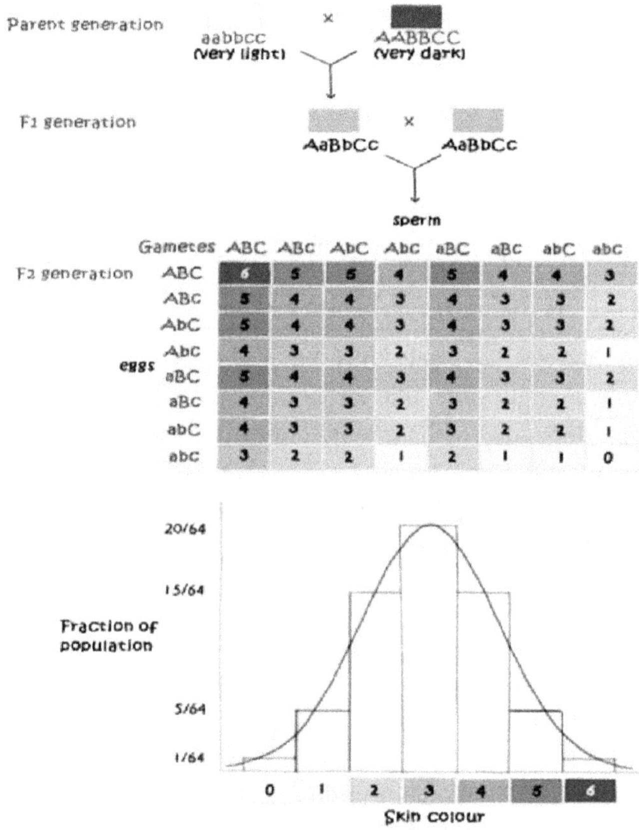

Fig. 2. Example of the variation that can be obtained for a trait with only three genes involved: 64 genotypes are possible, resulting 6 different phenotypes

The middle phenotype (number 3) occurs most frequent and both extremes are seen the least frequent. The more genes are involved in the expression of a trait, the more the frequency plot will resemble a smooth bell-shape. This bell-shape form is very common in frequency distributions of traits with discrete values.

A general assumption in animal breeding is, that traits are determined by an infinite number of genes, each having a very small effect, the bell shape curve will look smooth. It is also assumed that this infinite number of gene effects are all additive. The model underlying this assumption is called the infinitesimal model.

In reality, of course, the number of genes involved in expression of a trait is not infinite. But recent research has shown, that the general assumption that many genes are involved, each having very small effect, is often true. This facilitates the work considerably. The set of statistical rules of normal distributions can be applied which makes predictions easier.

And this is what animal breeding does: Predict genetic potential of animals and predict how the next generation will improve, if a certain proportion is used as parents. This topic will be explained in more detail in the chapter about ranking of animals.

VARIANCE COMPONENTS

The variation in a population can be quantified using the statistical model of Normal Distribution. It is expressed as variance component, the common symbol used for it in statistical models is s_2. The phenotypic variance is denoted s_2^P, the statistical sign for genetic variance s_2^G, and to indicate the environmental variance s_2^E is used.

The equation

$$P = G + E \qquad (6)$$

is also applicable to variance components:

$$s_2^P = s_2^G + s_2^E + 2\text{cov}G,E \qquad (7)$$

$$= s_2^G + s_2^E \qquad (8)$$

The covariance between G and E is assumed to be 0. This means, there is no correlation between genotype and environment, or vice versa. The genotype does not change if the environment changes.

The covariance between G and E is assumed to be 0. This means, there is no correlation between genotype and environment, or vice versa. The genotype does not change if the environment changes.

This assumption generally is justified because usually only a single type of environment is considered when variance components are estimated.

To estimate these variance components, the fact that a trait is heritable is used as starting point. This means, that brothers and sisters perform more alike than unrelated individuals. The phenotypic information on animals is combined with their genetic relationships (i.e. the pedigree). The only missing component is information about the environment.

Certain components of the environment, like housing and nutrition can be identified easily, but environmental influence starts much earlier, already with conception. Because of that and due to the fact that there are also components which are beyond awareness (like the potential influence of the weather three weeks ago) it is hardly possible to know each single environmental factor.

s_2^E can be estimated by subtracting s_2^G from s_2^P

$E = P - G.$

Due to environmental influences it is not a very accurate way to estimate the variance. This variance component is therefore called error variance, rather than environmental variance.

Simplify the genetic model

The G in the equation P = G + E is quite complex because it has a number of underlying components. This can be modelled as:

Genotype = additive effect + dominance effect + epistatic effect

$$\text{or } G = A + D + I \tag{9}$$

To start at the end of the equation: the epistatic effects indicate that there are genes interacting with each other. This is, for example, the case if one gene needs the product of another gene to come to expression, resulting in so-called gene-pathways. Expression of one gene thus depends on the allele combination in another gene.

The dominance effects indicate that expression of the gene itself depends on the allele combination in that specific gene. Two recessive genes will result in a different expression from one recessive and one dominant allele.

The additive effects indicate the effect of the gene without the dominance and epistatic effects, irrespectively of the allele combinations of the gene itself or of other genes. What remains are effects which can be added up.

Large-Scale Mutation Screens

As the name might imply, indirect approaches attempt to randomly make mutations in animal models' genomes. Then, the animals are screened in an attempt to determine which ones show phenotypes that are similar to human diseases. Thus, instead of being driven by the disease mutation, these methods are based on screening the phenotypes.

Two of the most effective ways to generate mutations are by exposing organisms to X-rays or to the chemical N-ethyl-N-nitrosourea (ENU). X-rays often cause large deletion and translocation mutations that involve multiple genes, whereas ENU treatment is linked to mutations within single genes, such as point mutations. ENU can produce mutations with many different types of effects, such as loss and gain of function, and it is frequently employed in screens in model organisms such as zebra fish. These types of models are particularly useful for identifying new genes and pathways that contribute to disease.

Transgenesis

As opposed to the use of X-rays and ENU, transgenesis is a directed approach. Transgenic animals are generated by adding foreign genetic information to the nucleus of embryonic cells, thereby inhibiting gene expression. This can be achieved by either injecting the foreign DNA directly into the embryo or by using a retroviral vector to insert the transgene into an organism's DNA. The first mouse gene transfers were performed in 1980; however, at that time, the methods for transgenesis were not optimal. For instance, the foreign DNA was incorporated into only a small percentage of embryos and was inconsistently passed to the next generation.

Also, small transgenes were inserted into random sites in the genome, and depending on their location, they weren't always expressed. More recently, scientists have developed a way to increase the size of the DNA fragments used in transgenesis by cloning them in yeast or bacterial artificial chromosomes (YACs or BACs, respectively). These larger transgenes are more likely to contain regulatory sequences necessary for normal gene expression and are usually more comparable to the endogenous gene.

As a result, the use of transgenic mice has dramatically increased in the past two decades, and this type of animal model has contributed greatly to our knowledge of disease development.

Single-Gene Knock-Outs and Knock-Ins

Both knock-out and knock-in models are ways to target a mutation to a specific gene locus. These methods are particularly useful if a single gene is shown to be the primary cause of a disease. Knock-out mice carry a gene that has been inactivated, which creates less expression and loss of function; knock-in mice are produced by inserting a transgene into an exact location where it is overexpressed. Over the years, more than 3000 genes have been knocked out of mice, and most of these genes have been related to disease.

Both knock-out and knock-in animals are created in the same way: a specific mutation is inserted into the endogenous gene, and then it is conveyed to the next generation through breeding. The use of embryonic stem (ES) cells is required for this technology. This is because ES cells can contribute to all cell lineages when injected into blastocysts, and they can be genetically modified and selected for the desired gene changes.

Homologous recombination creates the mutations; this is a process that physically rearranges two strands of DNA for the exchange of genetic material. Many types of mutations can be introduced into a model gene in this way, including null or point mutations and complex chromosomal rearrangements such as large deletions, translocations, or inversions. Many knock-out and knock-in mice have similar, if not identical, phenotypes to human patients and are therefore good models for human disease.

Conditional Gene Modifications

One drawback to using transgenic, knock-in, and knock-out mice to study human diseases is that many disorders occur late in life, and when genes are altered to model such diseases, the mutations can profoundly affect development and cause early death. These effects would preclude using animal models to study adult diseases. Thankfully, new technology has made it possible to generate mutations in specific tissues and at different stages of development, including adulthood.

To do this, mice with two different types of genetic alterations are needed: one that contains a conditional vector, which is like an "on switch" for the mutation, and one that contains specific sites (called loxP) inserted on either side of a whole gene, or part of a gene, that encodes a certain component of a protein that will be deleted. A conditional vector for the gene is made by inserting recognition sequences for the bacterial Cre recombinase (loxP sites) using homologous recombination in ES cells.

The vector contains a drug-resistant marker gene that allows only the targeted ES cells to survive when exposed to the drug. Thus, the mutant ES cells can be selected and injected into the host mouse embryo, which is implanted into a foster mother. The resulting offspring are chimeras and have multiple populations of genetically distinct cells.

Chimeric offspring are then crossed, and the resulting generation of offspring has the recombinase effector gene. The mice containing the Cre recombinase under the control of tissue-specific or inducible regulatory elements are crossed to the mice with the desired loxP sites.

When Cre is expressed, recombination occurs at the loxP sites, which delete the intervening sequences, and the resulting mutation is induced in specific regions and times. These conditional mutant models are becoming increasingly popular, and international initiatives have been created to accommodate their demand.

Chromosomal Rearrangement

The aforementioned advances in ES cells and Cre/loxP conditional mutations have helped pave the way for the creation of models for complex human diseases involving chromosomal rearrangements. Mouse models of these disorders can be created using indirect approaches, such as radiation, but their usefulness is restricted because pathological endpoints are unpredictable and undefined. Using the Cre/loxP recombination system overcomes these setbacks by allowing site-specific mutations necessary to produce accurate models of defects caused by human chromosomal rearrangements. These mutations can include chromosome deletions, duplications, inversions, and translocations, as well as nested chromosome deletions.

TRANSMISSION MODEL FOR NEXT GENERATION

Dominance and epistatic effects depend on allele combinations. They are broken in the gamete production and established again in the offspring, but how this happens cannot be predicted. The additive effects, however, are predictable because they do not depend on specific combination of alleles.

To be able to project the additive genetic effects, another model needs to be developed which describes the transmission of genetic potential from both parents to their offspring.

In Fig. 3 this is illustrated on a family of rabbits. Each parent has two different copies of each gene, but passes only 1 on to its offspring. Which one, is not known. For each gene there are two alleles per parent, and four different combinations of those alleles are possible in the offspring.

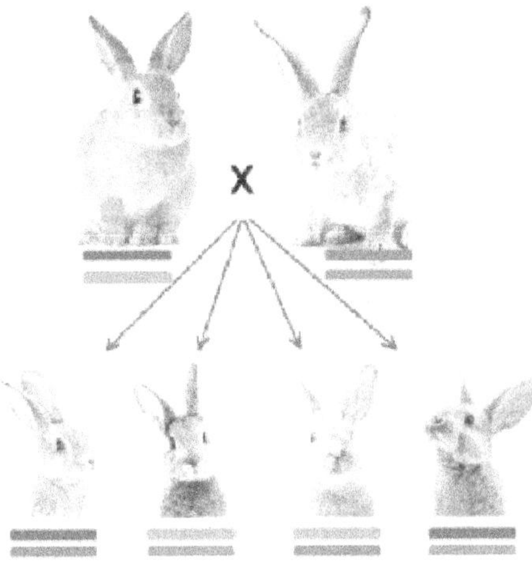

Fig. 3. Family of rabbits illustrating that offspring receive half of their genes of their parents; which half, is a matter of chance.

HERITABILITY

In animal breeding only the prediction of A is used, and not the one of G. The equation can be simplified: from P = G + E to P = A + E. The value of E in the second equation is higher because E also contains the D and I components which cannot be estimated. It now becomes more obvious why s_2^E is called the error variance: it contains more than only the effect of the environment.

$$h^2 = s^2_A / s_2^P \quad (10)$$

It is possible to estimate the heritability for a trait in a population if phenotypes and genetic relationships (pedigree) are available. A h^2 of 0.3 means that 30% of the observed variation in phenotypes is due to additive genetic differences between the animals. If ALL phenotypic differences are due to genetic differences, h^2 will be 1.0. By definition the value cannot be larger than 1.0. Similarly, if the differences between animals are NOT determined by their genetics, then $h^2 = 0.0$, which is by definition the smallest possible value.

RESTRICTIONS TO ESTIMATES OF THE HERITABILITY

The estimated heritability is always specific for a trait, but also for a particular population in a particular environment. This has two important reasons. First, the influence of the environment will naturally depend on the environment. Second, as demonstrated in the example of genetic variation in human hair colour, genetic variation for a trait may vary between populations.

If phenotypes are recorded in more than one environment, but for the same population, then there may be a third reason for difference in heritability: Prerequisites for performance with respect to the trait under consideration could vary between environments. As a consequence, different genotypes would be superior in each of the environments under consideration.

For example, if the global Holstein-Friesian cattle population is considered as a single population, milk production levels between The Netherlands and Bangladesh could be compared. Obviously, this is not a sound comparison. To be a top producer in The Netherlands and in Bangladesh do not require the same qualities. The genetic variation will be different because partly different genes are important for producing at top level. The environmental variation will also be different because the circumstances vary. Therefore, the heritability for the trait under selection should always be estimated for a specific population in a specific environment.

The estimating of the heritability: parent-offspring regression

There are methods to accurately estimate the variance components, corrected for a number of systematic effects. These variance components can be used to calculate the heritability.

For accurate estimates of the variance components a rather large number of records (animals with observations and pedigree) are required which might not always be possible. If only a limited number of observations is available, or good pedigree of the animals do not exist, a 'quick and dirty' way can be used to get an impression of heritability: The parent-offspring regression. Parents pass half of their genes on to the offspring. If the trait under consideration is determined by genetics only, the regression coefficient would therefore be 1 when the average performance of both parents (also called the mid-parent) on the X-axe is plotted against the performance of the offspring on the Y-axe. If the trait is to some extent influenced by the environment but also by genetics, the regression coefficient would be smaller than 1, but larger than 0.

This regression coefficient is an indicator of how much parents and offspring are alike. The assumption is that the only factor that makes them alike is their common genetic background i.e. the regression coefficient reflects the heritability. There are situations where only information of one parent is available. This would be the case for traits which come to expression in either males or females. Then, the regression coefficient does not reflect the complete heritability, but only half of it. The estimated regression coefficient (i.e. heritability) is 0.64. The estimated intercept of 0.56 suggests that the parents are systematically larger than the offspring which could be a sign of a change in environment between both generations. This may be the case if the data was collected on one stud farm. However, it could also be a matter of inaccuracy of measuring the height at withers. It has no value in explaining the results.

It is important to keep in mind that method this is not an accurate way of determining the heritability. If some families were kept in an optimal and others in a poor environment, this fact will influence the results and will have an increasing effect on the regression coefficient, and thus the heritability. Similarly, if parents are kept in environments of very different quality to that of their offspring, there will be less relation between performance in parents and offspring and the regression will be low. There are statistical techniques to take these systematic environmental influences into account.

Misconceptions about the heritability

There are a number of misconceptions about the heritability. Some of it are discussed below.

Misconception 1."A heritability of 0.40 indicates that 40% of the trait is determined by genetics"

This is a very common error which is based on a misunderstanding of the definition of the word "heritability". A heritability of 0.40 indicates that 40% of all the phenotypic variation in the trait is due to variation in the respective genotypes. This has a very different meaning from the definition that in each animal 40% of the expression of the trait is due to genes and this is caused by other influences.

Misconception 2. "A low heritability means that traits are not determined by genes"

A heritability larger than 0 always indicates that genes have an effect on the expression of the phenotype. The heritability is determined by the proportion of genetic variance relative to the phenotypic variance.

A low heritability indicates that the genetic variance is low. For example, the number of fingers on a hand is genetically determined, but because most people have five fingers on each hand, the genetic variance is very low.

Misconception 3. "A low heritability means that genetic differences are small"

A low heritability does not automatically indicate that the genetic variance is small. It can also mean that the error variance is large. The reason for this could be a large influence of the environment, but also inaccurate phenotype recording. For example: resistance to a certain infection will depend on the genetic potential to withstand that infection. The question is how to measure this potential. If sheep living in a herd are measured for infection with nematodes, only those which are at this specific point in time contagious will be identified. For all the others it will not be possible to distinguish between the ones that either have not been infected yet, had already recovered, or are resistant to nematode infections.

Observations therefore will not be very accurate. Because the correct phenotype cannot be assigned to each animal, the error variance will be relatively large and heritability will be low. The recording of nematode infections could be improved by more frequent measures and/or by improvement of the measurement methodology. Recording of sheep which are able to withstand nematode infection would be more accurate and data about genetic and environmental variance for this trait would be more reliable. The heritability can still remain low if there is not much genetic variation, but at least it is no longer due to inaccurate phenotypes.

Misconception 4. " A heritability is a fixed value"

Heritability reflects the relative weight of the genetic variance component in the phenotypic variance in a specific population. It is based on observations that were taken on a specific moment in time. The extent of the heritability depends on genetic variance in a population, the influence of the environment and on the accuracy of observations (see misconception 3).

The genetic variance in one population may be (somewhat) different from variance in another population. Especially if the other population is of a different breed. Within a population the heritability can also change over time. For example, if a new set of phenotypic observations is collected using a more accurate recording method or the housing system has been changed since the last recording. In these cases, the influence of the environment is different compared to previous measures. Heritability has therefore to be re-estimated at regular intervals.

IMPLICATIONS FOR BREEDING PROGRAMS

All additive models for predicting CP rely on phenotypic data collected from crossbred animals. This can be problematic in situations where the crossbred animals are not individually identified and thus such data collection pipeline is not implemented. This is likely the case on many farms housing crossbred animals. While additive models require phenotypes from crossbred animals, this is not the case for dominance models because the breeding values for CP can be derived from additive and dominance effects that are predicted in the pure breed, and from the allele frequencies in the opposite breed. Researchers proposed therefore to use dominance models for selecting purebred animals for CP based on purebred phenotypic and genotypic information only. They did a simulation study and estimated the marker effects with Bayesian LASSO. The results showed that the gain in CP was higher when the purebreds were selected for CPs, which demonstrated the feasibility of the method even when no crossbred data is available. Moreover, combining several related lines into a single reference population increased the prediction accuracy. However, training on crossbred animals leads to a higher selection response than training on purebred animals. A likely explanation is, that the level of heterozygosity was higher than in the purebred data.

Although genomic selection for CP is a promising strategy to increase selection response for CP in the short and medium term, researchers found that genomic selection for CP leads eventually to lower CP in the long term than genomic selection on PP. This hold regardless of whether training was on purebred or crossbred animals.

KEY ISSUES OF GENETIC MODELS

1. The phenotype is determined by the genotype and the environment.
2. The environment consists of any influence that occurred between conception and the moment of phenotype recording.
3. In breeding only the additive genetic effects are of interest because they are transmitted to the offspring.
4. The variation in phenotype can be expressed as phenotypic variance.
5. The phenotypic variance consists of additive genetic variance and error variance.
6. The error variance consists of variance due to environmental effects, but is also a waste bin containing dominance and epistatic effects, errors in the phenotypic measurements, etc.
7. The breeding value of the offspring consists of half the breeding value of the sire and half of the dam.
8. The Mendelian sampling term indicates the part of the additive genetic component in the offspring that cannot be predicted: which half of the sire was transmitted to the offspring and which half of the dam?
9. The heritability indicates what proportion of the phenotypic variance is due to additive genetic variance in the population. It is indicated with h^2.
10. The common environmental variance is the variance due to the fact that animals shared a common environment during (part of) their development.

    For example, were raised in the same litter or pen. The proportion of the phenotypic variance which is due to common environment is indicated with c^2.
11. The maternal effect is the effect of the environment created by the mother on the development of the offspring. Part of this maternal effect can be due to genetics of the mother.
12. An indirect genetic or social genetic effect is the effect that others have on the performance of an individual.

9

GENETIC DIVERSITY AND INBREEDING

Genetic diversity is the product of recombination of genetic material in the process of inheritance. It changes with time and space.

Sexual reproduction is important in maintaining genetic diversity as it gives unique offspring by combining genes of parents.

Mutation of genes, genetic drift and gene flow are also responsible for genetic diversity.

Enetic drift, also called genetic sampling error or Sewall Wright effect, a change in the gene pool of a small population that takes place strictly by chance. Genetic drift can result in genetic traits being lost from a population or becoming widespread in a population without respect to the survival or reproductive value of the alleles involved. A random statistical effect, genetic drift can occur only in small, isolated populations in which the gene pool is small enough that chance events can change its makeup substantially. In larger populations, any specific allele is carried by so many individuals that it is almost certain to be transmitted by some of them unless it is biologically unfavourable.

Genetic drift is based on the fact that a subsample (i.e., small, isolated population) that is derived from a large sample set (i.e., large population) is not necessarily representative of the larger set. As might be expected, the smaller the population, the greater the chance of sampling error (or misrepresentation of the larger population) and hence of significant levels of drift in any one generation. In extreme cases, drift over the generations can result in the complete loss of one allele in an allele pair; the remaining allele is then said to be fixed.

IMPORTANCE OF GENETIC DIVERSITY

- Genetic diversity gives rise to different physical attributes to the individual and capacity to adapt to stress, diseases and unfavourable environmental conditions.
- Environmental changes that are natural or due to human intervention, lead to the natural selection and survival of the fittest. Hence, due to genetic diversity,

the varieties that are susceptible, die and the ones who can adapt to changes will survive.

- Genetic diversity is important for a healthy population by maintaining different varieties of genes that might be resistant to pests, diseases or other conditions.
- New varieties of plants can be grown by cross-breeding different genetic variants and produce plants with desirable traits like disease resistance, increased tolerance to stress.
- Genetic diversity reduces the recurrence of undesirable inherited traits.
- Genetic diversity ensures that at least there are some survivors of a species left.

GENETIC DIVERSITY EXAMPLES

- Different breeds of dogs. Dogs are selectively bred to get the desired traits.
- Different varieties of rose flower, wheat, etc.
- There are more than 50,000 varieties of rice and more than a thousand varieties of mangoes found in India.
- Different varieties of medicinal plant Rauvolfia vomitoria present in different Himalayan ranges differ in the amount of chemical reserpine produced by them.

CONSERVATION OF GENETIC DIVERSITY

Activities like specific selection for harvesting, destruction of natural habitats lead to loss of diversity.

Genes which get lost might be having many benefits, so it is important to conserve diversity for human well-being and to protect a species from getting extinct.

In cases of drought or a sudden outbreak of disease when the whole crop is destroyed, it is possible to grow genetically diverse and disease-resistant species by conserving diversity.

There are various methods to conserve biodiversity:

- In situ conservation: It is impossible to conserve the whole of biodiversity, so certain "hotspots" are identified and conserved to protect species that are endemic to a particular habitat and are threatened, endangered or at high risk of getting extinct. E.g. wildlife sanctuaries, national parks.
- Ex-situ conservation: Threatened plants and animals are taken out from their natural habitat and kept in a special setting to give them special care and protection. E.g. botanical gardens, zoos, wildlife safari etc.
- Using cryopreservation techniques, gametes of threatened species are preserved in viable and fertile conditions for a longer period of time.

- Eggs can be fertilised in-vitro and plants can be propagated through tissue culture.
- Genomic library is a recent advancement to conserve genetic diversity.

CHANGES TO AN INDIVIDUAL'S DNA ARE CALLED MUTATIONS

A change in an organism's DNA. This can be a change of a single letter or a much bigger change of hundreds of letters at once. Mutations can arise when mistakes are made while cells are copying DNA, like making a spelling mistake when copying a word. These mutations make up a species' genetic diversity. Over generations, more and more mistakes are made, leading to more mutations. Most mutations are either harmful or have no impact at all, but sometimes these mutations can cause changes that are helpful for a species. The individuals that have these helpful mutations might have greater chances of survival, and have more babies as a result.

The process of a species changing in order to better survive in its environment.. When a mother and a father have babies, the DNA of their baby is a mix of the parents' DNA. Babies have two copies of every gene in their DNA, one from each parent. Copies of the same gene with different mutations are called allelesDifferent variations of a gene caused by mutations. Many species have two alleles for every gene, one copy from each parent.. When parents make a sperm or an egg, alleles in each parent are shuffled and recombined, and only one allele of a gene ends up in each sperm or egg cell. When the reshuffled alleles from a mother and a father are combined when sperm and eggs join, new mixes of alleles are created in the babies. The mixing of alleles allows for new combinations of mutations and characteristics, adding to a species' genetic diversitys.

Not all species need a mother and a father to make a baby. Bacteria can clone themselves (Fig. 1) and directly pass their alleles from a parent to its identical clone. Any mistakes in the parent's DNA will be passed on to the clone. Amazingly, bacteria can also give alleles to each other, even if they are not related! This is a unique way simple species like bacteria can increase their genetic diversity, without relying on the mixing of alleles between a mother and a father.

Genetic variation occurs mainly through DNA mutation, gene flow (movement of genes from one population to another), and sexual reproduction. Due to the fact that environments are unstable, populations that are genetically variable will be able to adapt to changing situations better than those that do not contain genetic variation.

DNA Mutation: A mutation is a change in the DNA sequence. These variations in gene sequences can sometimes be advantageous to an organism. Most mutations that result in genetic variation produce traits that confer neither an advantage or disadvantage. Mutations lead to genetic variation by altering genes and alleles in a population. They may impact an individual gene or an entire chromosome. Although mutations change an organism's genotype (genetic makeup), they may not necessarily change an organism's phenotype.

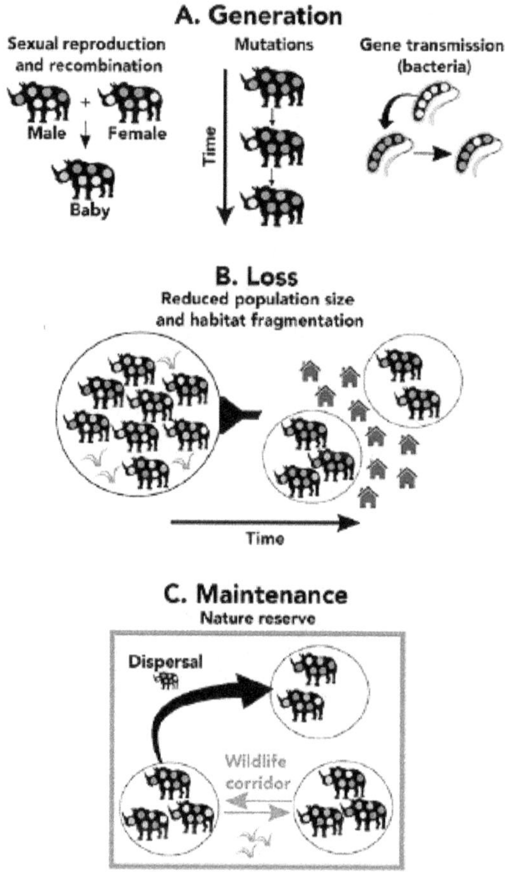

Fig. 1(A) Genetic diversity is generated when mutations create new alleles over time. Mixing alleles from parents creates new combinations of alleles in their babies. Organisms that can clone themselves, like bacteria, can pass alleles to each other. Each coloured dot represents a different allele. (B) Genetic diversity can be lost when habitat loss divides populations or when buildings or highways isolate populations. (C) Creating protected areas where individuals from different populations can migrate and spread their genes can help a species to maintain its genetic diversity.

Gene Flow: Also called gene migration, gene flow introduces new genes into a population as organisms migrate into a new environment. New gene combinations are made possible by the availability of new alleles in the gene pool. Gene frequencies may also be altered by the emigration of organisms out of a population. The immigration of new organisms into a population may help organisms better adapt to changing environmental conditions. The migration of organisms out of a population could result in a lack of genetic diversity.

Sexual Reproduction: Sexual reproduction promotes genetic variation by producing different gene combinations. Meiosis is the process by which sex cells or gametes are created. Genetic variation occurs as alleles in gametes are separated and randomly united upon fertilization. The genetic recombination of genes also occurs during crossing over or the swapping of gene segments in homologous chromosomes during meiosis.

Favorable genetic traits in a population are determined by the environment. Organisms that are better able to adapt to their environment survive to pass on their genes and favorable traits. Sexual selection is commonly seen in nature as animals tend to select mates that have traits that are favorable. As females mate more often with males considered to have more favorable traits, these genes occur more often in a population over time.

A person's skin color, hair color, dimples, freckles, and blood type are all examples of genetic variations that can occur in a human population. Examples of genetic variation in plants include the modified leaves of carnivorous plants and the development of flowers that resemble insects to lure plant pollinators. Gene variation in plants often occurs as the result of gene flow. Pollen is dispersed from one area to another by the wind or by pollinators over great distances.

Examples of genetic variation in animals include albinism, cheetahs with stripes, snakes that fly, animals that play dead, and animals that mimic leaves. These variations enable the animals to better adapt to conditions in their environments.

FORCES THAT INFLUENCE GENETIC DIVERSITY

There are a number of forces that influence genetic diversity. Some can be influenced by us, others occur by coincidence. At population level there are forces that increase genetic diversity, and forces that decrease it. Mutations are events that create new alleles. When it happens in germ cells it has an increasing effect on genetic diversity. Also migration may have an increasing effect, but only immigration (new animals moving into the population).

Emigration (animals moving out of the population) usually has a decreasing effect on genetic diversity, especially when the population size is small. Also selection has a decreasing effect: only animals with a specific genetic make-up are allowed to breed, at the expense of others. This will have an effect on allele frequencies, away from the equal frequencies. A final force with a decreasing effect on genetic diversity is the force of coincidence (genetic drift), and related to that is inbreeding. Genetic drift cannot directly be influenced by our selection decisions.

Forces that influence genetic diversity	**Direction of change in genetic diversity**
Genetic Drift and inbreeding	-
Selection	-
Migration	- or +
Mutation	+

Loss of genetic diversity: genetic drift

Genetic variation describes naturally occurring genetic differences among individuals of the same species. This variation permits flexibility and survival of a population in the face of changing environmental circumstances. Consequently, genetic variation is often considered an advantage, as it is a form of preparation for the unexpected. But how does genetic variation increase or decrease? And what effect do fluctuations in genetic variation have on populations over time?

Mating patterns are important

When a population interbreeds, nonrandom mating can sometimes occur because one organism chooses to mate with another based on certain traits. In this case, individuals in the population make specific behavioral choices, and these choices shape the genetic combinations that appear in successive generations. When this happens, the mating patterns of that population are no longer random.

Nonrandom mating can occur in two forms, with different consequences. One form of nonrandom mating is inbreeding, which occurs when individuals with similar genotypes are more likely to mate with each other rather than with individuals with different genotypes. The second form of nonrandom mating is called outbreeding, wherein there is an increased probability that individuals with a particular genotype will mate with individuals of another particular genotype. Whereas inbreeding can lead to a reduction in genetic variation, outbreeding can lead to an increase.

Random forces lead to genetic drift

Sometimes, there can be random fluctuations in the numbers of alleles in a population. These changes in relative allele frequency, called genetic drift, can either increase or decrease by chance over time.

Typically, genetic drift occurs in small populations, where infrequently-occurring alleles face a greater chance of being lost. Once it begins, genetic drift will continue until the involved allele is either lost by a population or is the only allele present at a particular gene locus within a population. Both possibilities decrease the genetic diversity of a population.

Genetic drift is common after a population experiences a population bottleneck. A population bottleneck arises when a significant number of individuals in a population die or are otherwise prevented from breeding, resulting in a drastic decrease in the size of the population. Genetic drift can result in the loss of rare alleles, and can decrease the size of the gene pool. Genetic drift can also cause a new population to be genetically distinct from its original population, which has led to the hypothesis that genetic drift plays a role in the evolution of new species.

Distribution

How does the physical distribution of individuals affect a population? A species with a broad distribution rarely has the same genetic makeup over its entire range. For example, individuals in a population living at one end of the range may live at a higher altitude and encounter different climatic conditions than others living at the opposite end at a lower altitude. What effect does this have? At this more extreme boundary, the relative allele frequency may differ dramatically from those at the opposite boundary. Distribution is one way that genetic variation can be preserved in large populations over wide physical ranges, as different forces will shift relative allele frequencies in different ways at either end.

If the individuals at either end of the range reconnect and continue mating, the resulting genetic intermixing can contribute to more genetic variation overall. However, if the range becomes wide enough that interbreeding between opposite ends becomes less and less likely, and the different forces acting at either end become more and more pronounced, and the individuals at each end of the population range may eventually become genetically distinct from one another.

Migration

Migration is the movement of organisms from one location to another. Although it can occur in cyclical patterns (as it does in birds), migration when used in a population genetics context often refers to the movement of individuals into or out of a defined population. What effect does migration have on relative allele frequencies? If the migrating individuals stay and mate with the destination individuals, they can provide a sudden influx of alleles. After mating is established between the migrating and destination individuals, the migrating individuals will contribute gametes carrying alleles that can alter the existing proportion of alleles in the destination population.

Here is an example of migration affecting relative allele frequency:

The overall effect

How do populations respond to all these forces? As relative allele frequencies change, relative genotype frequencies may also change. Each genotype in the population usually has a different fitness for that particular environment. In other words, some genotypes will be favored, and individuals with those genotypes will continue to reproduce. Other genotypes will not be favored: individuals with those genotypes will be less likely to reproduce. What type of genotype would be unfavorable? Unfavorable genotypes take many forms, such as increased risk of predation, decreased access to mates, or decreased access to resources that maintain health. Overall, the forces that cause relative allele frequencies to change at the population level can also influence the selection forces that shape them over successive generations.

For example, if moths with genotype aa migrate into a population composed of AA and Aa individuals, they will increase the relative allele frequency of a. However, if the aa genotype has a clear disadvantage to survival (e.g. vulnerability to predation), eventually the changes brought about by the initial migration will be reversed.

MENDELIAN SAMPLING EFFECT ON GENETIC DRIFT

Another reason for allele loss by coincidence has a clear relationship with Mendelian sampling. Even though animals are selected for breeding and mated and they do produce offspring, it is still uncertain which alleles are passed on to the offspring. And in case of multiple offspring: in what proportion they are passed on. Especially in smaller populations allele frequencies are sensitive to this type of genetic drift.

Purely by chance allele frequencies change from generation to generation. The smaller the population, the larger the fluctuation in allele frequencies due to genetic drift. Even if all animals participate in breeding, alleles with low frequency run the risk of extinction just because they are not passed on to the offspring by chance. Strangely enough, this can also involve alleles with a positive effect that are under selection!

Especially if these alleles have a dominant effect so that heterozygous animals also express the preferred phenotype. At low frequencies most animals that carry the desired allele will be heterozygous. Purely by chance they can all pass on the undesirable allele to their offspring. It sounds strange, but it really happens! Effects of genetic drift can have influences on allele frequencies that are larger than that of selection.

Effect of genetic drift is especially important in small populations, where genotypes of individual animals have an influence on the allele frequencies, but it plays a role in populations of all sizes.

Types of Genetic Drift

Bottleneck Effect

In the bottleneck effect, the population size severely decreases due to competition, predators, or diseases.

The frequency of certain alleles in a population change because the organisms that carry them are eliminated. The others increase in number because they are the only alleles left.

This is observed during natural disasters like volcanic eruptions, earthquake, etc. leading to the death of most of the population.

Founder Effect

In the founder effect, a new population is founded in a new location due to physical or geographical barriers.

The new population formed does not interact and mate with the original population.

As a result, the allelic frequencies of the new population will be different from the original population.

There are many species that are found only on a particular island. This is due to the founder effect, e.g., two birds of the same species reach an island. Their alleles will be responsible for the diversity on that island.

These alleles will dominate and mutations in the population will lead to the formation of new species. The new population will diverge to such an extent that they will no longer interbreed.

What Causes Genetic Drift?

Genetic drift usually occurs in smaller populations. In a small population with many alleles, any of the alleles can become extinct. In a population with many organisms, there is less chance of losing an entire allele. This is because many organisms contain the alleles and all the alleles cannot be wiped away.

If the allele affects the organism such that it causes more reproduction of DNA, the allele frequency increases. If the allele harms the organism, the allele frequency decreases. When the allele frequency increases or decreases because of its presence in some random organism that survived, it is known as genetic drift.

GENETIC DRIFT EXAMPLE

Genetic drift can be observed in the following examples:

The American Bison was once hunted to such an extent that it became endangered. The population which have recovered today show very little genetic variations.

Consider a population of rabbits with brown fur and white fur, white fur being the dominant allele. Due to genetic drift, only the brown population might remain, with all the white ones eliminated.

A couple with brown and blue eyes have children with brown or blue eyes. Even if there is a 50% chance of having blue eyes, brown eyes being the dominant allele, all the children might have brown eyes in the future generations as a matter of chance.

A bird has an allele for two different sizes of beaks. Genetic drift might eliminate one of the beak sizes from the population, thus reducing the genetic variations of the gene pool of birds.

Hypothesize a plant that produces blue or yellow flowers. If the yellow flowers are destroyed in a fire and the blue allele is the dominant one, the plant will produce only blue flowers.

GENETIC DRIFT VS GENE FLOW

Gene flow is the movement of genes between the populations, species, or organisms. E.g., bacteria can transfer genes between different cells. On the contrary, genetic drift refers to the random selection of genes in a population.

When individuals from one population migrate to some other population and breed there, gene flow occurs.

Unlike genetic drift, gene flow does not evaluate the allele frequencies.

Genetic Drift Consequences

What is the role of Genetic drift in evolution? Genetic results in loss of diversity in the genetic pool where fixation of certain genes may be similar to its initial frequency in the population. Another consequence of genetic drifting is the increase in differentiation among populations where different the population of the same species may have different alleles due to genetic drifting, this occurs if the frequency of one allele is fixed in a population, while its frequency decreases in another population since the frequencies of alleles in the genetic pool proceed in different directions.

Sampling error can cause more changes in small populations' allele frequencies than the large ones. In small populations, alleles are fixed more rapidly than large populations since the gene pool of large populations tends to be more stable.

However, Large populations are affected by genetic drift since they become small as a result of a natural disaster that decreases the population size greatly until the conditions improve to allow the regrowth of the population (bottleneck effect) or when a small population leaves the group to establish a new colony when the population is threatened (founder effect). In order to protect a small population from extinction, genetic diversity should be maintained, consequently, genetic drift should be minimized and mutation should be maintained to facilitate adaptation.

GENETIC DRIFT VS GENE FLOW

Gene flow is the flow of alleles from one generation to another by means of migration or dispersion, some populations do not usually experience migration or dispersion while others are more flexible, for example, plants and fungi send their pollens or spores away from their population to colonize in different environments. Even though some populations may seem stable, however, they are not as stable as they seem, such as lions that leave their mothers after development to search for a female that is not related to their population. This flow of genes among populations contributes to the change of the gene pool of every population as well as the introduction of new genes to continue the evolutionary process.

Gene drift is counteracted by gene flow since a population does not usually stay small for a long time to be influenced by genetic drift. However, gene flow can counteract the effect of genetic drift only if the population's gene flow is sufficient to increase the frequency of alleles lost by gene drifting. Gene flow may occur as a result of passive seed dispersal or active migration, studies have shown that only one migrant per generation can increase the genetic differentiation among the population it can also prevent the genetic drifting effect in decreasing the genetic variation among populations. Note that this rule applies only for ideal populations, while the nonideal populations may require more than one migrant to counteract the genetic drift effect.

GENETIC DRIFT IN EVOLUTION

Genetic drift contributes to the increase or decrease of a certain allele in each population; therefore, the effect of genetic drift is canceled over the long run in normal populations, however, the effect of genetic drift cannot be canceled if an allele frequency has reached zero unless a mutation produced this allele again. Genetic drifting is important in evolution since it determines the fate of a mutation, it determines whether it will disappear or becomes fixed in the population after a few generations. For nonideal populations Small in size), genetic drift is important even for the common genes.

Normally, if an allele is fixed in one generation it is most likely to increase in the following generations. However, in terms of genetic drifting, what occurs in one generation does not necessarily occur in the following generations, so if one allele increases in one generation, it may increase or decrease in the next generations.

A subdivided population adaptation is a process consisting of two phases, the first phase is genetic drifting where the loss or fixation of some alleles randomly occurs by chance which in turn helps the population to explore new genes, the second phase is characterized by natural selection of the most beneficial genes that were introduced in phase one, these genes are exported to other populations by migration. The genetic drift theory has a significant role in the evolutionary process of individuals where the balance between mutations and gene drifting creates a state in genetic variation. Since mutations introduce new alleles while gene drifting may eliminate or fix the new alleles.

Loss of genetic diversity: selection

Selection favours some alleles over others. That is the intention of animal breeding! Obviously this has consequences for the allele frequencies in the next generation. Unlike genetic drift, selection has a systematic and directional force on the change in allele frequencies. The frequency of the favourable allele increases at the expense of the less favourable allele. Consequently, more animals will become homozygous for the favourable allele and genetic diversity decreases.

Exception to this rule are traits where heterozygous animals are favoured. Selection in that case has an increasing effect on genetic diversity. This, for example, is the case with sickle cell anaemia in humans. Sickle cell anaemia is a hereditary disease where red blood cells obtain a sickle shape and lose their flexibility, resulting in various life threatening complications. The disease is caused by a mutation in the haemoglobin gene. People that are homozygous usually die of the complications at fairly early age. In the sub-saharan region the frequency of the allele causing sickle cell anaemia is higher than elsewhere. Important reason for this is that people who are heterozygous for this gene are less affected by malaria infections. Malaria is an important cause of death in that part of the world and carrying a single allele thus has a clear selective advantage. Another example where the heterozygote is favoured is with the Dutch cattle breed the Witrik.

The special type of colour marking only occur when they are heterozygous for the gene involved (Fig. 2).\

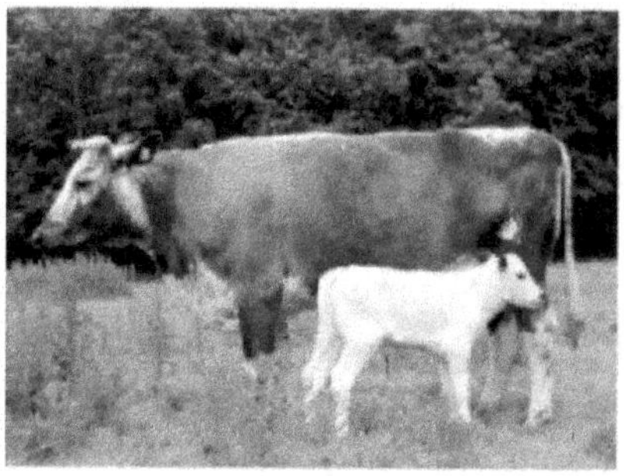

Fig. 2: A heterozygous witrik cow with her homozygous witrik calf

Natural selection

Natural selection not only occurs in natural populations. It represents forces of selection that are not decided on by us. Natural selection acts on alleles that contribute to survival and reproductive success, also called fitness. For example, animals that have reduced potential to survive until adult age have a lower fitness (natural selective advantage) than animals that are very fit and healthy and will survive until late age. Also, animals with reduced reproductive capacity will have a lower fitness compared to very fertile animals. In domestic animal species the circumstances in which the animals live generally are quite controlled. Resistance to, for example, food shortage is less essential than it can be in natural populations. Still natural selection also works on domestic animal species. The environment the animals are kept in will require some degree of adaptation. For example, animals that are kept indoors need to be able to withstand the lack of sunlight, whereas animals that are kept outdoors will need to be able to withstand the variation in climate and a potentially larger infection pressure. Not being able to cope with the situation results in reduced fitness. If the selected animals require and receive assistance to get pregnant, for example, this will work against the mechanisms of natural selection.

The bottleneck effect

The bottleneck effect is an extreme example of genetic drift that happens when the size of a population is severely reduced. Events like natural disasters (earthquakes, floods, fires) can decimate a population, killing most individuals and leaving behind a small, random assortment of survivors.

The allele frequencies in this group may be very different from those of the population prior to the event, and some alleles may be missing entirely. The smaller population will also be more susceptible to the effects of genetic drift for generations (until its numbers return to normal), potentially causing even more alleles to be lost.

How can a bottleneck event reduce genetic diversity? Imagine a bottle filled with marbles, where the marbles represent the individuals in a population. If a bottleneck event occurs, a small, random assortment of individuals survive the event and pass through the bottleneck (and into the cup), while the vast majority of the population is killed off (remains in the bottle). The genetic composition of the random survivors is now the genetic composition of the entire population.

The founder effect

The founder effect is another extreme example of drift, one that occurs when a small group of individuals breaks off from a larger population to establish a colony. The new colony is isolated from the original population, and the founding individuals may not represent the full genetic diversity of the original population. That is, alleles in the founding population may be present at different frequencies than in the original population, and some alleles may be missing altogether. The founder effect is similar in concept to the bottleneck effect, but it occurs via a different mechanism (colonization rather than catastrophe).

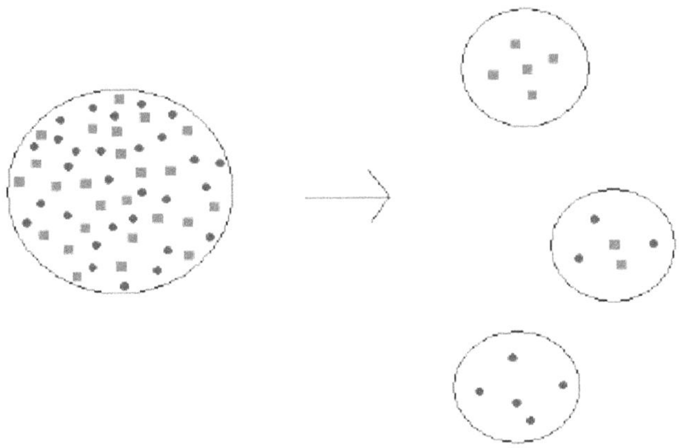

Fig 3. A population made up of equal numbers of squares and circles.

Random groups that depart to establish new colonies are likely to contain different frequencies of squares and circles than the original population. So, the allele frequencies in the colonies (small circles) may be different relative to the original population. Also, the small size of the new colonies means they will experience strong genetic drift for generations.

Increase in genetic diversity: mutation

Mutations are changes in the genetic sequence, and they are a main cause of diversity among organisms. These changes occur at many different levels, and they can have widely differing consequences. In biological systems that are capable of reproduction, we must first focus on whether they are heritable; specifically, some mutations affect only the individual that carries them, while others affect all of the carrier organism's offspring, and further descendants. For mutations to affect an organism's descendants, they must:

1. Occur in cells that produce the next generation, and
2. Affect the hereditary material.

Ultimately, the interplay between inherited mutations and environmental pressures generates diversity among species.

Although various types of molecular changes exist, the word "mutation" typically refers to a change that affects the nucleic acids. In cellular organisms, these nucleic acids are the building blocks of DNA, and in viruses they are the building blocks of either DNA or RNA. One way to think of DNA and RNA is that they are substances that carry the long-term memory of the information required for an organism's reproduction. This article focuses on mutations in DNA, although we should keep in mind that RNA is subject to essentially the same mutation forces.

If mutations occur in non-germline cells, then these changes can be categorized as somatic mutations. The word somatic comes from the Greek word soma which means "body", and somatic mutations only affect the present organism's body. From an evolutionary perspective, somatic mutations are uninteresting, unless they occur systematically and change some fundamental property of an individual—such as the capacity for survival. For example, cancer is a potent somatic mutation that will affect a single organism's survival. As a different focus, evolutionary theory is mostly interested in DNA changes in the cells that produce the next generation.

Are Mutations Random?

The statement that mutations are random is both profoundly true and profoundly untrue at the same time. The true aspect of this statement stems from the fact that, to the best of our knowledge, the consequences of a mutation have no influence whatsoever on the probability that this mutation will or will not occur. In other words, mutations occur randomly with respect to whether their effects are useful. Thus, beneficial DNA changes do not happen more often simply because an organism could benefit from them. Moreover, even if an organism has acquired a beneficial mutation during its lifetime, the corresponding information will not flow back into the DNA in the organism's germline. This is a fundamental insight that Jean-Baptiste Lamarck got wrong and Charles Darwin got right.

However, the idea that mutations are random can be regarded as untrue if one considers the fact that not all types of mutations occur with equal probability. Rather, some occur more frequently than others because they are favored by low-level biochemical reactions. These reactions are also the main reason why mutations are an inescapable property of any system that is capable of reproduction in the real world. Mutation rates are usually very low, and biological systems go to extraordinary lengths to keep them as low as possible, mostly because many mutational effects are harmful. Nonetheless, mutation rates never reach zero, even despite both low-level protective mechanisms, like DNA repair or proofreading during DNA replication, and high-level mechanisms, like melanin deposition in skin cells to reduce radiation damage. Beyond a certain point, avoiding mutation simply becomes too costly to cells. Thus, mutation will always be present as a powerful force in evolution.

Types of Mutations

So, how do mutations occur? The answer to this question is closely linked to the molecular details of how both DNA and the entire genome are organized. The smallest mutations are point mutations, in which only a single base pair is changed into another base pair. Yet another type of mutation is the nonsynonymous mutation, in which an amino acid sequence is changed. Such mutations lead to either the production of a different protein or the premature termination of a protein.

As opposed to nonsynonymous mutations, synonymous mutations do not change an amino acid sequence, although they occur, by definition, only in sequences that code for amino acids. Synonymous mutations exist because many amino acids are encoded by multiple codons. Base pairs can also have diverse regulating properties if they are located in introns, intergenic regions, or even within the coding sequence of genes. For some historic reasons, all of these groups are often subsumed with synonymous mutations under the label "silent" mutations. Depending on their function, such silent mutations can be anything from truly silent to extraordinarily important, the latter implying that working sequences are kept constant by purifying selection. This is the most likely explanation for the existence of ultraconserved noncoding elements that have survived for more than 100 million years without substantial change, as found by comparing the genomes of several vertebrates.

Mutations may also take the form of insertions or deletions, which are together known as indels. Indels can have a wide variety of lengths. At the short end of the spectrum, indels of one or two base pairs within coding sequences have the greatest effect, because they will inevitably cause a frameshift (only the addition of one or more three-base-pair codons will keep a protein approximately intact). At the intermediate level, indels can affect parts of a gene or whole groups of genes. At the largest level, whole chromosomes or even whole copies of the genome can be affected by insertions or deletions, although such mutations are usually no longer subsumed under the label indel. At this high level, it is also possible to invert or translocate entire sections of a chromosome, and chromosomes can even fuse or break apart. If a large number of genes are lost as a result of one of these processes, then the consequences are usually very harmful. Of course, different genetic systems react differently to such events.

Finally, still other sources of mutations are the many different types of transposable elements, which are small entities of DNA that possess a mechanism that permits them to move around within the genome. Some of these elements copy and paste themselves into new locations, while others use a cut-and-paste method. Such movements can disrupt existing gene functions (by insertion in the middle of another gene), activate dormant gene functions (by perfect excision from a gene that was switched off by an earlier insertion), or occasionally lead to the production of new genes (by pasting material from different genes together).

Effects of Mutations

A single mutation can have a large effect, but in many cases, evolutionary change is based on the accumulation of many mutations with small effects. Mutational effects can be beneficial, harmful, or neutral, depending on their context or location. Most non-neutral mutations are deleterious. In general, the more base pairs that are affected by a mutation, the larger the effect of the mutation, and the larger the mutation's probability of being deleterious.

To better understand the impact of mutations, researchers have started to estimate distributions of mutational effects (DMEs) that quantify how many mutations occur with what effect on a given property of a biological system. In evolutionary studies, the property of interest is fitness, but in molecular systems biology, other emerging properties might also be of interest. It is extraordinarily difficult to obtain reliable information about DMEs, because the corresponding effects span many orders of magnitude, from lethal to neutral to advantageous; in addition, many confounding factors usually complicate these analyses. To make things even more difficult, many mutations also interact with each other to alter their effects; this phenomenon is referred to as epistasis.

However, despite all these uncertainties, recent work has repeatedly indicated that the overwhelming majority of mutations have very small effects. Of course, much more work is needed in order to obtain more detailed information about DMEs, which are a fundamental property that governs the evolution of every biological system.

A mutation is a change in DNA, and thus creates a new allele and increases genetic diversity. The frequency at which this occurs is small, but differs between species. In humans the mutation rate is estimated at 10-5 per gene per meiosis (generation). Mutations tend to occur especially on specific regions on the genome: mutation hotspots.

A lot of mutations are deleterious. A dominant mutation often results in mortality (abortion) of the embryo. Recessive mutations hide in heterozygous state and spread through the population. They only come to expression in homozygous state. Some mutations are harmless, and some are positive. Positive mutations will be subject of selection and thus may increase in frequency more efficiently.

Not all mutations result in a change in function of the gene, these are called silent mutations. Many of the SNP (single nucleotide polymorphism) are such silent mutations and are used as genetic markers.

INBREEDING

Technically, various mating schemes of animals are classified under two broad categories — inbreeding and outbreeding. Classification depends on the closeness of the biological relationship between mates. Within each category, a wide variation in intensity of this relationship exists.

A very fine line separates the two categories. Mating closely related animals (for example, parent and offspring, full brother and sister or half brother and sister) is inbreeding. With less closely related animals (first cousins, second cousins), people disagree about where to draw the line between inbreeding and outbreeding.

Technically, inbreeding is defined as the mating of animals more closely related than the average relationship within the breed or population concerned. Matings between animals less closely related than this, then, would constitute outbreeding. These two systems of mating, with varying intensities in each, are described in Table 1. Matings indicated within the inbreeding category are self-explanatory.

Table 1. Degrees of inbreeding and outbreeding arranged according to biological relationship between indicated mates. (In reading from top to bottom, biological relationship between mates steadily decreases.)

Inbreeding or outbreeding	Coefficient of relationship between mates	Biological relationship between mates
Inbreeding	50 percent	Parent × offspring; full sibs
Inbreeding	25 percent	Half-sibs; double first cousins; aunt × nephew; uncle × niece
Inbreeding	12½ percent	First cousins
Inbreeding	6¼ percent	Second cousins
Inbreeding	?	Linebreeding1
Inbreeding/ outbreeding	0 percent	Random mating within breed or population2
Outbreeding	0 percent	Outcrossing
Outbreeding	0 percent	Breed crossing
Outbreeding	0 percent	Species crossing
Outbreeding	0 percent	Genus crossing

1. In a linebreeding program, the coefficient of relationship between mates is usually low; however, it can be quite variable.
2. Random mating within a breed or population means that mates are chosen by chance. It should be understood that under this circumstance it is possible that either inbreeding or outbreeding could occur.

Biological relationships between animals

Individuals are considered to be biologically related when they have one or more common ancestors. For practical purposes, if two individuals have no common ancestor within the last five or six generations, they are considered unrelated.

Biological relationship is important in animal breeding because the closer the relationship, the higher the percentage of like genes the two individuals carry. Closeness of relationship is determined by three factors:

- How far back in the two animals' pedigrees the common ancestor appears
- How many common ancestors they have
- How frequently the common ancestors appear. It is also influenced by any inbreeding of the common ancestor or ancestors

Causes of inbreeding

There are two causes of inbreeding: inbreeding due to genetic drift and inbreeding due to nonrandom mating. Or in other words: inbreeding due to coincidence and inbreeding on purpose, inevitable and evitable inbreeding.

Genetic drift causes a loss in genetic diversity due to loss of alleles, which leads to an increase in homozygosity and this is also called inevitable inbreeding. Imagine that at some moment in history a mutation occurred. You may assume that this mutation only occurred in a single animal, as it is unlikely that exactly the same mutation also occurred in another animal. Animals that carry the allele today, therefore, must be related because they have that original animal as common ancestor. This is the case for all mutations, even if the animal in which the mutation occurred lived a VERY long time ago. Given the definition that inbreeding is the result of mating related individuals, animals that are homozygous for the allele must be inbred. Homozygosity in a population is an indication of size of allele frequencies. If all animals are homozygous, the other allele(s) is/are lost from the population. Inbreeding due to genetic drift results in a permanent loss of genetic diversity because alleles are lost for ever.

Non-random mating can cause inbreeding, but this is evitable. Mating closely related animals on purpose, like brother and sister or father and daughter matings, results in an increased probability that the offspring of the mating will receive the same allele from both parents. This results in increased homozygosity, and thus in inbreeding. However, this is a temporary loss of genetic diversity because if you would stop mating closely related animals on purpose, but use random mating instead, this cause of inbreeding would disappear.

Inbreeding & how to manage it

Inbreeding is the practice of mating two genetically related animals. To a degree this is inevitable within any long-term selection programme involving a closed population.

Breeders will sometimes deliberately inbreed specific bloodlines to fix certain characteristics in the herd, increasing the frequency of favourable genes – or more rarely to expose recessive genes.

Inbreeding may have a place in a breeding strategy as in some instances it will bring a number of favourable genes together. However, it will also tend to increase the number of recessive or deleterious genes being expressed – leading to a reduction in fitness and productivity; this is referred to as "inbreeding depression".

The Challenge to Avoid Inbreeding

To make fast genetic progress in any particular attribute a small number of bulls and cows that excel in that attribute tend to be mated together. If this approach is taken to an extreme, it can quickly result in an increase in the level of inbreeding within the herd.

Modern livestock breeding programmes can be susceptible to increases in inbreeding due to the widespread use of AI & ET, fast generation turnover, selective use of specific family lines and the tendency for a relatively small number of different sire families to dominate within certain breeds. Increases in inbreeding are observed in both recording and non-recording herds.

Breeders need to strike a balance to optimise rates of genetic gain, whilst controlling increases in levels of inbreeding.

Calculating Levels of Inbreeding

The level of inbreeding is calculated as the probability of two alleles being identical by descent. This value is called the "inbreeding coefficient".

Typical inbreeding percentages are as follows, assuming no previous inbreeding between any parents

- Father/daughter, mother/son or brother/sister - 25%
- Grandfather/granddaughter or grandmother/grandson - 12.5%
- Half-brother/half-sister - 12.5%
- Uncle/niece or aunt/nephew - 12.5%
- Great-grandfather/great-granddaughter or great-grandmother/great-grandson - 6.25%

Should Breeders Completely Avoid Inbreeding?

Complete avoidance of inbreeding is almost impossible and a balance has to be struck between the genetic superiority of a specific bull and the level of inbreeding he creates in the future herd. Low levels of inbreeding (<6.25%) are often considered an acceptable compromise. Levels higher than that should be avoided.

The best solution to the inbreeding challenge is to measure the level of inbreeding between individuals and make recommendations based on this information.

Summary

Maternal Sheep Breeding Index

New breeding indexes for dual purpose maternal and crossing breeds

Two new breeding indexes have been generated to aid breeders and buyers in the selection of the most profitable rams for commercial sheep enterprises.

- A Maternal Index has been developed for Charmoise Hill, Easycare, Exlana, Jacob, Lleyn, Romney Marsh, Roussin, Tefrom, Wiltshire Horn.

  This index aims to reward maternal ability (milk production), prolificacy, early lamb growth rates and carcase quality; while limiting increases in ewe mature weights.

- A Blue Faced Leicester (Crossing) Index has been developed for the Blue Faced Leicester breed, which places less emphasis on prolificacy and more emphasis on early lamb growth rates and carcase traits.

  This index aims to reward well flesh breeding lines, with good maternal characteristics; while again trying to limit increases in ewe mature weights.

These indexes aim to enhance the efficiency of commercial ewes; making them more productive without increasing mature size and thus the cost of keeping them or compromising their working lifespan.

So what are the index weightings in the Maternal Indexes?

In general terms the index weightings are as follows

The raw weightings are shown in Table 2, but these mean little in isolation as traits have different heritability values and genetic correlations to each other.

Table 2. Raw Index Weightings

	Maternal Index Raw Index Weightings	**BFL Crossing Index Raw Index Weightings**
Eight Week Weight	1.2	1.5
Scan Weight	0.4	0.1
Muscle Depth	2.5	4
Fat Depth	2	2
Litter Size Born	6	1
Litter Size Reared	8	2
Maternal Ability	6	9
Mature (Shearling) Wt	None at present	None at present
Ewe Mature Size	See below	See below
Ewe BCS	None at present	None at present

In addition to these weightings two further penalties are applied within the index

- A non-linear penalty on sheep with very high/low litter born EBVs
- A non-linear penalty on the ~10% heaviest ewes

A better way to assess expected progress

A better way to assess the expected genetic change is to look at the relative change expected through selection.

Table 3. Emphasis in maternal breeding indexes

Emphasis	Maternal Index	BFL Crossing Index
Eight Week Weight EBV	27.2%	32.6%
Scan Weight EBV	23.8%	5.7%
Muscle Depth EBV	24.8%	37.9%
Fat Depth EBV	3.4%	3.2%
Litter Size Born EBV	3.2%	0.5%
Litter Size Reared EBV	4.3%	1.0%
Maternal Ability EBV	13.3%	19.1%

Understanding where you are going....

Now having said that; "weightings" and "emphasis" still don't always show the overall expected direction of travel in a breed programme. A trait could have very little weighting – but change a great deal because it is related to other traits that are being heavily selected for.

So if you really want to understand "direction of travel" in your flock then export your breeding values into a spreadsheet and plot each breeding value against the index, this shows you the degree to which EBVs are likely to increase under index selection.

Changing direction....

Don't forget Signet is working on "Index customisation software" that will enable breeders to test different sets of index weightings and determine the impact they would have on their breeding programme. So for breeders with very specific breeding objectives this will be another useful breeding tool for them to consider.

Updating existing EBVs

EBVs for lambing ease, birth weight, litter size, maternal ability and faecal egg count have all been updated using the latest research to make them more informative to commercial farmers.

Brand new EBVs

New estimated breeding values have been developed for the following breeding objectives

Parasite resistance

- Serum IgA EBV
- Parasite Plus (SI) – a sub-index to aid selection for worm resistance

Assessing Ewe Efficiency

- Ewe Mature Weight (at mating) EBV
- Body Condition Score (at mating) EBV

Assessing carcase traits using data derived from the abattoir

- Days to Slaughter EBV
- Carcase Weight EBV
- Carcase Conformation EBV
- Fat Class EBV

Publication of these traits will be influenced by the amount of data collection in the breed.

EBVs and Indexes set to a new base

All Estimated Breeding Values have been reset to a 2015 base, making EBV interpretation easier and more relevant to commercial ram buyers. Changes to the model mean that new, unrecorded breeding stock entering the analysis now do so with a fairer starting point.

Comparing performance between flocks

To enable the comparison of EBVs between flocks, there needs to be genetic linkage between the flocks i.e. some related sheep born in each flock. New online tools are being developed to show the degree of linkage between Signet-recorded flocks to show where comparisons can be made.

10

INHERITANCE OF MONOGENIC

TRAITS

Monogenic inheritance refers to the kind of inheritance whereby a trait is determined by the expression of a single gene or allele, not by several genes as in polygenic inheritance. It is a form of a Mendelian inheritance, which is defined as a type of biological inheritance that conforms to the set of principles proposed by Gregor Mendel. Gregor Mendel is an Augustinian monk and botanist who formulated the laws of heredity based on his careful breeding experiments on garden pea plants. He formulated laws regarding the transmission of genetic characters from parent organisms to their offspring based on breeding experiments on pea plants. These laws are now referred to as "Mendel's laws of inheritance", particularly the Law of Segregation, the Law of Independent Assortment, and the Law of Dominance.

According to the Law of Segregation, the paired alleles separate during gamete formation. As a result, each gamete would contain a single copy of every paired unit factors. In the Law of Independent Assortment, it states that for every pair of unit factors, each would assort independently into the newly formed gametes. As for the Law of Dominance, in the two alleles of a heterozygous pair, the allele that is expressed is the dominant allele whereas the allele that is not expressed is the recessive allele. A monogenic disease or monogenic disorder would thus result when a single pair of genes is involved.

Monogenic disorders (monogenic traits) are caused by variation in a single gene and are typically recognized by their striking familial inheritance patterns. Examples include sickle cell anemia, cystic fibrosis, Huntington disease, and Duchenne muscular dystrophy.

By contrast, complex disorders (complex traits) are those in which multiple genes play a role, often together with environmental factors. These include many complex disorders such as cardiovascular disease, asthma, diabetes, and cancer susceptibility.

CHARACTERISTICS OF MONOGENIC TRAITS

To repeat briefly: the loci for a monogenic trait may contain identical alleles: the animal is homozygous for this trait. It got an identical allele from the sire and from the dam. A loci also may contain two different alleles: the animal is heterozygous for this trait. It got an allele from the sire and a non-identical from the dam.

Homozygous implies that all offspring of an homozygous animal will get a similar allele from this animal when it is used for breeding and heterozygous implies that offspring gets either one of the two alleles with a chance of 50 %. In heterozygous animals we may have concern with intermediate inheritance (the value for the trait of the heterozygous lies just in between the values of the two homozygous forms) or with dominance/recessiveness.

Then the heterozygous animal cannot be distinguished from one of the homozygous forms based on their phenotypes; they are not different.

MONOGENIC GENETIC VARIATION

Genetic differences between animals are a result of differences in their DNA. If a trait is determined by only a single gene, such as for example in the case of having horns in cattle or not, then the phenotype depends on the combination of alleles for that single gene.

Having horns only occurs in case of homozygosity for the recessive allele h. Being polled (having no horns) is a dominant trait, so both Hh and HH animals are polled, and only hh cattle have horns. Especially in dairy cattle the calves are de-horned when they are still very young. However, also in the Holstein-Friesian some animals are naturally polled because they carry the H-allele.

Some aspects of coat colour are also determined by only a single gene with two alleles. But that may result in more phenotypic variation than in the example of having horns or not in cattle. In chestnut horse, for example, horses with no dilution factor (DD) are chestnut (brown coat and brown mane and tail).

But if they have a single dilution allele (Dd) they are palomino (lighter manes and tail, slightly lighter coat), and with a double dilution allele (dd) they are cremello (almost white in coat and mane and tail, and also lighter eyes). S

It may seem that monogenic traits are never influenced by the environment, so P = G. This is not always the case. An example of a gene that is influenced by the environment is the gene that causes phenylketonuria or PKU in humans.

It is a rare recessively inherited metabolic disorder. Only if two carriers have a child, that child can have PKU. In the Netherlands 1 in 18,000 children has it, but all are tested for it as newborn baby in the blood collected with the heel pinch. In people with PKU the enzym Phenylalaninehydroxylases is not present or not functioning, so that it cannot break down the amino acid Phenylalanine. This is thus accumulating in the blood and the spinal fluid, which causes damage to nerve cells, eventually resulting in brain damage.

Patients with untreated PKU are usually mentally retarded with behaviour problems, and often suffer from skin diseases. The treatment is very basic: a life-long diet with very little protein and no intake of aspartaam as that contains phenylalanine. Patients do get amino-acid additives to prevent deficiencies. Thus, the expression of this monogenic traits can be influenced by the environment, by the diet in this example.

For simply inherited traits one allele completely masks the expression of the other allele when the alleles are heterozygous for the gene. This results in heterozygous animals having the exact same phenotype as homozygous dominant animals. This is the type of dominance we see in red/black coat color, where black is dominant to red.

Cattle that have two black alleles are black (homozygous dominant), cattle that have one black and one red allele are also black (heterozygous), and red animals are the result of having two red alleles (homozygous recessive).

When dealing with traits with complete dominance, heterozygous animals are often called carriers because they are carrying the recessive allele and can pass it to their offspring even though they do not express the recessive phenotype themselves. That is why it is possible to breed two black animals and get a red calf; each parent was a red allele carrier.

Coat color is a good trait to demonstrate how alleles interact in a trait with complete dominance. For this example, we will mate an Angus bull to Hereford cows. The Angus bull is homozygous dominant, which means he has two black alleles (BB). The Hereford cows are homozygous recessive, which means they have two red alleles (bb). When mated, all offspring will be heterozygotes (Bb). The Punnett Square in Fig. 1 illustrates this mating. Cow gametes are egg cells, and bull gametes are sperm cells.

		Bull Gametes	
		B	B
Cow Gametes	b	Bb Black	Bb Black
	b	Bb Black	Bb Black

If we were to breed these heterozygous heifers back to a Hereford bull, we would get fifty percent heterozygous black (Bb) calves and fifty percent homozygous red (bb) calves (Fig. 2).

If we were to mate the Hereford x Angus heifers to Hereford x Angus bulls then we would get all three possibilities: homozygous black (BB), heterozygous black (Bb) and homozygous red (bb) (Fig. 3). The ratio would be 25%:50%:25%, respectively. The phenotypic ratio would be 75%:25% black to red.

		Bull Gametes	
		b	b
Cow Gametes	B	Bb Black	Bb Black
	b	bb Red	bb Red

Fig. 2. Punnett Square for coat color when mating a homozygous red bull to heterozygous black cows. The joining of the gametes shows the potential offspring and their color.

		Bull Gametes	
		B	b
Cow Gametes	B	BB Black	Bb Black
	b	Bb Black	bb Red

Fig. 3. Punnett Square for coat color when mating a heterozygous black bull to heterozygous black cows. The joining of the gametes shows the potential offspring and their color.

Traits controlled by one gene, with complete dominance, are easy to understand, but can cause problems because of the possibility of carriers of recessive genetic defects. For some traits, the only way to detect carriers is through progeny testing, which is costly and time consuming. However, with advancements in molecular technologies, carriers can be identified for many traits by conducting a DNA test on a tissue sample.

The simplest way to avoid having homozygous recessive calves is to always breed to a homozygous dominant bull. With this breeding strategy, even if you have the undesirable allele in your herd it will never be expressed because only homozygous dominant or carrier calves will be produced. This strategy can improve markets in the case of the red and horn allele, and increase reproductive rates when lethal alleles are involved.

MONOGENIC TRAIT MAPPING

As has been the case for older experimental methods of gene mapping, the greatest successes in identifying genes using GWA have been for monogenic traits. For instance, researchers discovered that mutations in the pigmentation-related gene MITF cause white spotting in dogs. To map this gene they used two breeds, boxers and bull terriers, in which the white spotting trait was segregating, and then used common haplotypes between the two breeds to increase the precision of mapping.

In cattle, researchers used GWA to identify three genes harbouring mutations causing three recessive abnormalities. This study was particularly efficient because the low Ne in cattle means that, typically, calves suffering from a fatal recessive disorder are homozygous for a large chromosome segment containing the causative gene, allowing this segment to be detected using moderately dense markers. For complex traits much larger numbers of animals would be needed, but the basic strategy seems applicable.

COMPLEX TRAIT MAPPING

For complex traits the results generally indicate many mutations, suggesting that the individual mutations each have a small effect. For example, reported 196 SNPs in

Canadian Holstein bulls with significant associations with traits describing the size and shape of cows. In the same breed, found 144 significant SNPs for milk protein yield, researchers found significant SNPs for feed conversion efficiency, and researchers found significant SNPs for a genotype × environment interaction for milk yield at the level of herd production. In chickens, SNPs with significant associations with mortality in broilers have been reported, both associations across environments and associations that differentially affect mortality in two different hygiene environments. Another study in chickens researchers reported 21 SNPs linked to 19 genes associated with resistance to Salmonella enterica colonization.

Validating SNP associations

However, in none of these cases were the significant SNPs confirmed in an independent sample. There are three reasons for this. First, the effect size of each association is small, even in the original GWA study. However, when you account for the so-called researchers, the true effects are even smaller and so a very large confirmation experiment is needed to have the required power to confirm the effect. Second, the lD between the SNP and the QTl may be present in the original sample of animals but not in other samples from a different breed or even from different families within the same breed. Third, the false discovery rate is often high, and so most of the significant associations are just those expected by chance when so many SNPs are tested.

In our own unpublished GWA studies, we find that SNP associations are most likely to be confirmed when the original GWA study used a large number of animals (>1,000) that were widely sampled from one breed, when the SNPs were highly significant, and when the confirmation was carried out in a large sample of the same breed.

By contrast, GWA studies in humans have found many confirmed associations with complex traits, such as height and susceptibility to disease. However, recently published papers have used consortia of scientists to amass GWA studies with tens of thousands of subjects and confirmation samples of approximately equal or greater size.

COLOUR GENES IN CATTLE

As in many mammals, coat colour in cattle results from the relative presence of eumelanin (black-brown pigment) and phaeomelanin (red-yellow pigment), the two basic pigments produced by melanocyte cells. Pigment production takes place in the melanosomes, organelles containing the enzymes directly involved in pigment biosynthesis. Tyrosinase (TYR) is the rate-limiting enzyme in the melanogenesis pathway. High levels of this enzyme are required for the production of eumelanin, whereas low enzyme levels result in the production of phaeomelanin. Tyrosinase activity is regulated by the melanocortin 1 receptor (MC1R or α-MSHR), whose stimulation by α-melanocyte-stimulating hormone (α-MSH) leads to the production of eumelanin. Phaeomelanin is produced in absence of α-MSH stimulation, either as result of a non-functional MC1R receptor or in the presence of the Agouti protein, which is secreted by cells adjacent to melanocytes and acts as an antagonist of the α-MSH action by blocking the MC1R. In addition to the genes coding for these proteins essential for pigmenta-tion, work in mice has uncovered more than 120 genes involved in colour variation. These include genes involved in the biosynthesis of melanin (Tyrp1, Tyrp2), the biology of melanocytes and melanosomes (e.g. ePomc1, Mitf, Silver, Ap3, Mlph, Myo5a, Rab27a) and migration and survival of melanocytes during development (e.g. Kit, Kitl, Edn3 and Ednrb). This information provides a number of candidate genes that may also affect coat colour in other species, including cattle.

In cattle, the Extension locus (MC1R), located on chromosome 18, plays a major role in the regulation of the synthesis of eumelanin versus phaeomelanin. The most common alleles at this locus are the dominant E^D allele and the recessive e allele, which are responsible for the black and red colour, respectively, and code for a receptor which is not affected by the Agouti protein. Breeds with a mix of red and black hairs (wild-type colour) carry Agouti-receptive alleles (E^+, E^1 and E^2). In contrast to mice, the role of the bovine locus for the Agouti protein (ASIP) in colour variation seems limited as no allelic variants have been found in the coding sequence.

In some cattle breeds, such as Dexter, Galloway, Charolais, Highland and Simmental, a lightening or dilution of the base colour defined by the Extension locus is observed. A wide range of colours results from this dilution phenomenon (white, cream, dun, gold, yellow, pale red, grey or brown). The gene responsible of the dilution seems to vary between breeds: e.g. the pale (dun) coat colour observed in Dexter cattle is due to the gene coding for the TYRP1 (tyrosine related protein 1), but this gene has been excluded as being responsible for dilution in other breeds. The silver (SILV) gene, which codes for a type I integral membrane protein in the pre-melanosome matrix (PMEL17), and which is essential for melanosome development, has been found to be responsible for coat colour dilution in Highland cattle.

The Charolais breed exhibits the most extreme case of dilution, as pure-bred Charolais individuals have a uniform white coat colour, despite the e/e Extension genotype of most Charolais cattle. Therefore, the characteristic coat colour of this breed results from a phaeomelanin dilution over the entire body. Charolais cattle are thought to be homozygous for a dilution mutation (Dilution Charolais, Dc/Dc), that in heterozygotes (Dc/dc^+) produces an intermediate phenotype: grey colour if the dilution applies to eumelanin (e.g. in a Black Angus × Charolais cross) or pale red or yellow if the background pigment is phaeomelanin.

Using an F2 Holstein × Charolais population, researchers recently reported an association between dilution of black pigment (eumelanin) and a region on bovine chromosome 5 including the SILV gene. However, these authors did not include animals of red background in their analysis, and therefore it remains to be shown whether the locus affecting the dilution of phaeomelanin, typical of the Charolais breed, co-locates with the linkage association reported by these authors.

We performed a genome scan to localise the genetic locus responsible for the dilution phenotype using a Charolais × Holstein experimental population obtained through a F_2 and balanced Backcross design. The linkage analysis included individuals with both black and red coat colour background, and therefore addressed the localization of the major locus involved in the dilution of the phaeomelanic pigment in the Charolais breed.

MONOHYBRID CROSSES

Overview

In the 1850s and 1860s, Gregor Mendel investigated inheritance by performing monohybrid crosses in pea plants. He crossed two plants that were true-breeding for different traits. Based on his observations, Mendel proposed that organisms inherit two copies of each trait, one from each parent, and that dominant traits can hide recessive traits. These results formed the basis of two fundamental principles in genetics: the Principle of Uniformity and the Law of Segregation.

Monohybrid Crosses Reveal Dominant and Recessive Traits

Over eight years spanning the 1850s and 1860s, an Austrian monk named Gregor Mendel carried out seminal breeding experiments with pea plants. These experiments demonstrated the fundamental principles of inheritance, earning him the moniker "the father of modern genetics." Mendel's experiments focused on seven pea plant characteristics, each manifesting as one of two traits that are determined by a single gene locus.

Mendel noticed that, when some of his pea plants reproduced by self-fertilization, their progeny always displayed the same trait. In other words, they were true-breeding. For example, some plants with yellow pods only produced offspring with yellow pods. When crossed with other plants that bred true for yellow pods, these plants also produced only progeny with yellow pods. Similarly, Mendel observed true-breeding pea plants that produced only offspring with green pods.

At the time, inherited traits were thought to be some mixture of parental features. Mendel instead observed discrete phenotypes, like green and yellow pods. He proposed that, rather than traits mixing in offspring, discrete factors (now known as genes) are inherited from parents and remain separate in the offspring. In cases where a trait skips a generation, Mendel proposed that the visible trait merely masks the presence of the other inherited trait. In other words, inheritance is particulate, and dominant traits hide recessive traits. To determine which trait was dominant, Mendel conducted monohybrid crosses. Monohybrid crosses combine two true-breeding organisms that differ by a single trait. All offspring of such crosses are monohybrids, or heterozygotes, and display the dominant trait.

For example, Mendel crossed pea plants that bred true for yellow pods with those that bred true for green pods to determine the dominant pod color. This parental generation (P_0) produced offspring, the first filial generation (F_1), that were all monohybrids with green pods. Repeatedly observing these findings established green pods as the dominant trait and demonstrated Mendel's principle of uniformity: heterozygotes for a single gene trait display the same phenotype.

Parental Alleles are Randomly Distributed to Gametes

Mendel then induced self-fertilization in the F_1 plants, producing the F_2 generation. F_2 pea plants with green pods outnumbered those with yellow pods by a ratio of 3:1. Mendel repeatedly observed this 3:1 inheritance pattern for each of the seven pea plant characteristics.

Mendel's law of segregation explains this recurring ratio. The law of segregation states that an organism distributes one of its two gene copies to each gamete (egg or sperm cell). Importantly, this distribution is random, such that a heterozygote (Gg) is equally likely to produce gametes with dominant (G) and recessive (g) alleles.

If a heterozygote self-fertilizes (Gg x Gg), the parental alleles can combine in four possible ways: paternal G with maternal G (GG), paternal G with maternal g (Gg), paternal g with maternal G (Gg), and paternal g with maternal g (gg). Three outcomes produce green pods (the GG and Gg genotypes) and one produces yellow pods (the gg genotype), a 3:1 ratio. Thus, if all outcomes are equally likely, self-fertilizing heterozygotes will produce three offspring with green pods for every one with yellow pods. This is remarkably close to the phenotypic ratio that Mendel observed, confirming his proposed law of segregation.

Dominant Traits are Not Always Common

Unlike green pods, green peas are recessive, whereas yellow peas are dominant. Why, then, are the peas we regularly encounter green? In short, people prefer green peas over yellow ones. As Mendel's experiments demonstrate, homozygotes produce offspring with the same trait, or phenotype, when self-fertilized or crossed with other homozygotes. If farmers continue to exclude yellow peas from their crop crosses, they will continue producing only green peas. This example illustrates another important point: dominant traits are not necessarily the most common traits. Harmful dominant traits, for example, may be selected against.

VALUE OF GENETIC MARKERS IN TESTING PARENTS FOR GENETIC DEFECTS

Parentage testing is based on the principle of exclusion, that is, a DNA profile of an offspring is compared to that of its parents and if matches can not be made the parent is excluded, however if matches are made, at each DNA marker evaluated, then the parent is said to qualify. A DNA profile—which provides information for several genetic markers—is obtained, and parentage analysis is performed. A variety of sample types can be utilized for routine testing, including blood, hair, semen, buccal swabs, and FTA cards. Non-routine sample types include bone, teeth, saliva, dried blood, urine, and feces. DNA is extracted from the samples, and the process of establishing a DNA profile begins with the PCR procedure. After which, the DNA profile of the offspring is compared to those of the presumed parents. A parentage specialist analyzes and reviews the results, performs several quality control experiments, and sends the final report. If a listed parent or parents are initially excluded, additional analysis is performed including retesting of samples and the possible use of additional DNA markers to confirm the exclusion.

Detailed DNA Parent Verification Information

Since the late 1950's parentage verification has been utilized in animal registration programs. Breeder experiences have proven that parentage testing, in combination with well run breeding programs, can ensure accurate pedigrees which preserves the integrity of animal breeds. This article will explain the basis of the DNA-based parentage test performed at the Veterinary Genetics Laboratory (VGL) and address the role of parentage analysis in animal breeding programs.

DNA and Microsatellite Structure

Understanding the DNA based parentage test requires a brief explanation of DNA structure. The DNA molecule contains four variations of a chemical structure called a base. These variants are referred to in shorthand as A, C, G and T. Chromosomes are comprised of millions of these four bases arranged in a linear fashion called a DNA strand. The sequence of these four bases at specific sites along the chromosomes is what determines the genetic code for each individual animal. Also found throughout animal genomes are specific sequences of bases repeated in a tandem fashion and referred to as microsatellite DNA markers. The most common microsatellite markers contain a two base sequence repeated in tandem, hence they are also referred to as short tandem repeats or STRs for short. An example of this is a CA sequence repeated ten times but flanked by unique sequence: (...TCAGGTCTACACACACACACACACACACATG CTTATGTACT...) The genomes of mammalian species contain thousands of these microsatellite markers.

Genetic Variation and DNA Analysis

The number of tandem repeats found at any given microsatellite marker will vary between individual animals. Places in the DNA where there are differences from one individual to the next are known as genetic variation. Genetic variation at the microsatellite level has been exploited by molecular biologists for a variety of functions. Microsatellite markers are the basis for individual identification, in forensics application for example, and are also used for the majority of animal parentage testing done today. The various forms of a given microsatellite that are identified by differences in the number of repeats are referred to as alleles and these are inherited in a Mendelian fashion. Meaning, an animal may possess only two alleles for a specific microsatellite, one inherited from its dam and the other from its sire. So if we consider the example above where for this particular allele the repeat length was ten (.....TCAGGTCTACACACACACACA CACACACATGCTTATGTACT.....) genetic variation may exist in a population where some individuals have 12 repeats (.....TCAGGTCTACACACACA CACACACACACACACATGCTTATGTACT......) and others might have 14 repeats (..... TCAGGTCTACACACACACACACACACACACACACACATGCTTATGTACT.....). The size of the alleles possessed by an offspring must correspond to those of the presumed parents. Thus if the sire had the allele with ten repeats and the dam had he allele with 14 repeats the offspring would have one allele with ten and one allele with 14 repeats. With an increase in the number of repeats there is a proportional increase in the allele size. Thus part of developing the DNA profile is to detect these size variations DNA. We do so by isolating the DNA from the sample, amplify several microsatellites by the Polymerase Chain Reaction (PCR) and at the same time tag these PCR products with a fluorescent dye. The dye-labeled alleles are detected by laser excitation and their size determined by gel electrophoresis and computer analysis. To have accurate parental exclusions several microsattelite markers are evaluated (typically 12-18) but the number needed is depends on several factors including the genetic diversity that exists with in a population.

Parentage Case Scenarios

The typical animal parentage case, as seen with most domestic species, includes a dam, offspring and one or more sires. Generally the identity of the dam is fairly certain. As mentioned earlier, in order to qualify to a set of parents an offspring must possess the same allele sizes as the parents. Outlined below are a few examples of the types of animal parentage cases submitted to the VGL. The numbers represent the allele sizes, which are the number of DNA base repeats, determined by PCR and gel electrophoresis.

Typical Parentage Case

One dam and three possible sires. For simplicity only four markers are shown.

Marker	A	B	C	D
Dam	86/112	150/164	202/206	224/260
Offspring	86/112	150/156	202/204	224/226
Sire 1	86/116	156/168	204	226/242
Sire 2	96/120	156/158	194/202	222/242
Sire 3	102/116	152	202	226

In this case the dam and sire 1 qualify as possible parents. Sires 2 and 3 are excluded at several markers without consideration of the dam. The alleles that have excluded sires 2 and 3. For example, at Marker A the offspring's DNA type is 86/112 and Sire 2's type is 96/120; there are no alleles in common. Sire 2 and the offspring also have no alleles in common at Marker D and Sire 2 is again excluded.

Mating Exclusion Case

Sire 4, below, is used to illustrate such a case. The dam, offspring and sire 1 are from example I.

Sire 4	86/128	150/164	188/202	224/228

The offspring possesses a Marker B 156 allele, a Marker C 204 allele and a Marker D 226 allele that are not possessed by either the dam or sire 4. This data indicates that one of the parents is incorrect. The offspring could have inherited the Marker B 150 allele, the Marker C 202 allele and the Marker D 224 allele from either parent. Therefore, neither parent can be definitively excluded so the mating must be excluded.

In the majority of cases, if all available microsatellite markers are utilized, one parent will be positively excluded from the mating. However, the outcome of a mating exclusion case can change significantly if only one parent is provided. In this case without knowledge of the dam's genetic contribution, both sire 1 and 4 would appear to qualify as a parent, which demonstrates the importance of providing both a dam and sire in a parentage case.

Nowadays for a lot of monogenic traits, genetic markers are available. Many of these genetic markers are not directly testing the presence of the allele responsible for the monogenic trait. But these markers are establishing the presence of a variable piece of non-functional DNA, an allele at a locus close to the locus of the functional allele. These genetic markers are extremely valuable to detect heterozygous animals, heterozygous for recessive alleles.

But these markers always have the risk that, through recombination effects between the marker and the locus of the monogenic traits in the meiosis, the relation between the marker and the functional allele is disrupted.

Thus, once a genetic marker closely located to the recessive functional allele on a chromosome is detected, the relation between the marker and the allele should be checked regularly in future generations. The closer the

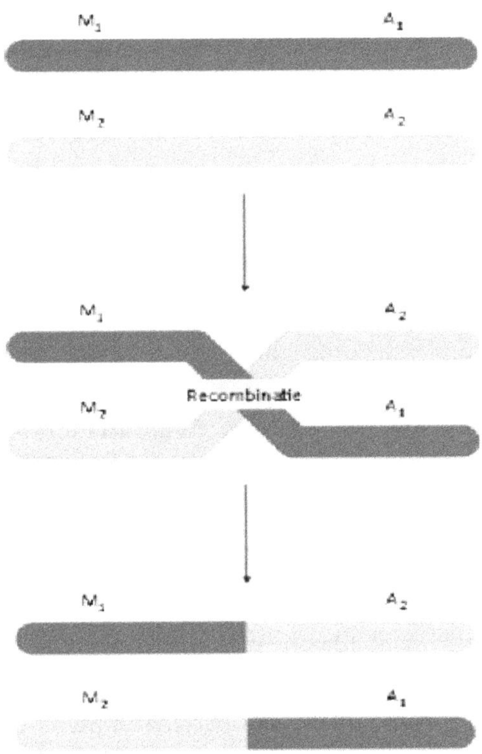

Fig. 4: Recombination disrupts the relationship between marker M1 and allele A1 and betwee n marker M2 and allele A2

marker is situated to the functional allele, the lower the chance for recombination and the higher the accuracy of the genetic marker.

Accuracy of Parentage Analysis

Parentage testing identifies individuals that, due to a specific combination of marker alleles, could qualify as a parent for a particular offspring. Accurate parentage testing requires breeders to identify possible parents since if considering a randomly selected large group of individuals there could be more than one that qualifies as a parent. As an example, human paternity testing was originally developed as a means to verify that a named individual could or could not be the father of a given child. At most it was meant to determine if one of several men could be the father of a child. The same rules hold true for animal parentage testing. A good application for animal parentage testing is verification that the dam is correct and which of the sires on a particular farm are the actual sire.

Finally, it is important to remember that while parentage exclusions are 100% accurate, parentage qualifications are not. The accuracy of most animal parentage tests is greater than 99% when both parents are included in the analysis and drops to around 95% when only one parent is included in the analysis. However, this accuracy will decrease when the potential parents are part of a large group of closely related animals. Again, an animal closely related to an actual parent could possess marker alleles that make it appear to be the correct parent. To prevent erroneous parentage qualifications, breeders need to submit samples from all possible parents when first requesting parentage verification. If more than one sire and one dam qualify as parents of an offspring, the laboratory can then test with additional DNA markers to sort out the actual parents.

Breeding aspects of genes

Molecular genetics can contribute to complex traits by identifying causal genes, understanding the regulatory mechanisms of gene expression, identifying genetic networks and pathways and understanding the role of ”other” genomic structures and mechanisms, e.g., structural variations, microRNAs, metagenome and epigenome.

Genetic improvement in domesticated animal populations through conventional livestock improvement programmes mainly involves selection of males and females that, when mated, are expected to produce progeny that perform better than the average of the current generation. Performance usually includes a combination of multiple characteristics, or traits, most of which are quantitative in nature.

Quantitative traits that are controlled by multiple to many genes (>100 to perhaps thousands), affected by environment, in livestock include traits such as milk yield, fat yield, protein yield in dairy animals and growth rate, fatness and feed intake in meat producing animals. The main criteria that are used to identify individuals to be used for breeding are estimates of their breeding values for the traits of interest.

The breeding value of an individual is defined as the sum of the additive effects of all loci that contribute to the trait (quantitative trait loci or QTL), deviated from the population mean. To date, extensive data bases of recorded phenotypes for traits of interest, or for traits that are genetically correlated to traits of interest, have been used as the main source of information to estimate the breeding value of selection candidates. To this end, sophisticated statistical methods based on best linear unbiased prediction (BLUP), mixed linear model methodology has been implemented.

These methods capitalize on information contained in the recorded phenotypes of not only the individual itself but also that of its relatives, in order to maximize the accuracy of the resulting estimated breeding value (EBV). Although selection programs based on EBV estimated from phenotype have been very successful, they also face a number of limitations. These primarily relate to the ability to routinely record phenotypes on selection candidates and/or their close relatives in a timely manner, such that accurate selection decisions can be made at an early age to reduce generation intervals.

Cost of phenotype recording also plays an important role here. Unfortunately, some traits of interest are only recorded late in life (e.g. longevity), only on one sex (e.g. milk yield in dairy cattle), require animals to be sacrificed (e.g. meat quality), or require animals to be exposed to conditions that would hamper the ability to market or export their germplasm (e.g. disease resistance). These phenotyping constraints limit the amount of genetic progress that can be made through conventional selection and breeding method.

Molecular genetics is the study of the genetic makeup of individuals at the DNA level. It is the identification and mapping of genes and genetic polymorphisms. By the use of molecular genetics techniques it is possible to identify genes that are involved in variety of traits. Armed with this information it would be possible to select improved livestock on the basis of their genetic makeup.

If applied with care, the use of molecular information in selection programmes has the potential to increase productivity, enhance environmental adaptation and maintain genetic diversity. The use of molecular genetics technologies potentially offer a way to select breeding animal at an early age (even embryos); to select for a wide range of traits and to enhance reliability in predicting the mature phenotype of the individual.

Beginning of Use of Molecular Genetic Techniques in Animal Breeding

Starting in the 1970's, the advent of the era of molecular genetics provided new opportunities to improve breeding programs in livestock by allowing the use of DNA markers to identify genes or genomic regions that control traits of interest.

For quantitative traits, these advances promised the identification of QTL and the development of DNA tests that could be use to select animals at an early age to help selection decision through marker-assisted selection (MAS), i.e. selection on a combination of information derived from genetic markers associated with QTL and the traditional phenotypic information.

To this end, large numbers of candidate gene and QTL mapping studies were conducted. This resulted in the discovery of substantial numbers of QTL and marker-phenotype associations and some causative mutations.

Advantages of Molecular Approach over Traditional Approach

1. Assuming no genotyping errors, molecular genetic information is not affected by environmental effects and therefore has heritability equal to 1.
2. Molecular genetic information can be available at an early age, in principle at the embryo stage, thereby allowing early selection and reduction of generation intervals.
3. Molecular genetic information can be obtained on all selection candidates, which is especially beneficial for sex-limited traits, traits that are expensive or difficult to record, or traits that require slaughter of the animal (carcass traits).
4. Molecular approach helps us to select for a wide range of traits which in turn saves time and efforts.
5. Molecular genetic information enhances reliability in predicting the mature phenotype of the individual.

APPLICATION OF ADVANCED MOLECULAR GENETICS TECHNIQUE IN ANIMAL BREEDING AND GENETICS

Use of Genetic Markers in MAS (Marker Assisted Selection) as a Tool in Breeding Programs

The fast development of molecular techniques has opened up foundation of genes to animal breeding that were not available before through conventional breeding, creating a lot of interest about MAS (Marker Assisted Selection). The advance use of molecular genetic technologies prospectively presents the way to select the breeding animals at an early stage (even embryo); to select for a superior variety of traits.

Animal researchers are currently formulating their trust on genetic markers. To discover the effect of the genes on the phenotype of animals, we can follow the inheritance of these markers in families of animals and see whether inheritance any of these is associate with the develop performance. If they are, then we presume that one or more genes in this region of marker are associated with beneficial effects. Then we use the information on the genetic markers to make future selection decisions, so the any animal that inherits the marker will also inherit the valuable effect correlated with it, this is known as marker assisted selection (MAS). In genome wide association studies (GWAS), both the candidate gene and QTL (quantitative trait loci) mapping strategies have been widely utilized in domestic animals for the finding of genetic markers appropriate for MAS.

Assisted Reproductive Technology (ART) in Animal Breeding

Advances in assisted reproductive technologies (ART) like artificial insemination, In vitro production, superovolution, embryo transfer, trangenesis and cloning have become significant in livestock breeding. These techniques have been introduced initially to overcome reproductive problems but have significant impact on livestock breeding.

All these technologies able to speed up genetic changes due to shorter generation interval and improving accuracy in selection program. Artificial insemination (AI) and embryo transfer (ET) are probably the most well known methods that have been adopted in developed and developing livestock production.

The recent advances in biotechnology technologies in reproduction included production of transgenic animals and cloning. RT has prolonged effects on animal breeding in the future, as it increases the rate of reproduction and decrease the generation time. The most successful reproductive technologies like AI and ET necessitated applying on large extent, some emerging biotechnologies such as Multiple Ovulation and Embryo Transfer (MOET), In Vitro Fertilization (IVF) and cloning provides prevailing tool for rapidly changing the animal populations genetically.

USE OF TRANSGENIC TECHNOLOGY IN ANIMAL BREEDING

Transgenic animal technology is in the progress of revolutionizing the manner we domesticate the livestock. The transgenesis means transfer of foreign gene (gene of interest) into the genome of other species in a way that it stably passed from generation to generation. It has been a potential way in accelerating and facilitating genetic improvement in livestock. The process to produce transgenic animals initiated with the purpose of producing better breed lines, which are strong, more carcass, high growth rate and increase milk production.

In breeding, transgenic animals are created to improve qualitative and quantitative traits in livestock and to reduce susceptibility to diseases. This technology uses the transgene encoding a particular trait is clone into a vector which may be synthetic, virus or plasmid DNA, and hybrid vector is inserted into the genome of the host organism. A variety of methods have been developed to produce transgenic animals, some have had much success and others are being further researched. There are several methods have been introduced to create transgenic animals, in these the most common method is the microinjection of a transgene into pronucleus of a newly fertilized egg, the introduction of desired gene into embryonic stem cells and the transgenic somatic cell nuclear transfer (TSCNT) which is the variant of SCNT.

Pronuclear Microinjection

The microinjection into pronucleous is the most common method known in microinjection of exogenous DNA into the pronucleus of a newly fertilized egg (zygote). This technique is used to produce transgenic sheep and pigs and also transgenic cattle.

Sperm Mediated Gene Transfer (SMGT)

Sperm mediated gene transfer (SMGT) is an alternative technique using natural ability of spermatozoa as a vector to transfer exogenous DNA into the egg at fertilization.

DNA Recombination in Embryonic Stem Cells

ES cells are derived from inner cell masses (ICM) of embryo at blastocysts stage. This type of embryo manipulation is used when inserting a transgene into a specific location in the genome. Two complementary strategies have been considered for the insertion of transgene in ES cell- homologous recombination and integrase mechanisms.

With the introduction of homologous recombination the scientists and researchers are able to restore gene function (knock-in animals), take out gene function (knock-out animals), inactivated, or introduce any alteration in gene of interest. In vitro the gene of interest is inserted into ES cells by microinjection, viruses, electroporation or chemicals.

Cloning Technology in Animal Breeding

Cloning is an asexual reproduction of genetically identical organism can be achieved by nuclear transfer (NT) or by embryo splitting. Cloning is a significantly useful breeding tool, considering a perfect way to improve the performance of farm animals. One of the principle purposes of cloning is to increase the number of species in a population with superior characteristics.

Cloning technology has concerned the interest of breeders for many years. Animal cloning is the most topical development of selective assisted breeding in livestock.

Cloning has been used to replicate elite breeding animals (Plume, 2009). As Dolly the sheep was the first animal to be cloned in 1996 by somatic cell nuclear transfer (SCNT). Since that time many other species have been cloned by the same process. According to researchers there are around 6000 farm animals' clones worldwide.

The cloning technology has been applied in the breeding of elite cattle, goat, pig, buffalo, camel, Rabbet and other pet species like dog, cat, rat, ferret, mouse. High cost of cloning is the factor that limited the use of this technology in practical animals breeding.

DNA Microarray Technology for Assisting in Breeding Decision

A variety of techniques have been available to identify difference in gene expression including subtractive hybridization, differential display, serial analysis of gene expression and microarray hybridization. Among these microarray technology has become one of the significant tools for scientists and animal breeders to monitor genome wide expression levels of genes in livestock.

DNA microarray also known as DNA/RNA Chips, BioChips or GeneChips are a collection of DNA segments, immobilized on a solid surface (e.g. glass, plastic or silicon chip) which allow the quantitative and high throughput analysis of several genes through hybridization to a set of specific probes. Each particular hybridization reaction on an array is referred to as a spot or feature, and a characteristic array may include thousands of spots.

Microarray is novel technology that has attracted a huge deal of attention from animal geneticists and breeders. It has been used for large scale gene expression studies. The high throughput system of microarray makes genotyping efficient and low cost, particularly for single nucleotide polymorphism (SNP) and indel polymorphisms. DNA microarrays are widely applied in genome wide genotyping for identifying variation.

Whole genome genotyping tools based on SNP markers are now available as microarray based genotyping arrays. These arrays are now allocated genotyping for the entire genome with tens of thousands of SNP markers in a single hybridization step, so it appreciably increasing the throughput and decreasing the cost of current gel based techniques for molecular mapping. These expression studies have been carried out to compare gene expression between breeds. Relatively apart from gene expression profiling to established fingerprint of an animal with desirable characteristics, direct genotyping of DNA for variants associate with genes that produce desirable traits will be of interest.

The DNA microarray used for this purpose would be allow the large scale screening of many hundred of such markers in a sole experiment, allowing selection based on multiple traits. The newly genomic approaches such as DNA microarray, SNP discovery and genotyping are hopeful tools for improving and advancing farm animal breeding.

Sex Determination of Offspring/Embryo sexing by the Help of Molecular Markers

Molecular markers can be applied in the determination of sex of pre-implantation embryos. This can be achieved by using as probes, Y-chromosome-specific (male-specific) DNA sequence. Researchers reported that using the PCR-based method of sex determination has the advantage of being carried out in less than five hours with almost 100% accuracy. The sexing of pre-implantation embryos can serve as an important tool for improving a herd for a desired purpose.

Although embryo sexing may not have dramatic effects on rates of genetic gain it can have considerable increases in efficiency. It is concluded from a study that an all-female heifer system using ET was 50% more efficient than the highest achievable in a traditional system. It has been suggested that, if multiple sexed-embryo transfer became a routine operation such as AI, beef operations based on this system could become competitive with pig and poultry production in terms of efficiency of food utilization.

Use of High-Density SNP Genotyping for Whole-Genome Selection

For most livestock species, commercial platforms are currently available that allow the genotyping of an individual for tens of thousands of SNP across the genome at a reasonable cost (<$150 per individual, depending on volume). The first such high-density SNP genotyping platform available in livestock was the 50k bovine illumina SNP panel.

To date, tens of thousands of dairy and beef bulls and cows have been genotyped using this platform.

Similar SNP panels of 40 to 65 thousand SNP are now available for other livestock species, including pigs, poultry, sheep, and horse. Recently, panels with over 700k SNP have become available in cattle and such higher density panels are also under development in other species. In dairy cattle, the main use of high-density SNP genotyping has been to implement genomic or whole-genome selection.

Genomic selection involves estimation of the effect of each SNP on the high-density panel using models that fit all SNP simultaneously, with their effects treated as random variables. Once estimates of the effect of each SNP are obtained, they can be used to estimate the breeding value of selection candidates based on their SNP genotypes across the genome.

Alternatively, the high-density SNP genotypes can be used to construct a so-called genomic relationship matrix among all individuals in the population and use it instead of the traditional pedigree-based relationship matrix in the BLUP mixed model procedures that are routinely used to estimate breeding values in livestock.

This procedure, known as GBLUP, has been shown to be equivalent to the Bayesian SNP effect estimation method in which the prior distribution of SNP effects assumes that the genetic variation for the trait is equally distributed across all SNP on the panel, similar to the infinitesimal model of quantitative genetics.

Thus, in contrast to the phenotype-based models for prediction of breeding values, methods that utilize genomic data do depend on having some knowledge of the genetic architecture of traits.

Alternatively, non- or semi-parametric methods have been advocated for use in genomic selection. Methods to combine data on genotyped individuals with phenotypic data on individuals that have not been genotyped have been developed also.

Estimation of breeding values using high-density SNP data has been implemented in dairy cattle breeding programs in several countries and research to implement genomic selection in other livestock species is underway. In dairy cattle, this has resulted a substantial increase in the accuracy of EBV at a young age (increases of 35% on average and up to 50%, depending on the trait and size of the data set used for training).

The availability of genome-enhanced breeding values (GEBV) at a young age is having a major impact on breeding programs in dairy cattle, in particular by allowing young bulls to be selected for breeding prior to the availability of extensive progeny data. This is expected to substantially increase (up to double) the rate of genetic improvement by reducing generation intervals and by enhancing opportunities to select for traits with low heritability, e.g. fertility. Reduction or removal of the need for progeny testing also has the potential to substantially reduce the cost of breeding programs in dairy cattle.

In the last decade there have been massive advances in genotyping technology, but due to technological limitation, approximately all genotyping is partial, through these technologies only a small fraction of an individual genotype is determined rather than the whole genome' genotype. In the near future the new innovative e.g. Illumina's Human-1 Bead Chip or mass sequencing technologies have promise the whole genome's genotyping.

Multicolor fluorescence detection ability of CE (capillary electrophoresis) instrument such as ABI PRISM genetic analyzer have a leading role in STR genotyping, the effort is going to develop microchip platform to perform high resolution DNA genotyping. In addition mass spectrometries (MS) with matrix assisted laser desorption/ionization (MALDI) and elctrospary ionization (ESI) techniques have been used for STR typing without allelic ladder.

There are a number of genotyping techniques available, capillary electrophoresis based genotyping techniques includes AFLP®, ISSR (inter simple sequence repeat) analysis, Relative Fluorescence Quantification, Resequencing Heterozygote Detection, Single Sequence Conformation Polymorphisms (SSCP), Polymerase Chain Reaction, Confronting two pair primers (PCR-CTPP), Melting Curve Analysis of SNPs (McSNP®) and Copy Number Analysis (CNA) have been play their role.

Use of High-Density SNP Genotyping for Genome-Wide Association Studies

The large amounts of high-density SNP data that are being generated for implementation of whole-genome selection can also be used for genome-wide association studies (GWAS) to identify genetic markers or genomic regions associated with traits based on population-wide linkage disequilibrium (LD). Several studies have capitalized on this to analyze the genetic architecture of traits of interest in animal agriculture. For GWAS, several alternate statistical methods have been used. Most studies have used single SNP models in which each SNP is fitted separately as a fixed effect, ideally in a BLUP animal model to properly account for the family structure of the data by fitting a polygenic effect with pedigree based relationships.

A problem of single SNP models is that they rely on the pair wise LD of a QTL with individual SNP. Single SNP models can also lead to excessive false positives if population structure is not properly accounted for. Researchers used mixed linear model methodology to estimate the proportion of genetic variance associated with each genomic region of 50 SNP from the Bovine 50k Illumina SNP chip for three quantitative traits in dairy cattle.

Fitting each region separately, their model simultaneously used two genomic relationship matrices, one based on 50 SNP in the region and one based on the rest of the genome, to separate genetic variance contributed by the region from variance contributed by the rest of the genome.

The Bayesian methods that have been developed for genomic selection have also been used for GWAS. In particular the Bayesian variable selection methods have been shown to be effective for GWAS in simulated and real data.

Several criteria have been used to identify important SNP or genomic regions using these methods, including the proportion of iterations of the MCMC chain that a given SNP or a set of SNP in a genomic region were given non-zero effects, or the proportion of variance that is explained by a given SNP or by a region of the genome.

An advantage of the genomic selection methods over the single SNP models is that all SNP are fitted simultaneously. This allows capture of all information if multiple SNP are in LD with a QTL and also implicitly accounts for any population structure that is present in the data, reducing false positives. In addition, by fitting SNP effects as random rather than fixed, estimates are shrunk towards zero depending on the amount of information that is contained in the data and the priors that are specified.

In July 2010, Illumina released two new genotyping SNP chips including a low-density chip (Bovine3K) having 2,900 SNP and a high density chip (Bovine HD) with 777,962 SNP and in January 2011 affymetrix released a high density chip with 648,855 SNP. Although such chips can provide genotypes that enhance the precision of genomic evaluation by better tracking of the loci responsible for genetic difference. SNP chips are currently available for human, ovine, bovine, canine, porcine and equine species.

Molecular Markers – A Tool for Exploring Genetic Diversity

Diversity among organisms is a result of variations in DNA sequences and of environmental effects. Genetic variation is substantial, and each individual of a species, with the exception of monozygotic twins, possesses a unique DNA sequence. DNA variations are mutations resulting from substitution of single nucleotides (single nucleotide polymorphisms – SNPs), insertion or deletion of DNA fragments of various lengths (from a single to several thousand nucleotides), or duplication or inversion of DNA fragments.

DNA variations are classified as "neutral" when they cause no change in metabolic or phenotypic traits, and hence are not subjected to positive, negative, or balancing selection; otherwise, they are referred to as "functional".

Mutations in key nucleotides of a coding sequence may change the amino acid composition of a protein, and lead to new functional variants. Such variants may have an increased or decreased metabolic efficiency compared to the original "wild type", may lose their functionality completely, or even gain a novel function. Mutations in regulatory regions may affect levels and patterns of gene expression; for example, turning genes on/off or under/over expressing proteins in specific tissues at different development or physiological stages. In the absence of reliable phenotype and QTN data, or to complement the existing data, the most rapid and cost-effective measures of genetic diversity are obtained from the assay of polymorphisms using anonymous molecular genetic markers.

Anonymous markers are likely to provide indirect information on functional genes for important traits, assuming that unique populations that have had a particular evolutionary history at the neutral markers (e.g. because of ancient isolation or independent domestication) are likely to carry unique variants of functional variations. Molecular techniques have also proved useful in the investigation of the origin and domestication of livestock species, and their subsequent migrations, as well as providing information on evolutionary relationships (phylogenetic trees), and identifying geographical areas of admixture among populations of different genetic origins.

Using Markers to Estimate Effective Population Size

Researchers suggested estimation of effective population size (Ne) using gametic phase disequilibrium of DNA polymorphisms. This estimation can be based on genotypes for linked markers (microsatellites or SNPs). The expected correlation of allele frequencies at linked loci is a function of Ne and the recombination rate. Ne can, therefore, be estimated from the observed disequilibrium. Researchers suggested a similar approach based on chromosome segment homozygosity, which, in addition, has the potential to estimate Ne for earlier generations, and therefore allows a judgment of whether an existing population was of increasing or decreasing size in the past. The study demonstrated, with example data sets, that the Holstein-Friesian cattle breed underwent a substantial reduction of Ne in the past, while the effective population size of the human population is increasing, which is in agreement with both census and pedigree studies.

Use of Mitochondrial DNA based Diversity and Phylogeographical Analysis in Livestock Breeding

Mammalian mitochondria contain a small circular DNA plasmid of 16.5 kb which codes for 37 genes required to be expressed within the inner mitochondrial membrane. The mitochondrial genome evolves 17 times faster than nuclear DNA; probably due to lack of DNA repair mechanisms. As a result, the mitochondrial DNA sequence can be used to monitor evolution on a shorter time scale than is possible with chromosomal DNA. Mitochondrial genome polymorphisms are therefore frequently used to analyse population structure and demographic history. Mitochondrial DNA is haploid, and so each individual has a single haplotype. It is maternally inherited as a result of the limited contribution to the zygote of mitochondria from sperm. This limits its use in relation to domestic species where gene flow through the male line forms an important determinant of evolution and population structure, for instance through artificial insemination, but provides the advantage that it allows introgression through the female line to be distinguished from that through the male.

The value of mitochondrial DNA for animal breeding is that it allows an understanding of population history and structure in time and space. For instance, a low level of mitochondrial DNA polymorphism within a species suggests it has survived a reduction in population size or bottleneck, whereas a high level of variation is characteristic of a large and well-established population. Mitochondrial DNA is extremely valuable in resolving important taxonomic questions when distinguishing subspecies and in identifying evolutionary significant units. Mitochondrial DNA bar coding has been suggested as an aid to assessment of biodiversity, but this has been questioned, particularly in species subject to parasite infestation or with a high incidence of symbiont infection. The general conclusion from large-scale analyses of livestock populations, which are perhaps the most informative for this purpose, suggests that variation in maternal lineages explain at most a small fraction of the variation in traits of commercial interest.

Use of mtDNA has broadened the perspective on the origin and evolution of domesticated cattle. Further, one of the persistent challenges in the analysis of population genetic data is to account for the spatial arrangement (nonrandom distribution of genetic variation among individuals within populations) of samples and populations. mtDNA data have been extensively used to understand the spatial distribution of genetic lineages within species allowing the historical factor with the highest effect on the lineages spatial patterns.

mtDNA has been used for the identification of maternal and paternal lineages as well as test hypothesis related to past genetic history and evolution of different species. The recognition of mitochondrial DNA molecule as a genetic marker in population and evolutionary biology derives in part from the relative ease with which clearly homologous sequences can be isolated and compared. Simple sequence organization, maternal inheritance and absence of recombination make mtDNA an ideal marker for tracing maternal genealogies.

Use of Cytogenetic and Molecular Methods for Screening of Genetic Defects in Livestock

Genetic diseases occur due to abnormalities in genetic material, at any nucleotide to chromosome level, of any kind of individual. Mostly genetic defects are rare in nature because of continuous natural selection against them. Although, all of the genetic defects do not culminate into a disease condition, but sometime, individual looking normal may have genetic defect in heterozygous condition and can act as carrier during inheritance. During recent time, we are now able to diagnose the genetic defect in the individuals. Now, biotechnology offers to diagnose genotypes, such as normal, carrier, or affected individuals. Understanding the molecular basis of a defect, the direct detection of the heterozygous carriers is thus possible even during embryonic stage. In livestock, genetic screening has become much essential in view of intensive selection in dairy and meat industry, which has predisposing only few of the high valued males.

In such circumstance, any individual with genetic defect may inherit the defective gene or chromosome to a larger number of progenies; thereby have more economic concern in livestock industry. Because most genetic diseases are inherited from the carriers, which generally produce no noticeable indications, the undesirable trait can proliferate extensively in absence of screening of genetic defects. Now a day, cytogenetic and molecular screening of all breeding males has been made essential in the new National Programme on Cattle and Buffalo breeding (NPCBB) to keep our farm animals free from genetic defects aroused by any chromosomal abnormalities or nucleotide mutations. Multiple congenital malformations are seen with many types of chromosomal abnormalities, particularly deletions and aneuploidy.

Animals with a balanced set of chromosomes will generally be normal phenotypically. If an individual does not have a balanced set of chromosomes, this will normally be visible through more or less deviation of phenotype from normality. Animals with a non-balanced set of chromosomes will most often be sterile and have low vitality. Chromosome deviations, in animals with a normal phenotype, are normally detected due to low fertility or complete sterility. The subfertility is caused by problems in chromosome pairing and segregation during meiosis. In general, however, it shows a substantial, often greater than 50% reduction in fertility.

Chromosomal fusion in heterozygote form causes a slightly lower fertility. The karyotype of a bull with low fertility has shown having a 1/8 translocation. In twinning of foetus with different sex, a mixture of stem cells is established for the white and the red blood cells by mixing the blood in the early foetal stage. If the mixing is too extensive the heifer in a mixed twin pair gets abnormal sexual organs and is infertile and called Freemartins.

The bull birthed from such twining generally has normal fertility, however, might show the genotype of the other twin. Cytogenetic screening i.e. by studying the chromosomes, we generally study the inheritance pattern from one generation to another. It also gives an opportunity to locate the genes and their arrangement on the chromosomes, which become important for the linked loci. Now a day's advanced molecular cytogenetics like Fluorescent In Situ Hybridization (FISH) and Comparative Genomic Hybridization (CGH) has also been come out, which is analyzing the chromosome with more refinement, however, limited use is there in routine due to high cost. Researchers reported that a particular RFLP in the Prion protein gene was responsible for the variation in host's response to the causative agent, and the incubation time of bovine spongiform encephalopathy (BSE). The PCR-RFLP assay has been used to identify carrier animals possessing the defective recessive allele in bovine leucocyte adhesion deficiency in cattle, hyperkalemic periodic analysis in horses and malignant hyperthermia in pigs (Fujii et al., 1991). Researchers identified carrier animals of weaver disease in cattle using microsatellite (TGLA 116) marker.

Use of Molecular Genetic Tools for Livestock Germplasm Conservation

The genetic resources of farm animals in India are represented by a broad spectrum of native breeds of cattle, buffaloes, goat, sheep, swine, equines, camels and poultry. The genetic biodiversity among this livestock has developed and stabilized over millions of years of evolution and endowed the indigenous breeds with capabilities to withstand hostile climate, epidemic pests and diseases, and to survive on inadequate quantities of feed, fodder and water. However, over the years due to many reasons the population size of many breeds is declining. As genetic diversity equips farmers and breeders to utilize a wide range of production environments and develop diverse products to meet the needs of local communities, the unavailability of such diversity in future may hamper sustainable development. Hence the need for conservation of animal genetic resources has been accepted in India as well as globally.

Conservation methods can be broadly categorized as in situ and ex situ. In situ conservation means that animals are kept within their production system, in the area where the breed developed its characteristics. Ex-situ conservation applies to situation where animals are kept outside their area of origin (herds kept in experimental farms, farm parks, within protected areas or in zoos) or more often, when genetic material is conserved and stored in gene banks in the form of semen, ova, embryo or DNA methods that include organized flocks/herds needs lots of space and infrastructure however ex situ conservation methods that include cryopreservation of embryos, somatic cell banking, epididymal sperms banking, cryopreservation of embryonic stem cell lines, cryopreservation of spermatogonial stem cell lines, storage of DNA, frozen semen are the advanced techniques which can be used for long time conservation of number of species and breeds in a small area.

Determination of Parentage by the Use of Molecular Techniques

The identification of parentage in segregating populations generally takes place by means of the exclusion principle. That is, presence at some genetic locus in the offspring of an allele not found in either of the putative parents effectively excludes the particular parental pair from biological parenthood. Highly polymorphic DNA fingerprinting markers have been reported to be very useful in parentage testing. Molecular markers can be employed for sire identification in Artificial Insemination programmes.

Use of DNA Barcoding Markers for Species Identification

A DNA barcode is a short DNA sequence from a standardized region of the genome used for identifying species. The essential aim of DNA barcoding is to use a large-scale screening of one or more reference genes in order to assign unknown individuals to species, and to enhance discovery of new species. Biological taxonomists apply this principle to species classification. The first application of using the DNA sequences in systematic biological taxonomy (also called DNA taxonomy) was conducted by researchers and then , Hebert et al., 2003 proposed the concept of DNA barcoding and suggested its use for a single mtDNA gene, mitochondrial cytochrome c oxidase I (COI), as a common sequence in animal DNA barcoding studies. DNA barcoding has a high accuracy of 97.9%, and provides a new, quick, and convenient identification strategy for animal genetic diversity.

HURDLES IN THE APPLICATION OF THESE MOLECULAR GENETICS TECHNIQUES

Economic Factors

According to researchers, "economics is the key determinant for the application of molecular genetics in genetic improvement programmes. The use of markers in selection incurs the costs that are inherent to molecular techniques." Developing costs (e.g. identifying molecular markers on the genome, detecting association between markers and the traits of interest) and running costs (e.g. typing individuals appropriate in the selection programme) are quite expensive. If the Developing and running costs of the technology is much high it may certainly out-weigh whatever benefits that could be derived from it for this the accessibility and affordability of the technology needs to be increased.

Need for Global Data Infrastructure

A global molecular data infrastructure needs to be built to share and access molecular data, in combination with performance traits between countries. This requires a re-think of how to redefine intellectual property rights.

Lab to Land Transfer of Techniques

"Dissemination Scenarios" must be developed on how to extend the genetic progress from lab to land. One could imagine that genomics selection is practised in a local nucleus herd from which selected sires (and surplus dams) are sold/ distributed to farmers. Given the unique local environmental challenges, it is important to maintain a local level of input into the selection programme.

Lack of Funds/Grants to Researchers

The researches involving molecular technologies are being hampered in developing nations due to the inability of researchers to access grants and funds. Many times researchers are denied opportunity to secure research grants because their institutions or their basic affiliations could not provide the basic equipment/facilities required to effectively carry out some researches. Sometimes when research grants are provided, the amount is hardly sufficient to procure all the necessary reagents and other consumables. For all this to happen, considerable funds need to be allocated both at national and international levels.

Lack of Adequately Trained Personnel

The application of molecular markers to the improvement of animal species is also being hampered by the non-availability of enough number of adequately trained personnel with the requisite practical experience in the universities. It is therefore advocated that training and re-training of personnel be carried out to forestall the problem of inadequate human resources.

MILK PROTEIN GENES

Genetics is the science of heredity which is concerned with physical and chemical properties of the hereditary material, how the material is transmitted from one generation to the next and how the information it contains is expressed in the development of an individual. Genetic make-up of animals control their structural configuration and productive abilities either via single genes or by multiple genes situated in different loci. Genes are compost of nucleotide sequences packaged into chromosomes in the nucleus. Milk production is largely affected by a combination of factors namely; genetic make-up in terms of the use of improved breeds selected for milk production, a favourable nutritional environment and improved managerial practices.

Consequently, genetic make-up of dairy animals plays a great role in the variation of milk yield and composition. Milk production is, therefore, a factor of genotype-environment interactions. It is important to balance selection for both production (e.g., milk yield and composition) and functional (e.g., fertility, disease resistance, feed intake and body weight) traits. Techniques applied in molecular genetics in conjunction with conventional animal breeding techniques could be used to optimize animal breeding programmes, resulting in higher yields (i.e., greater genetic gains), as it is possible to determine the potential of an animal, even before the trait is expressed phenotypically.

A genetic marker serves to favourably relate alleles for quantitative characteristics with information about the individual mode of action and their interaction of genes, helping to understand the quantitative variations and their practical use in animal husbandry. DNA markers present two possible future applications in animal selection; the combination of the best alleles of two or more breeds, and the selection of the best alleles within a breed or lineage. Commonly used genetic markers are the DNA-based markers; RFLPs and minisatellites, and PCR-based markers like microsatellites, and SNP. DNA-based markers are more direct molecular markers that survey DNA variation itself rather than rely on variations in the electrophoresis mobility of protein that the DNA encodes. They allow the number of mutations between different alleles to be quantified.

DNA containing genetic information identified to influence milk production traits can be artificially introduced into a dairy animal, using recombinant DNA technology, and then it must be transmitted through the germ line so that every cell, including germ cells, of the animal contain the same modified genetic material. Such techniques enable dairy animals to acquire desired milk production characteristics.

However, use of such transgenic techniques attracts ethical questions. Generally, genetic marker approaches is a promising tool for milk production improvement. It is imperative that genetic improvement for milk production is approached holistically, taking into consideration all the factors that may affect a breeding programme.

FUNCTIONAL TRAITS GENETICS

Functional traits are those traits that increase biological and economic efficiency not by higher outputs of products, but by reduced costs of production. Functional traits have become important for efficient breeding schemes in the dairy industries, due to increased costs of production relative to milk prices and consumers demand for safe, quality food and attention to animal welfare.

Since dairy animals are bred in a wide range of local production conditions, the list of candidate functional traits may be large, including components of milk feed efficiency (body weight, feed intake and body reserves), reproduction traits (sexual precocity, out-of-season calving/lambing/kidding ability, female fertility), calf/lamb/kid meat production (suckling ability, prolificacy), milking ability (udder morphology, milking speed), resistance to disease (mastitis, scrapie, internal parasites), adaptation to local breeding conditions (fitness, wool, longevity), and others. The relationships between milk production and functional traits are often null or antagonistic, illustrating the importance of knowledge of the genetic correlations between milk production and the functional traits of interest.

Functional traits that increase efficiency not by higher output of products but by reduced costs of input, might have a greater impact on the profit of dairy farmers and should, therefore, be included in breeding programmes. Apart from economic reasons for including functional traits in the breeding programmes, there are several non-economic reasons, for example ethical and consumer concerns, which are becoming increasingly important.

The inclusion of functional traits in breeding programmes will likely have a major impact on the expected selection response of the functional traits, and will result in only small losses of the expected selection response of the production traits. Depending on the number of functional traits included in a breeding scheme, the relative importance of production versus functional traits varies from 70:30 to 30:70, sometimes even more. Relative weightings for the two groups of traits, production and functional, for the Estonian Holstein population were 79:21.

In any of breeding scenarios tested, selection response in financial terms will come largely from production traits, because genetic parameters favour fat and protein yields (high heritability, high positive genetic correlation).

Smallholders, pastoralists and their animals often live in harsh environments which may be hot and dry, hot and humid, or high in altitude and cold. Moreover, these environments can be characterized by scarce feed and water resources and high disease pressure with large seasonal and annual variation. Adaptation to these factors is largely based on genetics, but animals can "learn" to live under such stressful conditions. To match genotype with the environment, breeders can follow two alternative strategies: adapt the environment to the needs of the animals as is the case in industrial animal production systems or keep animals that are adapted to the respective environment as is the case in low input smallholder and pastoral systems. Because of this, smallholders and pastoralists need different and diverse animal genotypes, species mix and types to enable animal husbandry in their specific physical environment locations and production systems.

Milk production traits genetic determinants

The phenotypic expression of milk production traits (e.g., milk yield and composition) are controlled by genes, which may or may not be transferred to the offspring. The genetic value of a trait indicates the likelihood that the genes responsible for that trait will be transferred to any offspring. Consequently, when dairy producers are selecting animals for breeding stock, they are typically more concerned with an animal's genetic value rather than its phenotypic value of a particular trait. The difference is that while the phenotypic value refers to the presence or absence of particular traits, the genetic value indicates the potential (or probability) that this animal, if bred, will give birth to calves with certain desired traits. The challenge of the dairy breeder is, therefore, to determine which cows and bulls to breed in order to obtain progeny with high quality milk production traits, as well as any other desirable attributes.

Two main reasons for the decline in fitness traits of cows associated with increased genetic merit for milk yield are: (i) fitness traits are ignored in the construction of selection indices because they are considered to have lower heritability or are not easy to record and (ii) use of inappropriate breeding programmes while the underlying genetic process (selection and inbreeding depression) is not well understood.

However, the low heritability of some fitness traits does not imply negligible genetic variance; often heritability is low because the phenotypic variance is rather larger than the genetic variance as evidenced by as high genetic coefficient of variation for fitness traits as for some production traits.

The appropriate strategy for any breeding programme would, therefore, be to set suitable selection goals that match the production system rather than ambitious performance objectives that cannot be reached under the prevailing environment. Area-specific approach utilizing the existing resources and taking into account the prevailing constraints appears to be the only reasonable sustainable solution. Such approach would also enable in situ conservation of farm animal genetic resources, the only viable and practical conservation method in less developed countries compared to ex situ or cryopreservation approaches. This would support the importance of identifying the most adapted genotype capable of coping with the environmental challenges posed by any particular production systems.

Researchers analyzed the impact of crossbreeding zebu with temperate cattle breeds for dairy improvement in Kenya using sector- and farm-level approaches. The agricultural sector model showed that a dairy technology that involved crossbreeding and complementary improvements in nutrition and management has had a positive impact on Kenyan economy and welfare but this approach ignored important social cost components of crossbreeding. The farm-level approach, however, indicated that farm performance was little improved by replacing the indigenous zebu with exotic breeds. Conversely, this analysis indicated that a breeding programme that concentrates on improving the local zebu breeds would improve the financial performance of the farm level with important implications for the conservation of farm animal biodiversity.

Molecular genetic technologies

Molecular genetics is the study of the genetic makeup of individuals at the DNA level; it is the identification and mapping of genes and genetic polymorphisms. There are opportunities for using molecular genetics to identify genes that influence milk production traits. Armed with this information, it would be possible to select improved livestock on the basis of their genetic makeup. If applied with care, the use of molecular information in selection programmes has the potential to increase productivity, enhance environmental adaptation and maintain genetic diversity. The first task is to understand the genetic control of the trait of interest and then to identify the genes and genotypes involved.

Molecular genetic technologies have been used to identify loci or chromosomal regions that affect single-gene traits and quantitative traits. Single-gene traits include genetic defects, genetic disorders, and appearance. For the purposes of quantitative traits loci (QTL) detection and application, quantitative traits can be categorized into (a) routinely recorded traits; (b) difficult to record traits (e.g., feed intake and product quality); and (c) unrecorded traits (disease resistance). Each of these can be further subdivided into traits that are (i) recorded on both sexes; (ii) sex-limited traits; and (iii) traits that are recorded late in life. The ability to detect QTL depends on the availability of phenotypic data and decreases in the order a, b, c and within each of those in the order i, ii and iii. For related reasons, genome scans, which require more phenotypic data than candidate gene analyses, are often used to detect QTL for traits in category a, whereas candidate gene approaches are more often used to identify QTL for traits that are not routinely recorded (b and c).

The use of molecular genetic technologies potentially offer a way to select breeding animals at an early age (even embryos); to select for a wide range of traits and to enhance reliability in predicting the mature phenotype of the individual. The broad categories of existing gene technologies based options include; molecular analysis of genetic diversity, animal identification and traceability, reproductive enhancement; transgenic livestock; germ line manipulation and; marker/ gene based trait selection; animal health: diagnosis, protection and treatment; ruminant and non-ruminant nutrition and metabolism.

GENETIC MARKERS

Recent developments in molecular biology and statistics have opened the possibility of identifying and using genomic variation and major genes for the genetic improvement of livestock. Molecular techniques allow detection of the existence of variation or polymorphisms among individuals in the population for specific regions of the DNA. These polymorphisms can be used to build up genetic maps and to evaluate differences between markers in the expression of particular traits in a family that might indicate a direct effect of these differences in terms of genetic determination on the trait.

Application of molecular genetics for genetic improvement relies on the ability to genotype individuals for specific genetic loci. Genetic markers can be used to identify specific regions of chromosomes where genes affecting quantitative traits are located, i.e., QTL (Davis and DeNise, 1998). These techniques can directly confirm the potential parent-to-offspring transfer of those genes associated with a desired trait. For these purposes, three types of observable polymorphic genetic loci can be distinguished: (i) direct markers: loci that code for the functional mutation; (ii) LD markers: loci that are in population- wide linkage disequilibrium with the functional mutation; and (iii) LE markers: loci that are in population wide linkage equilibrium with the functional mutation in outbred populations; linked markers can be used within families segregating marker and QTL alleles following the establishment of the phase relationship.

The LE markers can be readily detected on a genome-wide basis by using breed crosses or analysis of large half-sib families within the breed. Such genome scans require only sparse marker maps (15 to 50 cM spacing, depending on marker informativeness and genotyping costs; to detect most QTL of moderate to large effects. The LD markers can be identified using candidate genes or fine-mapping approaches.

Direct markers (i.e., polymorphisms that code for the functional mutations) are the most difficult to detect because causality is difficult to prove and, consequently, a limited number of examples are available, except for single-gene traits. Direct markers where a linkage analysis has been performed and a zero recombination rate found between the markers and the QTL, or where sequence data have verified the exact location of the genetic change in a number of individuals.

Direct markers can be used across families after prediction of an allelic effect for a given genetic background. Both markers can be used in MAS programmes that incorporate other pedigree and phenotypic information for the genetic evaluation of animals.

Direct markers can be identified by use of candidate gene approach. Candidate gene approach proposes that a significant proportion of quantitative genetic variation of a given trait is contributed by segregation of functional alleles of one or more of the candidate genes for the trait. Candidate genes are genes that play a role in the development or physiology of a trait of economic importance.

At the DNA level, a candidate gene comprises a contiguous tract of DNA, including introns, exons, and upstream and downstream regulatory regions concerned with biosynthesis of a single protein or via alternative processing to produce related proteins. Allelic variation at a candidate gene sequence can cause a change in protein production or efficiency in a metabolic process that will influence a specific trait. The candidate gene approach can be very powerful and can detect loci even with small effect, provided that the candidate gene represents a true causative gene. However, there are often many candidate genes for the trait of interest and it may be more time-consuming to evaluate all of these than performing a genome scan. Furthermore, the candidate gene approach might fail to identify a major trait locus simply because of the gap in knowledge about a gene function.

Candidate gene tests must be interpreted with caution because spurious results can occur because of linkage disequilibrium to linked or non-linked causative genes or because the significant thresholds have not been adjusted properly when testing multiple candidate genes. Once the chromosomal location of a trait locus has been determined, this information can be applied in breeding programmes by using Marker-Assisted Selection (MAS). Candidate genes can be sequenced and analyzed in animals manifesting divergent expressions of a given trait of interest. Sequence analysis provides highest resolution of DNA variation; provides the fundamental structure of the gene systems. It is a vital tool in the analysis of gene structure and expression.

Quantitative trait loci have been detected in experimental and commercial populations of cattle, swine and sheep. In dairy cattle, linked markers have been reported for milk and component yields and cheese yield.

CLONING ADULT DAIRY ANIMALS

Cloning an animal is the production of a genetically identical individual, by transferring the nucleus of differentiated adult cells into an oocyte from which the nucleus has been removed. This is known as "nuclear transfer" and is how the Dolly sheep was produced. In the case of Dolly, mammary gland cells in culture from a 6-year old donor ewe where subjected to a reduction in the concentration of serum and, consequently, obliged to enter in a quiescent state of the cell cycle (G0). Nuclear transfers to enucleated oocytes, was followed by electrical pulses for fusion of the donor cell nucleus and oocyte membranes and to activate division. Use of cloning in animal genetic improvement for milk production may increase the rates of selection progress in certain cases, particularly in situations where artificial insemination is not possible, like in pastoral systems with ruminants. Cloning is another technique that raises concerns both from the ethical and practical point of view. In animals, besides the very low success rates, some abnormalities should suggest that more information is required on the consequences of such practices in humans but also in animals, before its routine use.

MEAT QUALITY GENE

Meat quality is a composite concept as pointed out by Cameron and therefore it is difficult to measure meat quality in a simple and unique manner. Meat quality traits are complex characteristics of considerable importance to the producers, consumers and processing industry, and the measurement of these traits usually include measurements assessing backfat, intramuscular fat, marbling, loin eye area, water-holding capacity, pH, glycolytic potential, colour, tenderness, juiciness and flavour.

Meat quality is influenced by a large number of factors including muscle characteristics (fibre size and type, fat and connective tissue), production and environmental conditions [growth rate, nutrition, age, (pre-) slaughter conditions and post-mortem ageing] and the genetics of the animal (breed, genotype). Genetic effects play a crucial role in 'designing' pig carcass composition and quality, although the heritability of quality traits is quite low. Generally, between 10% and 30% of the variation in meat quality traits and meat products (ham), such as ultimate pH, colour, water-holding capacity, drip loss, tenderness, marbling, etc. is determined by the genetic background of the animal.

The traits determining meat quality are difficult to improve by traditional selection, because the heritability is quite low and the measure for the quality traits is difficult, expensive and only possible after slaughter. Moreover, the lack of knowledge on the number of genes for the single qualitative characteristics of meat, on the quantitative effects of the single genes and on their interactions represents a limit for the complete exploitation of the opportunities of a selection plan. Molecular genetics can overcome these limits, offering new opportunities to the improvement of meat quality, as it supplies tools to analyse the quantitative genetic variability directly at DNA level with the possibility of detecting the individual genes influencing the qualitative characteristics.

Meat quality traits are controlled by an unknown number of genes mapping in quantitative trait loci (QTL) regions and some of these individual genes may have large effects on a specific trait. The main goal of genome research in farm animals in general is to map and to characterize trait loci.

A lot of work has been carried out in this field to find potential genes or chromosome regions responsible for (or associated with) meat quality and processed meat products, but to date the knowledge of genes and their interactions that are involved in meat properties are very limited. As a consequence, the understanding of meat quality on a genetic basis is scanty. At the present time, the main task of genetics is to identify factors in the molecular or biological components of meat quality that will be useful for marker-assisted selection in breeding, giving the opportunity to 'design the meat' by genetic and molecular methods.

In pigs the halothane gene (located at chromosome 6) is known to influence the stress susceptibility and the meat quality. Research is focused on chromosome 6 in pigs were genes are located that influence the androstenone production in boars. Androstenone is responsible for (an awful) boar taint in the meat of intact boars. Up to now boars are castrated to avoid this boar taint, but selecting against boar taint is a better approach for the welfare of the boars.

FERTILITY GENES

In sheep several genes are described that have an influence on the litter size. An example is that of the Booroola gene present in the Australian Merino has a marked effect: the heterozygous carrier produces one lamb more and the homozygous carrier two lambs more per litter. This allele is now also present in the Dutch Texel breed by crossbreeding merino carrier rams of the allele with Texel ewes and backcrossing the crossbreds with Texel sheep.

GENETICS OF COAT COLOUR

The genetics of coat colour

A gene called the melanocartin 1 receptor is involved in the production of red/black coat colour in cattle. The melanocartin 1 receptor controls the levels of an enzyme called tyrosinase in skin cells. High levels of tyrosinase in the skin cells cause a dark colour (brown or black) while low levels of tyrosinase result in a light coat colour (red or yellow).

The two main alleles (or alternative forms) for the melanocartin 1 receptor gene are Black (ED) or, Red (e), while another allele, Wild Type (E+) is also present in a very small percentage of animals, including Angus cattle.

Each animal inherits two alleles for coat colour, one from each parent, with the Black allele being dominant over both the Red and Wild Type alleles. An animal can consequently be phenotypically, or visually Black but still carry one copy of either the Red or Wild Type allele, which can then be inherited and expressed by progeny. The Wild Type allele (E+) is considered to be neutral and can produce either a red or black coat colour depending on its interaction with other genes. The Red allele (e) is recessive and an animal must carry two copies of the Red allele to have red coat colour.

Breeding for coat colour – the theory

Because animals inherit two alleles for the base coat colour, it is possible that their phenotype, or visual appearance, does not reflect their underlying genotype. For example a phenotypically black animal may be either "homozygous" Black, meaning they have two copies of the Black allele (ie. ED ED), or "heterozygous" Black, meaning they have one copy of the Black allele and one copy of either the red or wild type allele (i.e. ED e or ED E+).

Consider the four mating combinations shown in Fig. 5 where only phenotypically black sires are used in a breeding program.

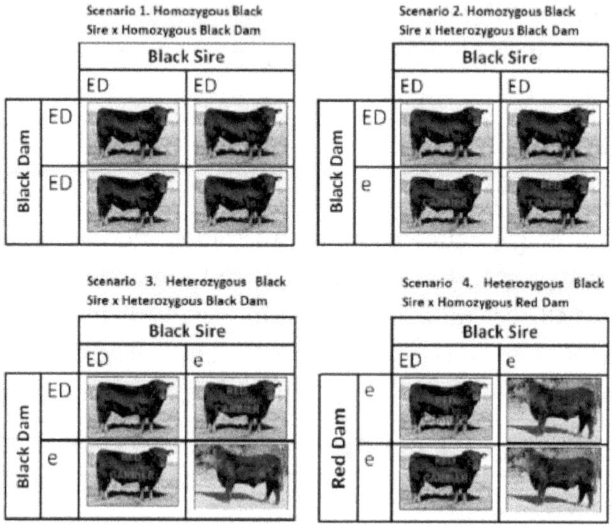

Fig. 5. Four mating combinations where phenotypically black sires are used in a breeding program.

In the first scenario, homozygous black dams (ED ED) are joined to a homozygous black sire (ED ED) with 100pc of the resulting offspring being homozygous black (ED ED).

In the second scenario, heterozygous black dams carrying the Red allele (ED e), are joined to a homozygous black sire (ED ED). The resulting offspring will all be phenotypically black, but 50pc will be heterozygous (ED e) and will carry one copy of the Red allele.

In the third scenario, heterozygous dams (ED e) are joined to a heterozygous sire (ED e), with 25% of the resulting offspring being homozygous black (ED ED), 50pc being heterozygous black (ED e) and 25pc being homozygous red (e e).

In the final scenario, homozygous red dams are joined to a heterozygous black sire. The resulting offspring will be 50pc heterozygous black carriers and carrying one copy of the Red allele, while the remaining 50% would be homozygous red.

The above scenarios not only apply to straight-bred Angus breeding programs, but also to crossbreeding programs where Angus animals may be joined to animals from another breed. For example, if a heterozygous Black Angus sire is joined to Hereford cows, who are homozygous red, 50pc of progeny would be black Baldies, while 50pc would be red Baldies, as per the final scenario.

DNA tests for coat colour

A number of DNA tests are available that enable breeders to determine whether a phenotypically black animal is carrying one copy of the Red allele, and therefore has the potential to produce a proportion of phenotypically red offspring if joined to other animals who also possess a Red allele.

DNA testing can be carried out as part of Angus Australia's DNA services as either a stand-alone test, as an individual add on to the HD50K for Angus or Angus GS genomic products, or as part of the full genetic test add-on panel to the HD50K for Angus or Angus GS genomic products.

Testing as a stand-alone test is available for $25.85 via both Zoetis and Neogen, whereas the cost if conducted as an individual add-on to HD50K for Angus or Angus GS is $8.25 or $11.00 respectively. The full genetic test add-on panel to both HD50K for Angus GS is available for $41.25 and includes all 8 genetic conditions recognised by Angus Australia, plus coat colour, myostatin and homozygous poll.

DNA test results for animals which have been tested for the Red allele are displayed on the "Genetic Tests" tab within the Angus Database Search and Angus SELECT facilities on the Angus Australia website.

In addition, a suffix of (RED) is displayed at the end of the name for any animals recorded with Angus Australia that are red in colour.

BREEDING FOR COAT COLOUR – THE PRACTICAL

While the majority of Black Angus animals are homozygous black, a proportion are heterozygous black, and if joined to other heterozygous black or homozygous red animals, can produce a proportion of calves that are red in colour.

Breeders wishing to minimise the incidence of calves that are red in colour should carefully consider and develop a management strategy that is suitable for their breeding program. This is particularly important in herds where there is a higher likelihood of breeding females carrying the Red allele, such as in straight-bred Angus herds that have a history of producing the occasional red animal, or commercial herds that have other breed content in their background, such as Hereford or Shorthorn.

In simple terms, animals that are red in colour can be prevented by avoiding mating a Red allele carrier sire to a Red allele carrier dam.

Only using sires that have been found not to be carrying the Red allele via DNA testing, or sires who are not expected to be carrying the Red allele from analysis of their pedigree, is sufficient in most circumstances.

Breeding for coat colour should always be balanced with selection for other traits of economic and functional importance within the breeding objective. Simply selecting for coat colour without consideration for other economically important traits may potentially compromise the genetics of animals for these other traits.

Colour genes in pigs

In pigs also the extension, agouti, roan and dilution gene determine the base colour. In addition a lot of genes are known, as in ruminants, that give cause to different colour patterns. A dominant allele at the roan locus is responsible for the complete white pigs we have at the moment in many commercial pig breeding programs.

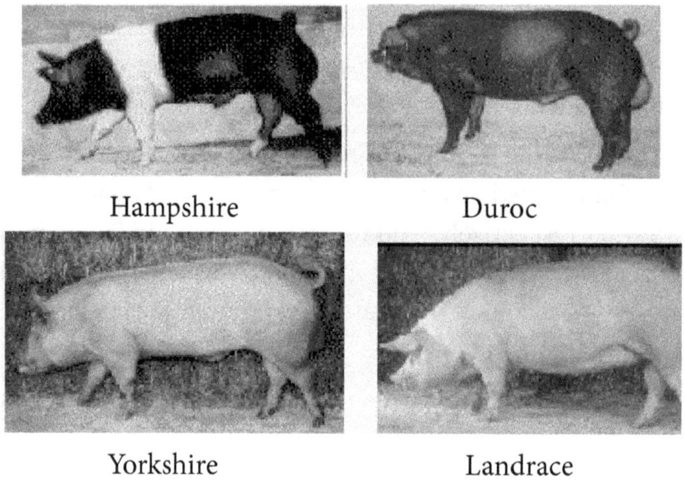

Fig. 6. The Landrace and Yorkshire are homozygote for dominant white, the Duroc is red and the Hampshire is black with a white belt

Colour genes in horses

The basic coat colors of horses include chestnut, bay, and black. These are controlled by the interaction between two genes: Melanocortin 1 Receptor (MC1R) and Agouti Signaling Protein (ASIP). MC1R, which has also been referred to as the extension or red factor locus, controls the production of red and black pigment. To date, there are three versions (alleles) of this gene that have been identified at the molecular level: E, e, and e^a. The e and e^aalleles are recessive to E and are considered to be loss of function mutations in MC1R. In homozygous individuals (e/e or e^a/e^a) only red pigment is produced, hence the name red factor. ASIP, also known as Agouti, controls the distribution of black pigment. The dominant allele (A) restricts black pigment to the points of the horse (mane, tail, lower legs, ear rims), while the recessive form (a) distributes black pigment uniformly over the body.

Currently, genetic tests for the three basic coat colors include: Agouti and Red Factor

Variability exists among the three basic coat colors. This variability has been described as shade. For example, some horses are a very dark chestnut known as liver chestnut while others are a much lighter yellow shade. While, over 300 different genes have been identified that contribute to mammalian pigmentation, for many of these their contribution to equine pigmentation variation remains unknown. The genetics behind the variability in shade in horses is something we still have a lot to learn about.

Dilution Genes

There are several genes that that have been shown to reduce the amount of pigment produced and/or reduce the amount transferred from the pigment cell to the hair follicular cells, and these are know as dilution genes. Some of these dilution genes affect only one type of pigment (red or black) while others affect both (red and black). Some dilute both the coat and the points (mane, tail, lower legs, ear rims), while others primarily dilute the points, and still others leave the points unaffected and only dilute the coat. Molecular characterization of six different dilution phenotypes in horses include Cream, Champagne, Dun, Pearl, Silver, and Mushroom. Cream is dominant and has a dosage effect in that a single copy of the cream allele (N/Cr) produces palominos on a chestnut background and buckskin on a bay background.

Two doses of the Cream allele (Cr/Cr) produce cremellos on a chestnut background, perlinos on a bay background, and smoky creams on a black background. Pearl is an allele at the same locus at Cream (SLC45a2) but is recessive; two copies of the Pearl allele (Prl/Prl) or one copy of Pearl and one of Cream (Prl/Cr, this is known as a compound heterozygote) are needed to see the dilution effect on the coat.

Champagne, Dun, and Silver are all dominant traits, and therefore only one copy of dilution causing allele is needed to produce the respective phenotypes. Silver is interesting because it primarily affects black pigment of the points (black and bay horses). Chestnut horses with the sliver mutation do not show a different coat color phenotype than those chestnut horses without the silver mutation, as silver does not dilute red pigment. Horses with the silver mutation, regardless of base coat color, have an ocular condition known as multiple congenital ocular anomaly or MCOA for short. Horses with two copies of silver (Z/Z) have a more severe phenotype than those with one (N/Z).

The mushroom allele (Mu) is recessive and dilutes red pigment. Chestnut horses who are homozygous for Mu will have a dilute sepia coat phenotype. Bay horses homozygous for the mushroom phenotype have a lighter shade of red body with black counter shading, suggesting that Mu increases black pigment production having the opposite effect on black pigment as it does on red.

White Spotting Pattern Genes

There are several genes responsible for white coat patterns in horses. These can occur on any base color and in combination with any dilution mutation. White spotting patterns can be divided into distributed white or patch white patterning. Distributed white patterns, in which white hairs are intermixed with colors hairs, include classic Roan and Gray. Both classic Roan and Gray are caused by dominant mutations. Classic Roan horses have fully or nearly fully pigmented faces but white hairs are distributed throughout the coat.

Grey horses will progressively loose pigment distributed in the coat as they age. Gray horses are at risk for melanoma. Patch white spotting patterns include Appaloosa, Dominant White, Sabino 1, Splashed White, Tobiano, and Overo. These all vary in the location of the white pattern. For example, Appaloosa white patterning tends to be symmetrical and centered over the hips, but the amount of white can vary from just a few white flecks on the rump to a horse that is almost completely white. Patch white patterns identified to date have all been caused by dominant mutations.

Some of these, like gray and silver described above, have pleiotropic effects; that is, a mutation in one gene can affect more than one body system. Homozygosity for the frame-overo allele (O/O) is lethal (Lethal White Overo syndrome). Horses with two copies of the Appaloosa mutation (LP/LP), also known as leopard complex, have an ocular condition known as congenital stationary night blindness, which means they are unable to see in low light conditions.

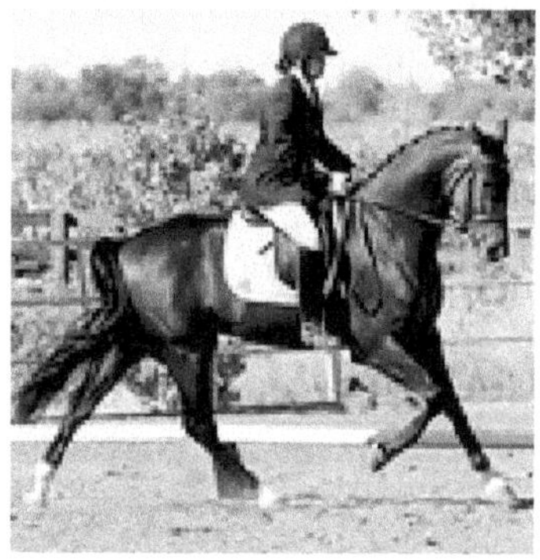

Agouti
A/A=Homozygous Bay
A/a=Heterozygous Bay
a/a=Black

Below you will find very simple images that represent the basic colors, patterns and modifiers of various horses. Should you like more detailed information, you'll find many links within the descriptors leading you to expanded and detailed information including scientific publications and images.

The ASIP gene, also known as agouti, controls the regional distribution of black pigment. Dominant agouti ("A") pushes the black base color ("E") to the edges (points) of the horse, resulting in black legs, mane, tail, and ear tips with a reddish body (the bay coat color). A horse needs two recessive "a" alleles to show black throughout the coat. Agouti only affects black pigment, and thus is not visible on a red (chestnut/sorrel) base.

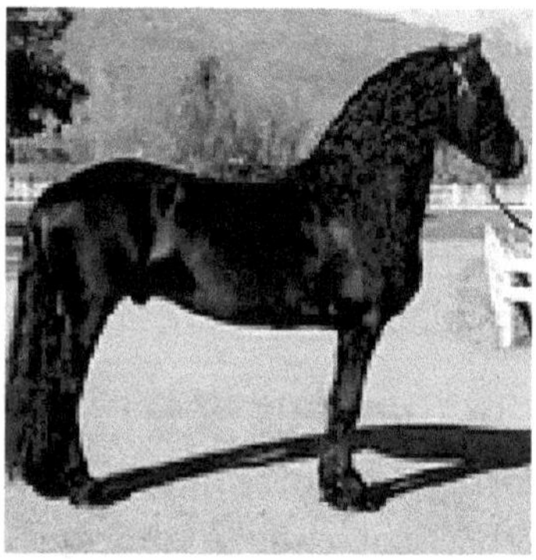

Red/Black Factor
E/E=Homozygous Black
E/e=Heterozygous Black
e/e=Red

The MC1R gene, also known as extension, determines whether a horse can produce black pigment. Black ("E") is dominant to red ("e"). Therefore, a horse with the genotype "E/e" (one black and one red allele) has a black base color, but can produce either black or red base offspring. Homozygous black (E/E) horses will always produce black based offspring.

Dominant white ("W") refers to a class of white spotting patterns in which a horse with one copy generally displays markings on 50-100% of the body. Unlike other extreme white patterns, this trait generally leaves the eyes dark.

A mutation in the MITF gene, the macchiato coat color was documented in a single Franches-Montagnes stallion. He displayed a dilute coat color, blue eyes, extended face and leg markings, and white on the body. He was also noted as being completely deaf and had low progressive sperm motility.

Frame overo (lethal white overo) is a white spotting pattern characterized by patches of white bordered or "framed" by normal pigmentation. It is usually accompanied by blue eyes, and generally white patterning does not cross the topline. While heterozygous horses (LWO/N) only have this white spotting pattern, homozygous foals (LWO/LWO) are born completely white and with megacolon, an abnormal dilation of colon which necessitates immediate euthanasia.

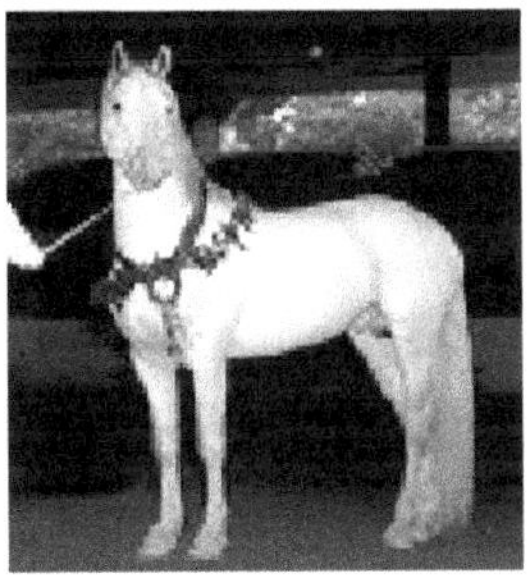	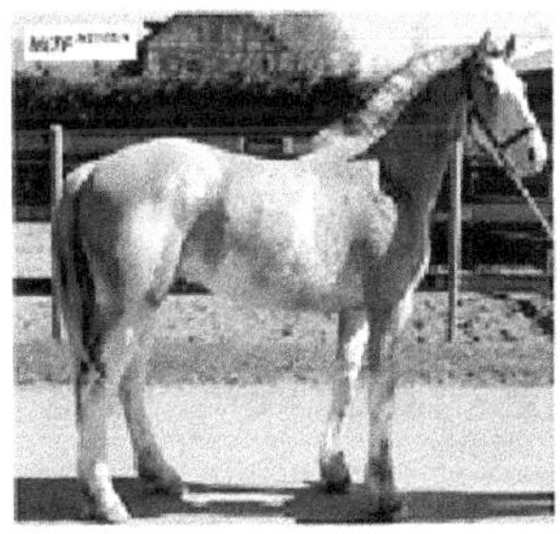
Dominant White W/W=Homozygous W W/N=Heterozygous W N/N=Non-W	Macchiato (fun fact!) M/M=Not observed M/N=Macchiato N/N=Non-Macchiato

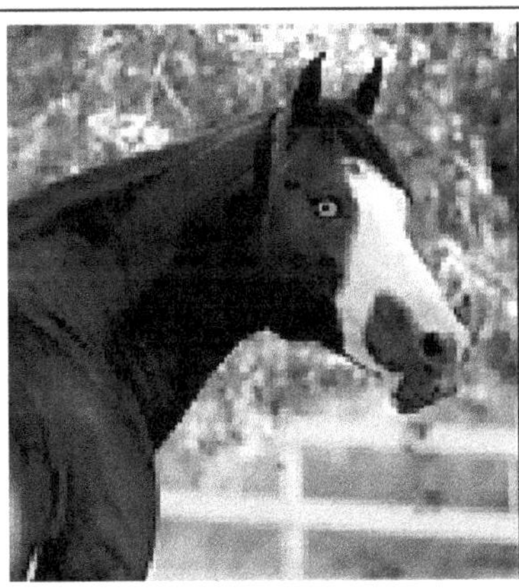	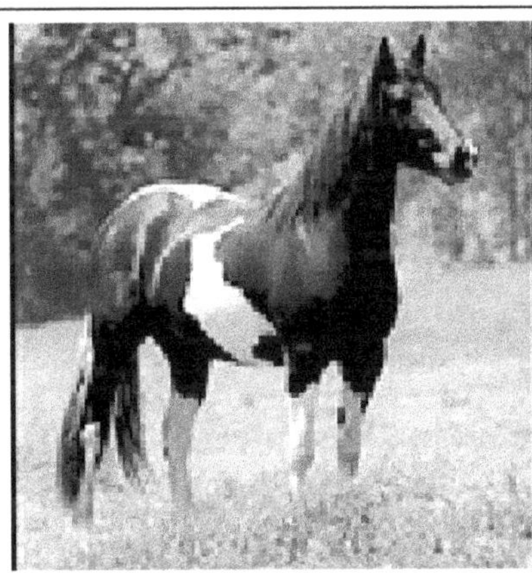
Frame Overo (Lethal White Overo) LWO/LWO=Lethal White LWO/N=Frame Overo N/N=Non-Frame Overo	Tobiano TO/TO=Homozygous Tobiano TO/N=Heterozygous Tobiano N/N=Non-Tobiano

Tobiano spotting is characterized by large white patches on the limbs and body. Often times, these patches have smooth edges, cross over the topline, and are accompanied by dark eyes. Expression can range from white present only on the legs, to horses nearly completely white. As this trait is dominant, horses with either one (TO/N) or two (TO/TO) copies will have a similar appearance.

It will be obvious that if two homozygous parents that have the same color, are mated, their off spring has the same color.

Some examples are:

Bay (AAEE) x black (aaEE) ® bay foal (AaEE)

Bay (AAEE) x chestnut (aaee) ® bay foal (AeEe)

black (aaEE) x chestnut (aaee) ® black foal (aaEe)

On top of the basic colors (B, A and E) some other genes can determine the color of a horse. One of these genes is the g gene. The letter G stands for gray. The GG or Gg genotypes overrule all other colors and cause the horse to become grey at later age. These horses are therefore not born as greys. There is a group of genes that dilute the basic colors. The C and C cr are examples of such dilution genes. They are responsible for coat colors like Isabel and cremello. Another group of genes causes the colors to not be equally distributed; patches of different colors or white spots can be the result. Overo and Tobiano genes are examples of this group.

Coat colours in dogs

Dogs have been selected to have more variation in size and body type than most species of domestic animals. Is it any wonder they also vary so much in coat colour (Fig. 7, p 235)? The genetics of coat colour in dogs, as well as other mammals, has been studied for many years.

Researchers both wrote books postulating a number of genes that could explain the inheritance of coat colour and pattern in dogs. Each based their hypotheses on breeding data. Both authors used letters to indicate various loci, some with only two alleles, some with more. Although they did not use the same letters, in general their hypotheses regarding the number of genes with various effects were very similar.

The melanocortin 1 receptor gene

Melanocortin 1 receptor (MC1R) was the first gene studied using molecular approaches in dogs. MC1R cM from was mapped to CFA5, 6 ZuBeCa6 (Schmutz *et al.* 2001a). Researchers published a loss-of-function mutation, 914C>T, which causes clear red coat colour in dogs (Fig. 7e,h,l). This mutation, which causes an arginine to be replaced by a premature stop codon (R306ter), is present in a wide range of dog breeds. Researchers called this the E or extension locus and therefore this allele was termed e and the wild type allele E (Table 1, pp236-237).

The agouti signal peptide gene

Agouti signal peptide (ASIP) has several alleles that are involved in coat colour in dogs. ASIP has been mapped to CFA24 between AHT 118 and AHT 125.

Photographs and selected genotypes of various dogs illustrating the variety of coat colours and gene interactions. (a) Brown-and-tan French Brittany ky/ky, E/E, b/b, at/at; (b) (left) brown German Shorthaired Pointer KB/KB, E/E, b/b and (right) black Large Munsterlander KB/KB, E/E, B/b; (c) Landseer Newfoundland KB/KB, E/E, B/B, s/s; (d) fawn masked Chinese Shar-Pei ky/ky, EM/E, B/B, ay/ay; (e) fawn French Bulldog kbr/ky, e/e, B/B, ay/ay; (f) brindle Staffordshire Bull Terrier kbr/ky, E/E, B/B, ay/at; (g) merle Australian Shepherd ky/ky, E/E, B/B, at/at, M/m; (h) (left) clear red Miniature Dachshund ky/ky, e/e, B/B and (right) black-and-tan Miniature Dachshund ky/ky, E/”, B/B, at/at; (i) blue Great Dane KB/”, E/E, B/B, ay/ay, d/d; (j) dilute fawn Italian Greyhound ky/ky, EM/E, B/B, ay/ay, d/d; (k) young Kerry Blue Terrier KB/KB, EM/E, B/B, D/D, G/G; (l) gold Viszla KB/KB, e/e, b/b.

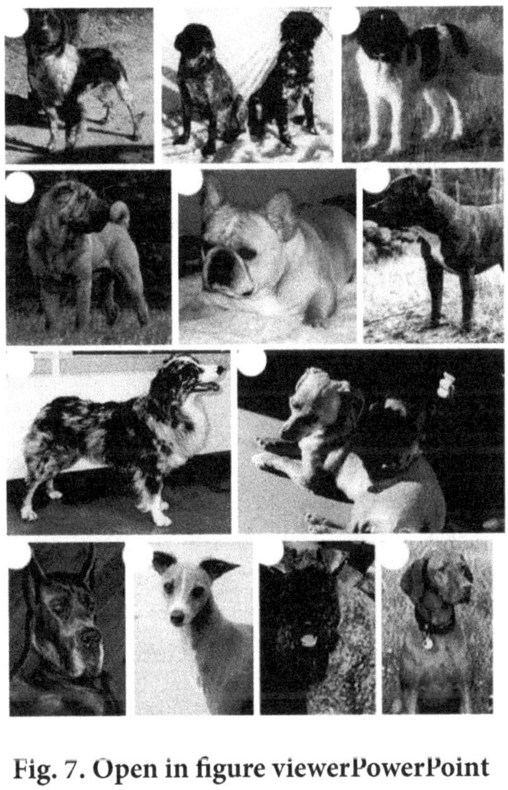

Fig. 7. Open in figure viewerPowerPoint

There are four alleles present in dogs in the dominance hierarchy $a^y > a^w > a^t > a$. The wild type allele (a^w) causes some hairs to have a band of eumelanin, phaeomelanin, eumelanin pigment from base to tip.

These banded hairs are typically along the dorsal region of the torso. The ASIP sequence of this allele has complete homology to the wolf sequence and the amino acid sequence of the coyote is also the same.

Table 1. Genes and loci discovered and predicted to be involved in dog pigmentation.

a	Recessive black
B	= (brown)tyrosinase related protein 1 (TYRP1) CFA11
B	Black eumelanin
b (b s, b d, bc)	Brown eumelanin
E M	Melanistic mask
E	Eumelanin (black, brown, blue) can be produced
e	Only phaeomelanin (red, yellow, cream) produced
K	(= (from 'dominant blacK')CBD103) CFA16
KB	Black, brown or blue (eumelanin pigmentation only)
kbr	Brindle (on body region that would be phaeomelanin pigmented otherwise)
DILUTED COLOURS	
D	= (dilutes eumelanin)melanophilin (MLPH) CFA25
D	Not diluted
d	Diluted pigmentation
d2?	Diluted pigmentation with skin problems
C ? gene	= (coloured)
C	Full pigmentation
c^{ch}	'Chinchilla' which causes paler eumelanin and phaeomelanin
c^{a}	Complete albinism
P	= (dilutes both melanins)P gene? (dominant/recessive)
P	Not diluted
p	Diluted but not to completely white
/?	gene (co-dominant) = (dilutes only phaeomelanin)
/	Intense, not diluted
/	Co-dominant decrease in intensity
G?	gene (dominant/recessive) = (progressive grey)
G	Greying at early age, progressive greying
g	Not greying
WHITE MARKINGS	
M	(= (merle)SILV) (M/m is the merle genotype) (co-dominant) CFA10
M	Not coloured
m	Coloured
S	(= (spotting)MITF) CFA20
S	Solid coloured
s^{i}	Irish spotting
s^{P}	Piebald

s^w	Extreme white
T ?	gene (dominant/recessive) = (ticking)
T	Ticked
t	Not ticked
R ?	gene = (roan)
R	White in homozygote
r	Coloured in homozygote
H ?	gene (dominant/recessive if = (Harlequin) M allele causing merle is present)
H	Harlequin if also M/m or M/M
h	Not Harlequin

The alleles are listed in their 'predicted' dominance hierarchy. Those in bold have been confirmed at the DNA level.

As in horses, there is a recessive allele which causes dogs to have a black coat. This R96C allele (a) (c.288C>T) occurs primarily, but not solely, in herding breeds.

It is the only cause of black in the German Shepherd Dog and Shetland Sheepdog but it occurs in some black Schipperke, Groenendael and Puli. This allele has also been identified in Samoyeds and American Eskimo Dogs, both of which are white. The occurrence of this allele in Samoyeds was perplexing but a review of the history of this breed suggests they were originally used to herd reindeer and then later used additionally as sled dogs. The American Eskimo Dog may include Samoyed ancestors based on this finding, but not all breed clubs suggest this is the history of this breed's development.

One of the most common alleles in domestic dogs is known as the a^y allele, inherited as the dominant allele in this series. The allele has two amino acid changes in comparison to the wild type, A82S and R83H (c.246G>T and c.250G>A). The coat colour is called fawn in most breeds (Fig. 7d,e,j), but sable in a few. This allele has been identified in over 22 breeds. In all 45 dogs of this phenotype for which complete exon 4 sequence was obtained, both mutations were present. Neither mutation was found in the wolf or seven coyotes for which sequence was obtained.

As residue 82 was conserved in more species than residue 83, the PCR-RFLP test to detect this allele was designed for this mutation. There is considerable variation in the number of black hairs intermingled in dogs with this a^y allele. Although it has been postulated that this variation may be due to the Mahogunin gene, this has not been proven.

A fourth allele, known as a^t, is believed to exist in dogs that are black-and-tan (Fig. 7a,h right). No differences have been observed in the coding sequence (exon 2–4) of dogs of this phenotype and dogs with the banded-hair wild-type phenotype. This putative allele must likely differ in one of the promoter regions. In other mammals such as mice, there are alternate dorsal and ventral promoters, but the ASIP promoters have not yet been identified in dogs. In many dog breeds, the extent of the ventral phaeomelanin varies amongst individuals, and also among breeds. Researchers were able to find an association with TBX15 mutations and variation in the relative proportion of black vs. tan in mice. Although some breeders have postulated a fifth allele, a^s for saddle tan, there is no evidence of such an allele at this time.

The beta-defensin 103 gene

The symbol K was chosen to denote the locus causing black coat colour which is inherited as a dominant because some dog breeders had adopted this, choosing the K from the last letter of black.

Researchers had postulated there was an allele 'A', for solid colour, at the agouti locus, but as discussed above, this allele does not seem to exist in dogs. A few breeds do have a loss-of-function mutation in agouti that causes black to be inherited as a recessive trait, as discussed above.

In the vast majority of dog breeds, in order for solid eumelanin coat colour (black, brown and grey) (Fig. 7a–c,i,k) to occur the dog must have at least one E or E^M allele at MC1R and at least one dominant allele at the K locus. Research on this locus has been led by Greg Barsh in collaboration with others.

The gene is beta-defensin 103 on CFA16. The gene at the K locus has not previously been described as having a function in the pigmentation pathway and therefore the mechanism by which it functions is of considerable interest.

There are also two other alleles at this locus. A single copy of the k^{br} allele in the presence of a k^y allele is sufficient to cause the dog to express the phenotype known as brindle. Brindle in dogs consists of alternate stripes of phaeomelanin and eumelanin of various shades (Fig. 7f).

In some dogs, there is such a preponderance of eumelanin that the dog appears virtually black whereas in other individuals the eumelanin stripes are very thin. Brindle occurs over the entire body in dogs with an a^y allele (Fig. 7f) but only on the ventral surfaces in dogs with an a^t/a^t genotype. Dogs with a k^y/k^y genotype at this locus could be fawn (Fig. 7d,j), wolf sable or eumelanin-and-tan (right Fig. 7a,h) depending on their genotype at ASIP.

DNA testing has successfully predicted eumelanin vs. phaeomelanin pigmentation in some breeds, such as Labrador Retrievers, using only MC1R genotyping. The reason is likely that this breed is virtually fixed with a K^B/K^B genotype and e/e is epistatic to both K^B and k^{br} (Fig. 7e).

However in other breeds, such as Great Danes (Fig. 7i), eumelanin vs. phaeomelanin pigmentation is controlled by K^B/" vs. k^y/k^y, as this breed appears to be fixed for the a^y/a^y gentoype in the presence of E or E^M.

Shades of the basic coat colours

The melanophilin gene

Many dog breeds have individuals that are grey or dilute in coat colour (Fig. 7i,j). However, blue is used to denote other phenotypes in various breeds. In some breeds, these blue individuals are born grey, whereas in other breeds individuals take several months to turn from black to grey. The latter characteristic was referred to as 'progressive greying' and attributed to the G locus. In some dog breeds this is called 'silver'. A few dog breeds have both types of grey occurring. Some Great Danes and all Weimaraners are born blue or dilute whereas Kerry Blue Terriers (Fig. 7k) and Old English Sheepdogs are born black and lighten as they grow into adulthood.

Both of these inherited traits cause modification of both eumelanin and phaeomelanin pigmented areas to a paler shade, although the phaeomelanin change is not as dramatic as the eumelanin dilution. Fawn dogs with a melanistic mask (Schmutz et al. 2003a) are easier to observe because their mask is grey instead of black. Dilute fawn dogs have charcoal instead of black nose leather and pads (Fig. 7j).

Dogs with an e/e genotype at MC1R or clear red phenotype, such as the two Beagles in our previous study were very difficult to detect as dilute. Dogs that are brindle and dilute, such as some Whippets and Greyhounds, have grey stripes on a pale fawn background.

Dogs, such as Weimaraners, that have two copies of the mutations in TYRP1 causing brown and two dilute alleles are a pale brown. The nose leather and pads of such dogs are a similar pale brown. In some breeds such as Chinese Shar-Pei, the dogs are called lilac and in Doberman Pinschers, they are called Isabella.

Recently, we reported that Doberman Pinschers, German Pinschers, Large Munsterlanders, and Beagles with a dilute phenotype, co-segregated with specific haplotypes of melanophilin (MLPH). A mutation in exon 2 of MLPH causes a splice junction problem in homozygous mice of the leaden phenotype.

The last seven amino acids of exon 2 are spliced out in leaden mice because a C-to-T transition introduces a premature stop codon. A human infant was reported to have Griscelli Syndrome Type III due to a R35W mutation near the end of exon 2. The hair colour of this child was not reported but this syndrome is considered a form of albinism.

We have now extended our study of MLPH to include approximately 20 dog breeds. Although a mutation that co-segregates with blue in some breeds has been found, no single mutation has been found that explains the blue in all these breeds. A couple of common mutations occur only in blue dogs. Our study to identify all the alleles causing blue is ongoing.

Progressive greying

We support the hypothesis that dogs with a progressive grey phenotype have a mutation distinct from the allele he refers to a 'd' at the D or dilute locus. The greying begins on different parts of the body and at different ages in the breeds that show progressive greying. Some such dogs had a localized reaction to vaccination or skin injury that caused hair in the affected area to revert to its dark juvenile pigment. Over the course of several months, this darker hair would typically lighten again. This would fit suggestion that the progressive greying trait is controlled by a separate locus he designated as the G locus.

A progressive greying phenotype also occurs in horses. This trait has been mapped to a region of ECA25q which corresponds to HSA9q. Based on reciprocal chromosome paints, the relevant section of HSA9, corresponds to canine chromosome 11. A search for the G locus in dogs, thought to be associated with progressive greying might be directed to this chromosome. Horses with the progressive greying phenotype show a propensity to develop skin tumours. This pleiotropic effect was not reported in any of the dogs in our study with a progressive greying phenotype.

Cream and/or white

There are several breeds of dogs that are born white or cream with pigmented nose leather and pads. This is another example demonstrating that pigment migration into hairs and keratinized skin is not entirely controlled by the same genes. One example of a breed fixed for white is the Samoyed. A limited number of Samoyeds were genotyped and all were e/e at MC1R and also a/a at ASIP. We have also genotyped white individuals in several other breeds and found that all were e/e at MC1R.

These included the Akita, Shar-Pei, Poodle, Puli, German Shepherd Dog, Caucasian Mountain Dog and the Miniature Schnauzer. Some individuals might more appropriately be called cream as a hint of phaeomelanin pigmentation existed, often on the ears. In the Akita, no littermates that had an E or E^M allele were ever cream, although some appeared fawn red because of an a^y/" genotype. This suggests that there is a gene that only pales individuals with an e/e genotype. In the Akita, Caucasian Mountain Dog, German Shepherd Dog, Miniature Schnauzer and Puli breeds, there are no individuals that are red, in turn, suggesting that these breeds are fixed for this allele that pales only and all individuals with an e/e genotype.

In some breeds, such as the Labrador Retriever and Golden Retriever, all dogs that are pigmented with phaeomelanin have an e/e genotype at MC1R. These dogs vary in shade from a golden yellow to a cream colour, but are not white. In a study of families which segregated for these shades, it would appear that the cream shade is inherited as an autosomal recessive. Cream did not co-segregate with polymorphisms in tyrosinase (TYR) nor with SLC45A2, formerly called MATP (unpubl. data). The first gene that is reported to dilute only phaeomelanin is SLC7A11 (Chintala et al. 2005). Although researchers found abbreviated mRNA products in mice with dilute phaeomelanin pigmentation, we obtained mRNA sequence from pale yellow dogs that appeared to be full length (GenBank EF143580).

However, in some breeds such as Afghans and Poodles, there are also individuals that are cream/white that have an E or E^M allele at MC1R. The genetic mechanism underlying this form of white is unknown at this time.

Spotting patterns and white markings

There are many types of white markings in dogs. Until 2006, none of the genes causing these patterns had been elucidated in dogs.

Spotting

Researchers were among the first to try to find a gene associated with spotting. They used a family of dogs from a study designed to map behaviour traits. They excluded both EDNRB and KIT as the gene causing the white underside markings seen in most Border Collies which segregated as an autosomal recessive trait in Newfoundland–Border Collie backcross families. Similarly, these genes were excluded for the white markings seen in Boxers.

The microphthalmia-associated transcription factor gene

Researchers at Iowa State University completed a candidate gene study of spotting in dogs and identified MITF as the candidate gene for random spotting, while excluding six other genes. Their study focused on beagle crossbreds and Newfoundlands (Fig. 7c). They found complete co-segregation with a SNP in intron 3 and recessively inherited, random or piebald spotting in these dogs.

In a simultaneous collaborative study between researchers at the Broad Institute and Swedish Agricultural University, one major gene involved in white markings has been identified. A genome scan identified CFA20 as harbouring the gene for white markings in Boxers. The candidate gene in this region was MITF. Their study focused on Boxers but also included Bull Terriers, Dalmatians and Cavalier King Charles Spaniels. Researchers had predicted that Dalmatians would have the same allele for white markings as Boxers as they were born white and the small black spots developed at a few weeks of age, under the influence of another gene.

Mutations in MITF apparently can affect melanoblast survival in the lineage derived from neural crest cells that ultimately cause coat pigmentation. Therefore, a lack of pigmentation or white markings could be anticipated. Several isoforms of MITF have been described in species such as mouse and human. MITF-M has been considered the major isoform expressed in melanocytes in most species. We had obtained MITF-M mRNA sequence, with and without the 18-bp exon 6A, from dog skin (GenBank AY240952).

The MITF protein is encoded by exons 5–9 and it is believed that the presence and absence of exon 6A in the product is related to different regulatory elements. Although some polymorphisms were detected in the coding region (GenBank DQ923322) and adjacent 32 -UTR sequence of exon 9, none of these occurred consistently in dogs with any particular form of white markings. However several mutations in MITF in mice cause spotting (reviewed by Goding 2000) and involve mutations outside the coding exons.

The markings in Boxers are often considered to fit a co-dominant inheritance pattern: no white (S/S), white undersides and facial blaze in the 'flashy' Boxers (S/s), predominantly white (s/s) and this was supported by the MITF data.

Although the white markings of a flashy Boxer and a typical Border Collie are phenotypically very similar, Border Collies are rarely predominantly white and only occasionally have no white. Although researchers postulated that there were four alleles at the locus for spotting (S, s^p, s^i, s^w), he also suggested that plus and minus modifiers caused a gradation of phenotypes such that distinct phenotypes of these alleles were not clear. Researchers also suggested modifiers but implied these would be at separate genes.

It is likely further research from Broad/Swedish collaborative group and the Iowa group, as well as others, will help determine how many alleles occur in MITF and which spotting patterns they explain, or if variability in spotting is affected by other genes.

Merle

Researchers have demonstrated that a SINE element and a run of thymidine nucleotides in intron 10 of the 11 exon SILV causes the merle pattern (Fig. 7g). This allele is typically known as the M allele. Researchers had postulated that merle would be caused by a transposable element because he had collected reports from breeders that some merle offspring were born to parents, neither of which were merle. He postulated that this was due to germinal reversion. Researchers had also mapped the merle trait to CFA10 in the region where SILV is located.

We have obtained normal mRNA product from Australian Shepherds heterozygous for this SINE insertion with the accompanying run of thymidines (GenBank EF090519) for part of exons 9, 10 and 11 through the stop codon, with no evidence of a mixed product. This suggests any improperly spliced product degrades quickly. It also illustrates how easy it would have been to miss this mutation if one studied only the coding sequence of dogs with the merle phenotype.

Several dog breeders consider they have a dog that produces merle pups, even though it is not merle and refer to such dogs as cryptic merles or phantom merles. Researchers litters but no pups that were merle. suggest that the SINE element alone, with no accompanying string of thymidines is the explanation for these cryptic merles. We have observed this SINE element alone in several dogs that do not exhibit a merle phenotype. One such tricoloured Shetland Sheepdog has sired 7

Since the mutation was discovered, we have been able to test dogs for the merle mutation of various coat colour genotypes at other loci. Dogs that are fawn show minimal merle markings. This can occur in fawn Dachshunds where the trait is called dapple, as well as in fawn Great Danes. As merle is the presence of dark eumelanin areas swirled amongst a paler colour, and dogs with an e/e genoytpe at MC1R do not produce any eumelanin pigment in their hair, such a dog would not exhibit a merle phenotype even though it carried the merle mutation (unpubl. data).

We had excluded KITLG as the gene causing merle during a study of this phenotype in Australian Shepherds. Recently, we genotyped these dogs for the SILV mutations and 27 dogs were found to be homozygous for the merle mutation of the SINE and run of thymidines. All were deaf by breeder observation and/or BAER testing. Only five reported serious eye anomalies such as microphthalmia, although several dogs had blue or hetero-chromatic iris colour.

Researchers reported that deafness did not occur in all Catahoula Leopard dogs that were homozygous for the merle mutation, however. Perhaps researchers hypothesis that merle would have more effects in dogs that also carry white spotting is the explanation for this difference between breeds, as all the Australian Shepherds we studied had white markings. Researchers demonstrated that mice with mutated MITF that lead to absence of melanoblasts, did not express SILV in their retinal pigmented epithelium either. This demonstrates that MITF and SILV interact.

Harlequin

Harlequin is the pattern that occurs in Great Danes that consists of ragged black patches on a white background. Authors such as researchers have postulated that this pattern requires one copy of the merle mutation and one copy of a second mutation, designated H, at another locus. Researchers confirmed that the Harlequin Great Danes they tested all had at least one copy of the merle mutation. We have studied a few candidate genes in segregating litters and have excluded MITF and EDNRB but PAX3 co-segregated with Harlequin in one small pedigree.

Ticking

Researchers described another type of spotting that consists of very small spots on a white background (Fig. 7a,b right). These are not present at birth but begin to appear within a few weeks. At the present time, no study of the gene causing ticking is available.

The type of spotting seen in Dalmatians is considered to be unique to this breed by some, although researchers provided some breeding data from a small number of litters which led him to conclude this was ticking. Researchers presented data to suggest that the gene associated with the atypical production of urea instead of allantoin by Dalmatians was in LD with the gene causing this pattern. It is possible that this gene is either closely linked to Dalmatian spotting, or even that this is the gene involved in this trait.

Roan

Roan is a pattern consisting of intermingled pigmented and unpigmented hairs (Fig. 7b left). Roan often occurs in dogs that also have ticking. Researchers questions whether roan is actually a separate pattern or if it is just a variation of ticking. Until such time as the gene causing ticking or roan is identified this cannot be supported or refuted. As roan in cattle was found to be caused by a mutation in KITLG, we studied this as a candidate gene but it did not co-segregate with ticking or roan in families.

Furthermore, some dogs are called blue belton which is a pattern of intermingled black and white hairs, often called roan in other animals. Researchers also suggested that this trait was called 'roan' and that it was inherited as an autosomal recessive. Australian Cattle Dogs, sometimes called Blue Heelers in North America often have this pattern.

Speculation regarding related phenotypes

Recently, the work on the differences during the domestication of foxes has been rediscovered. One trait he mentioned is the presence of white markings that became more prominent with more generations of domestication. He attributed this to the 'star gene'. Is this MITF? Is there a chance that a difference in neuroblast migration or development caused by mutations in MITF might affect docility?

Some breeds of dogs, such as Siberian Husky, have a characteristic facial pattern in which white extends up the muzzle and over each eye. Is this caused by another allele of the S locus or is this pattern caused by another gene? Is it coincidental that Siberian Huskies often have blue eyes into adulthood when this trait is not typical in any other breed?

There are some additional phenotypes that are known to dog breeders, but not yet tackled by molecular geneticists. Chow Chow and Chinese Shar-Pei (Fig. 7d) typically have a melanistically pigmented tongue, whereas the tongue of most other breeds is pink or not pigmented (Fig. 7k). Although nose leather, pad and eye rim pigmentation is influenced by the alleles at TYRP1, the tongue was not affected in most breeds. Does this suggest that the tongue is more keratinized in these Asian breeds or is there a mutation in another pigmentation gene?

The effects of TYRP1 mutations in the eumelanin pathway suggest that no dog should be able to simultaneously produce both brown and black pigment anywhere on their body. However, there is a colour called 'seal' in some breeds which gives the impression of a brown coat colour from a distance. Such dogs typically have black nose leather however. On closer examination, the coat of such dogs is composed of intermingled black and reddish hairs. Some of these hairs may be banded. Is this another expression of the K^{br} mutation or is this caused by another allele or another gene?

Ramifications of selection for coat colour

In some breeds only a single coat colour or a very limited range of coat colours are allowed within the standard. Hence, any other genes in this region would also be under inadvertent selection pressure because of the selection for coat colour. used an example of two breeds which separated relatively recently on the basis of brown (German Longhair) vs. black (Large Munsterlander) coat colour. Using a set of microsatellite markers on CFA11, they showed that there was a region spanning approximately 20

In recent years, there seems to bc an interest in breeding dogs to have colours uncommon in a particular breed. Is this simply selection of rare mutations or is it intentional introgression? At the present time, this is impossible to differentiate. The former is generally acceptable provided that the colour in question is allowed by the breed's standard, the latter is almost universally rejected as it does not conform to the regulations of the major registries.

DNA testing is currently used by many breeders to plan matings to obtain specific coloured pups. DNA testing is also used to exclude certain mates in order to avoid pups of undesirable coat colour.

Colour genes in poultry

The two categories of chromosomes are sex chromosomes and autosomes. The sex chromosomes carry the genetic material that determines the sex of an offspring. In humans, the sex chromosomes are referred to as X and Y. A human having the sex chromosomes XX is female, and a human having the sex chromosomes XY is male. In chickens, the sex chromosomes are referred to as Z and W. A chicken having the sex chromosomes ZW is female, and a chicken having the sex chromosomes ZZ is male. The sex chromosomes of mammals and birds are illustrated in Figure 8. Autosomes are all the chromosomes except the sex chromosomes.

Because chromosomes come in pairs, genes also come in pairs. Each parent contributes one gene in each pair of genes. The phenotype for a specific trait in a chicken depends on the makeup of the gene pair for that trait. If the genes are the same, the genetic state is referred to as homozygous. If the genes are different, the genetic state is referred to as heterozygous. A gene that can express itself in the homozygous state or the heterozygous state is referred to as a dominant factor. A gene that can express itself only in the homozygous state is referred to as a recessive factor.

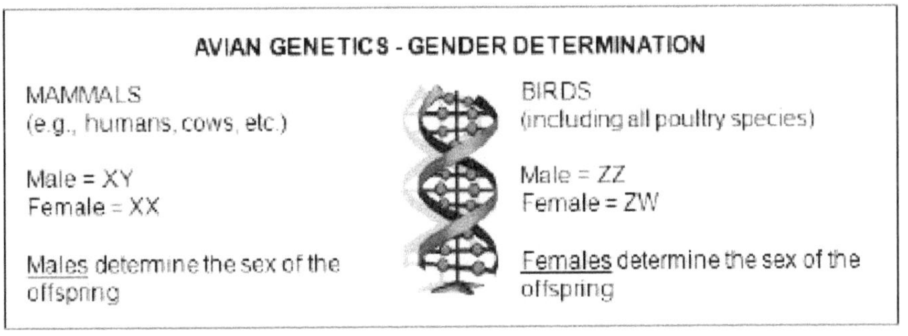

Fig 8. Sex chromosomes of mammals and birds

When dealing with a trait for which there is a dominant gene and a recessive gene, three conditions (combinations of the genes in the gene pair) can occur. The homozygous dominant condition occurs when both genes present are the dominant gene. The homozygous recessive condition occurs when both genes present are the recessive gene. The heterozygous condition occurs when one gene present is the dominant gene and the other is the recessive gene. (The two variant forms of the gene in such a gene pair are called alleles.)

Typically, in the heterozygous condition, the dominant gene is expressed over the recessive gene. In some gene pairs, however, each gene is capable of some degree of expression in the heterozygous condition. This phenomenon is referred to as codominance. The contribution from each gene in the pair can be equal, or the contribution can be dominated more by one gene than the other.

To confuse things further, not every trait is controlled by a single pair of genes. A particular trait can be controlled by numerous gene pairs. Such traits are called quantitative traits. Brown shell color in eggs, for example, is controlled by as many as 13 genes. The result is the range of brown color observed in eggs laid by different breeds of chickens.

Genetics of significant observable traits in chickens

When breeding chickens, it is helpful to understand why certain significant observable traits exist in certain chickens. These traits include comb type, feather color, shank/foot color, and skin color.

Genetics of comb type

Chickens have a variety of comb types, as shown in Fig. 8. The genetics of comb type of chickens is historically significant. Gregory Johann Mendel is considered the father of genetics. His work with peas resulted in the idea that genes control different physical characteristics. Building on this idea, William Bateson used comb type of chickens to show that genetics apply to animals as well.

Comb type in chickens basically is controlled by two different genes on two different chromosomes. One is the rose comb gene (represented by the letter R), and the other is the pea comb gene (represented by the letter P). A presence of the gene is represented by the uppercase letter; an absence of the gene is represented by the lowercase letter. Both the rose comb gene and the pea comb gene can express themselves in the heterozygous state. That is, only one copy of the rose comb gene or the pea comb gene is sufficient for that type of comb to occur. Therefore, both genes can be thought of as dominant genes.

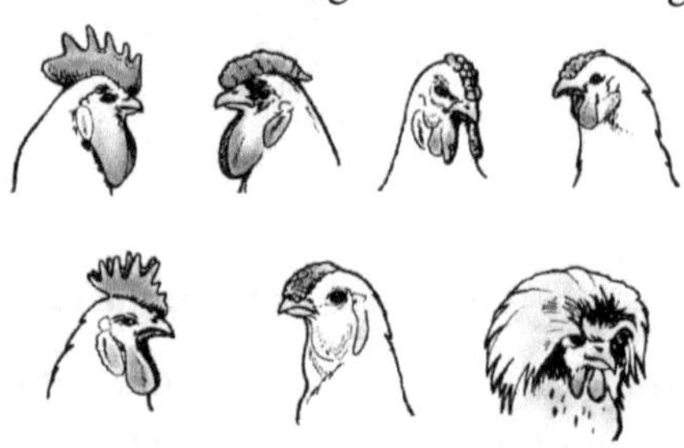

Fig. 8. Diagram showing the different comb types for chickens.

- When at least one copy of the rose comb gene is present and the pea comb gene is absent, the result is a rose comb. In other words, a chicken with a rose comb has one of two possible gene combinations: RRpp or Rrpp.
- When at least one copy of the pea comb gene is present and the rose comb gene is absent, the result is a pea comb. A chicken with a pea comb has one of two possible gene combinations: rrPP or rrPp.
- When at least one copy of each gene is present, the result is a walnut comb. A chicken with a walnut comb has one of four possible gene combinations: RRPP, RrPP, RRPp, or RrPp.
- When both genes are absent, the result is a single comb. A chicken with a single comb has the only possible gene combination: rrpp.

To further understand the genetics of comb type, consider the results of breeding certain chickens. For example, what happens if a chicken that breeds true for pea comb (that is, a chicken that has the gene combination rrPP) is crossed with a chicken that breeds true for rose comb (that is, a chicken that has the gene combination RRpp)? Considering that each parent contributes to the offspring one each of the two genes that control comb type, the only possible gene pair that the parent that breeds true for rose comb can donate is Rp. Similarly, the only possible gene pair that the parent that breeds true for pea comb can donate is rP. Consequently, as shown in Fig. 9, all offspring from such a mating would have the heterozygous state for both genes (that is, RrPp) and would thus have walnut combs. The offspring, however, would not breed true for walnut combs; that is, birds with walnut combs bred to birds with walnut combs could produce offspring with other comb types.

	Rp	Rp
rP	RrPp	RrPp
rP	RrPp	RrPp

Fig. 9. Gene combinations resulting from mating a chicken that breeds true for pea comb with one that breeds true for rose comb

Exploring further, if two of the offspring depicted in Fig. 9 are crossed, the number of possible combinations of genes increases. Each parent could contribute one of four possible gene combinations, resulting in 16 genetic combinations in the offspring. By considering the phenotype associated with each different genotype combination, you can calculate the odds of a particular comb occurring in the offspring. As shown in Figure 10, there would be a 9/16 chance for a walnut comb, a 3/16 chance for a rose comb, a 3/16 chance for a pea comb, and a 1/16 chance for a single comb.

GENETICS OF FEATHER COLOR

	RP	Rp	rP	rp
RP	RRPP Walnut	RRPp Walnut	RrPP Walnut	RrPp Walnut
Rp	RRPp Walnut	RRpp Rose	RrPp Walnut	Rrpp Rose
rP	RrPP Walnut	RrPp Walnut	rrPP Pea	rrPp Pea
rp	RrPp Walnut	Rrpp Rose	rrPp Pea	rrpp Single

Fig. 10. Gene combinations resulting from mating offspring of the cross depicted in the previous figure

To understand the genetics of feather color, it is necessary to understand how the different colors of poultry are achieved. In poultry, there are secondary and primary color patterns. A secondary pattern is a color pattern that appears on individual feathers. Single and double lacing, mottled, and so on are secondary patterns. Primary patterns are color patterns that involve the entire body of the chicken. An example is the Silver Columbian pattern. The Silver Columbian is a white chicken with some black in the neck, wing, and tail areas. Because the pattern does not manifest on individual feathers, it is referred to as a primary pattern.

To breed a chicken having a particular color scheme, one begins with the background color, which is controlled by the E-locus gene. The other color and (secondary) pattern genes essentially modify this background. Several different genes interact to determine feather colors and patterns. Considering white and black to be colors, there are three basic feather colors: black, white, and red (gold). (Technically, white and black are not colors: white is actually the result of all the colors combined, and black is the lack of reflection of light in the visible range.) The colors of chicken feathers are achieved by diluting and enhancing or masking black and red. For example, Rhode Island Reds have the gold gene with the dominant mahogany (red-enhancing) gene. A blue feathering is produced when a black-feathered chicken has the blue gene, which dilutes the black color. Two copies of the blue gene result in the splash effect. A white chicken can be achieved in a number of ways by inhibiting black and red pigmentation with combinations of genes (such as dominant white, recessive white, silver, Columbian, and Cuckoo barring).

Some perceived feather colors actually are due to the structure of the feather rather than to pigmentation. That is, the purple and beetle green sheens seen in some poultry are due to the way the feather structures reflect light rather than to the presence of pigments.

Genetics of shank/foot color

The visible color in the shanks/feet of chickens is the result of a combination of colors in the upper skin and deeper skin. Shank/foot color basically is controlled by three genes, one of which is sex-linked and located on the Z sex chromosome. T Remember that each chicken has two copies of each gene. The table is only a guide because other genes affect shank/foot color as well. For example, the sex-linked barring gene, B, is located on the Z sex chromosome and is a strong inhibitor of melanin pigment in the skin.

Barred Plymouth Rock chickens would not have light shanks if not for the fact that they have the sex-linked barring gene. Female Barred Plymouth Rocks (having the sex chromosomes ZW) tend to have darker shanks than the males (having the sex chromosomes ZZ) due to the dose effect of the barring gene in the male.

Genetics of dark skin color

The silkie chicken, is known for its dark skin color. Dark skin results from higher than normal levels of melanin. A pigment cell activator called fibromelanosis causes pigmentation of connective tissue. The inheritance of the dark skin phenotype is controlled by the fibromelanosis gene, Fm, as well as dermal melanin inhibitors, such as the sex-linked Id dermal melanin–inhibiting mutation. Chickens having the Fm gene but not the Id gene have dark skin and connective tissue. The combination of the Fm gene and the Id mutation results in a chicken with no visible skin pigmentation. Other dermal melanin inhibitors also may have an influence on the degree of melanization (pigmentation) caused by the Fm gene (or the degree of expression of the Fm gene). Moreover, some genes influencing plumage color also have an effect on skin color, such as the E-locus alleles, which may influence the expression of the Fm gene. However, fibromelanotic silkies exist with black, white, blue, and partridge feather patterns.

CONCLUSION

Numbers of molecular techniques together with conventional breeding methods are frequently making their impact in animal improvement in present era. Molecular techniques like detection of DNA-level polymorphism by restriction fragment length polymorphism (RFLP), AFLP, SNP and a number of molecular markers are in frequent use to improve animal performance from one generation to next, both knock-out and/or over-expression of a gene have provided us a better understanding of a given gene and its relevance with respect to overall animal physiology, RNA interference (RNA I) has been extensively leveraged to "silent" undesired disease specific genes in domestic animals and avian species, Mitochondrial DNA markers are particularly useful for studying evolutionary relationships among various taxa, DNA bar- coding based on mitochondrial genes has emerged as a powerful strategy for species identification. The origin and refinement of genetic markers clearly led to the development of innovative strategies against conventional breeding methods, which are slowly becoming obsolete. Standardized protocols are now followed to define, develop and bring into practice a successful method, which then becomes routine among global animal breeders. SNPs are beginning to influence and refocus our strategies, and certainly along with next-generation sequencing technologies, have major role to play in the near future. These later tools have given the animal geneticists a formidable opportunity to incorporate "desirable traits" at will, while simultaneously getting rid of undesirable elements in given animal populations.

These high-tech DNA techniques, such as PCR, DNA sequencing, SSR, SNP, etc., have revolutionised all aspects of molecular biology, particularly its use in animal breeding strategies and in the conservation of genetic diversity. Presently, the pace of development of molecular markers is tremendous, and the trend suggests that explosion in marker development will continue in the near future. It is obvious that molecular markers will continue to serve as a potential tool to geneticists and breeders to evaluate the existing genetic potential, and to manipulate it, to create animals as desired and needed by the farmers. It is not likely that these advanced molecular technology, will replace 'conventional' methods for genetic improvement. Instead, they probably will begin to be gradually incorporated into current genetic improvement programs that use efficiently classical improvement methods to achieve particular objectives.

In summary, for molecular genetic tools to make a positive contribution to sustainable livestock production we need a joined-up strategy addressing genetic progress as well as conservation overcoming all the hurdles in the application of molecular genetic techniques in routine use for animal improvement programmes.

11

SELECTION AND MATING

INTRODUCTION

Selection in breeding programs can be done by using phenotypes (phenotypic selection), pedigree relationship (breeding value selection) or molecular markers (marker assisted selection or genomic selection). All these methods are based on truncation selection, focusing on the best performance of parents before mating. In this article we proposed an approach to breeding, named genomic mating, which focuses on mating instead of truncation selection. Genomic mating uses information in a similar fashion to genomic selection but includes information on complementation of parents to be mated. Following the efficiency frontier surface, genomic mating uses concepts of estimated breeding values, risk (usefulness) and coefficient of ancestry to optimize mating between parents. We used a genetic algorithm to find solutions to this optimization problem and the results from our simulations comparing genomic selection, phenotypic selection and the mating approach indicate that current approach for breeding complex traits is more favorable than phenotypic and genomic selection. Genomic mating is similar to genomic selection in terms of estimating marker effects, but in genomic mating the genetic information and the estimated marker effects are used to decide which genotypes should be crossed to obtain the next breeding population.

Mating of good quality animals to produce highly productive and suitable animals for enhancement of overall performance in the subsequent generations and to augment production and profitability is termed animal breeding.

MATING

Mating designs have received less attention than selection methods, presumably because selection has the largest impact on long-term genetic gain. However, mating designs can be worthwhile. Choosing appropriate mating designs can increase long-term genetic gain. Any increases brought about by mating can be seen as an added benefit to breeding schemes as most mating designs can be implemented without extra costs or logistical constraints. This is because most of the information required to implement mating designs is collected to make selection decisions. Mating designs can increase long-term genetic gains by improving family structure.

They make ancestral contributions more independent by dispersing the contributions within breeding populations and increasing the number of ancestors that contribute to each descendent. This can have three consequences for long-term genetic gain.

First, it enables selection to align ancestors closer to exact threshold–linear relationships.

Second, it reduces rates of inbreeding, expression of inbreeding depression, and the risk of alleles being lost through genetic drift.

Third, it may reduce variation in the accuracy of breeding values between selection candidates by increasing 'connectedness'. All of this means, therefore, that mating designs are worth considering because they can increase long-term genetic gains without burdening breeding schemes with extra costs or logistical constraints.

Genomic information may enable us to develop mating designs that disperse genetic contributions within breeding populations more effectively than pedigree information. One possibility is to extend two designs that were developed using pedigree information: minimum-coancestry mating and mating by minimising the covariance between ancestral contributions (MCAC mating). Minimum-coancestry mating has long been recommended for practical breeding schemes because it minimises the variation of each ancestor×s contribution across allocated matings.

It could exploit genomic information by maximising the probability that all ancestors contribute chromosomal segments to all allocated matings. By comparison to minimum-coancestry mating, MCAC mating is a new design that may be particularly responsive to genomic information by maximising the number of combinations of chromosomal segments from ancestral animals in allocated matings. Both minimum-coancestry and MCAC mating can be extended to include genomic information by replacing their pedigree-relationship matrices with the single or multiple-relationship matrices that were proposed to control parental relationships and monitor losses of variation with OCS. So, genomic relationships could be used to develop mating designs that disperse genetic contributions within breeding populations more appropriately, leading to increases in long-term genetic gains.

Interacting components

Not only does genomic information impact on several components of breeding schemes, these components also interact for two reasons. First, available resources in breeding schemes are finite. Allocating resources to one component limits the resources available to other components, which implies that resources should be allocated to those components that realise the largest marginal returns in long-term genetic gain. Second, decisions made within components also impact on the outcomes of other components. The following highlights approaches to address five interactions between components that can have a major impact on long-term genetic gains.

i. Establish genotyping and phenotyping strategies simultaneously. This involves allocating available resources to collect genotypes and phenotypes, aligning genotypes with phenotypes to establish reference populations for traits included in the total-merit index, and allocating genotypes and phenotypes to available selection candidates. It could also involve the order in which genotypes and phenotypes are collected. The order generates a priori information that can be used to make subsequent genotyping and phenotyping decisions more informative.
ii. Align prediction models and genotyping and phenotyping strategies. Just as the performance of prediction models depends on the genotypes and phenotypes that have been collected , the most-suitable genotypes and phenotypes probably depend on the available prediction models. This implies that choosing a prediction model and developing genotyping and phenotyping strategies should be carried out simultaneously.
iii. Align OCS with genotyping strategy. The level of parental relationship that is deemed acceptable when using OCS can have a bearing on genotyping strategies. Breeders that will only accept low levels of relationship, implying risk-aversion, need to genotype more selection candidates than breeders with a disposition for risk. Genotyping more candidates increases the probability of capturing those animals that maximise the weighted-genetic merit with strict constraints on the level of parental relationships.
iv. Cater for new traits in total-merit indices by modifying phenotyping and genotyping strategies. Including new traits in the total-merit index modifies phenotyping strategies as we shift available resources to collect well-defined phenotypes for the new traits. It is also modifies genotyping strategies, particularly when new reference populations are required.
v. Modify the infrastructure of breeding schemes to cater for genomic selection. Not only does the infrastructure of breeding schemes determine whether it is worthwhile investing in genomic selection, the potential to increase long-term genetic gains using genomic selection could make it worthwhile modifying the infrastructure to realise these gains. There are two ways that this could occur. First, it could bring about the establishment of new infrastructures, including larger breeding schemes or the amalgamation of schemes, establishment of facilities and techniques to collect difficult-to-measure traits, and investments in reproductive technologies that increase selection intensity and amplify the genetic gains from genomic selection. Genetic gains are amplified by increases in selection intensity because selection intensity and accuracy have a multiplicative interaction in the breeder×s equation. Second, genomic selection could make established infrastructures obsolete. The most-notable example is the termination of progeny testing in dairy cattle, where bulls and heifers are increasingly being selected early in life to reduce generation intervals.

These interactions highlight that components of breeding schemes need to be optimised simultaneously if we are to design breeding plans that maximise long-term genetic gains. Clearly, addressing interactions between components is a logical step towards well-designed breeding plans for breeding schemes using genomic information.

Designing breeding plans using decision frameworks

Designing breeding plans that optimise components simultaneously is a complex task, particularly when the optimum breeding plan for individual breeding schemes is influenced by species, traits, management, effective-population size, genetic (co)variances, economic values, marker densities, and numbers of independent loci.

In more cases than not, breeding schemes, their components, and interactions between these components do not allow optimum breeding plans to be designed by mere reasoning. Designing breeding plans requires decision frameworks: testing sound hypotheses by designing and executing controlled experiments using decision tools, such as mathematical–statistical models. These decision frameworks, direct adaptions of conventional scientific method, have three advantages when designing breeding plans. First, they provide an objective and theoretical basis by which to make and validate breeding decisions. Second, they enable us to understand the underlying mechanisms of breeding schemes with genomic information. Third, they allow us to test practical implementation of breeding decisions against theoretical models. So, decision frameworks are essential to the design of breeding plans that maximise long-term genetic gains in breeding schemes using genomic information.

Decision frameworks require decision tools or virtual laboratories to test hypotheses related to breeding plans. In animal breeding, these models are typically simulation models, both deterministic and stochastic, that provide useful representations of practical breeding schemes. To be useful, these models must fulfil at least five criteria. First, they must be guided by the hypotheses being tested. Second, they must be founded on animal-breeding theory and genetic principles. Third, they must describe practical breeding schemes using mathematical equations, functional relationships, rules, variables, and/or parameters on temporal or spatial scales. Fourth, they must have an appropriate level of complexity in terms of constraints and simplifying assumptions. Models that are too simple fail to generate realistic trends. Too complex and we are unable to understand emerging trends. Fifth, we must be able to evaluate the extent to which the models behave in the same way as the practical breeding schemes they represent. Fulfilling each of these criteria ensures confidence and credibility with which we can apply breeding plans to practical breeding schemes. Therefore, developing decision tools that provide useful representations of practical breeding schemes is an important step in the design of breeding plans with genomic information.

MATING SYSTEM

There are two types of mating of animals for production of the progenies. These are

- **Natural propagation/mating :** Mating of animals by natural means.
- **Artificial insemination (AI) :** Mating is done through artificial means by collecting semen from male and the inseminating the females. This method help in use of outstanding males for mating of a large number of females thereby production of large number of highly productive and performing progenies.

SYSTEM OF BREEDING

Basically, there are two methods of breeding which are as follows:

1. Inbreeding : Breeding of the related animals as sire (male) and dam (female) are known as inbreeding.
2. Out breeding : Out breeding of unrelated animals as male and female is known as out breeding.

Inbreeding

- Inbreeding i.e. mating of related individuals often results in a change in the mean of a trait.
- Performance of inbred animals lowers down the reproductive efficiency and may have several disorders. Hence, this method of breeding is not practiced for livestock improvement.
- However, inbreeding is intentionally practiced to create genetic uniformity of laboratory stocks and to produce stocks for crossing (animal and plant breeding).
- But inbreeding is unintentionally generated by keeping small populations for breeding and during selection.

There are again two types of inbreeding which are:

a. Close breeding : This is most intensive breeding where animals are very closely related and can be traced back to more than one common ancestor. Examples: Sire to daughter Son to dam Brother to sister.

b. Line breeding : Mating animals that are more distantly related which can be traced back to one common ancestor. Examples: Cousins Grandparents to grand offspring, Half-brother to half-sister. Line breeding increases genetic purity amongst the animals of progeny generations.

Out breeding

Out breeding system i.e. breeding of unrelated animals is generally of two types:

1. **Crossbreeding:** Crossbreeding is the mating of two animals of different breeds. Superior traits that results in the crossbred progeny from crossbreeding are called hybrid vigor or heterosis.

2. **Grading up:**
   - Grading up is the breeding of animals of two different breeds where the animals of an indigenous breed/genetic group is mated by an improved pure breed for several generations towards attaining the superior traits of the improved breed.
   - Grading up is continuous use of purebred sires of the same breed in a grade herd. By fifth generation, the graded animals may reach almost purebred levels.

By following out breeding system i.e., crossbreeding, selective breeding and grading up according to the need, results in improvement in production performance of the crossbred/graded along with improvement in growth rate, reproduction and production.

General Considerations Regarding Crossbreeding Systems

- Good record keeping of the animals is required for selection good quality of male and females for breeding. Records on milk production and age at first calving are two important characters besides others.
- Calving difficulties may increase when crossing large breed sires with small breed dams and hence selection of animals/breeds should be done carefully.
- Fewer calving problems if large breed dams are used. However, large breed dams have higher maintenance costs.
- Artificial insemination allows access to better bulls which may be practiced.

Selection of breeding animals

- Selection of good quality improved animals for breeding is done by allowing some animals to have offspring while preventing the animals with inferior quality from reproducing.
- The process allows producing genetically superior animals. Emphasis has to be given on several traits when selecting breeding stock.
- The breeding of animals is under human control, and the breeders decide which individuals shall produce the next generation. The breeder makes a choice.

The breeding of animals is based upon the fact that certain qualities are genetic ,hence valuable qualities are passed on from parents to off -springs. The qualities can be maintained or improved in the next generation.

The performance of an animal is influenced by two major factors:

- Genetic potential
- The environment, which includes:

Feeding, Health, care and the ecological conditions.

The genetic potential of an animal is inherited from its parents.

In selection and breeding animals with superior characteristics are selected and allowed to mate.

In the process they transmit the superior characteristics to their offspring.

When this is done over a long period of time, it results in livestock improvement.

Reproduction and Reproductive Systems

Reproduction is the process by which off-springs are produced. All farm animals multiply by means of sexual reproduction.

It begins with fertilization which is the fusion of male and female gametes to form a zygote. Fertilization takes place internally in the body of the female. The embryo(zygote) formed develops inside body of mother, fed and protected until end of gestation period.

In poultry, the process is different in that eggs are fertilized internally but laid and development of the chick takes place outside during incubation.

In both male and female, certain organs are specialized for the process of reproduction.

Some of these organs secret fluids which are necessary for the movement and survival of the gametes(reproductive cells.)

Reproduction in Cattle

Male Reproductive System (Bull)

The male reproductive organs produce the male gametes,the spermatozoans.

These are introduced into female reproductive system, where they fuse with the sperm to form zygote.

The reproductive system(bull) iscompsed of the following parts:

i. Testes
ii. Epididymis
iii. Sperm ducts
iv. Accessory glands(Seminal vesicles and prostrate glands)
v. Penis

The testis

- There are two testes hanging loosely between hind legs.

  Enclosed by loose skin (scrotum)scrotum regulate temperature of testis for optimum production of sperms.

- Produce spermatozoa(sperms)which are stored in coiled tube called epididymis.

Epididymis: Storage of spermatozoa.

Sperm ducts:

- Conveys sperm from the testis and urine through the penis.
- sphincter muscles contract to allow each to pass separetly.

Seminal vesicles produce fluid called semen. Semen carries sperms out of penis in fluid form.

Semen contains nutrients to the spermatozoan.

Prostate gland -produce fluid that neutralize the acidic effects of urine in the urethra preventing death of sperms.

Accessory glands: Include seminal vesicles cowpers gland and prostate gland. **Urethra:** Conveys urine and semen.One sperm fertlizes ovum

Penis

- Surrounded by a sheath which is an extension of skin.
- It introduces sperms into the vagina of a cow through the vulva during mating.
- It is a copulatory organ, also used for urination.

The Female Reproductive System(Cow)

The reproductive systemm of a cow is composed of:

i. Ovaries
ii. Fallopian tubes

Ovaries and fallopian tubes(oviduct)

Two ovaries located in abdomen, left and right. Produce ova/eggs and hormones which control sexual cycle. Oestrogen produced by graafian follicle inside ovary induces oestrus i.e. Heat period so that the cow shows signs of heat. The hormone oestrogen is produced under the influence of other hormone called the Follicle stimulating hormone.

After every 21 days the ovary releases a mature ovum and the cow comes on heat. The ovum travels through the fallopian tubes to the uterus.

The release and movement of the ovum down to the uterus is called ovulation. If mating is done at this time, fertilization will take place.

The fertilized egg implants itself onto the endometrium(walls of uterus)and develops into foetus.

Fallopian tubes:

Fertilization takes place here. Also a passage for the egg from the ovary to the uterus.

The uterus:

Implantation takes place here and also embryo develops here.

The cervix of the uterus: Closes the uterus.

The vagina and Vulva:

Vulva is the external opening of female reproductive system.

It allows mating to take place so that sperms are deposited into the vagina.

The foetus and urine are removed through the vulva.

Pregnancy

is period between fertilization of ova and the expulsion of the foetus through the vulva. Also called gestation period. In cattle gestation period is 270-285 days. Ends with the birth of a calf.

The reproductive tract undergoes a period of rest during which it is repaired and returns to normal. During pregnancy, hormone called progesterone is produced by the placenta to maintain the foetus in the uterus.

Animal	Length of days
Cow	270-285 Days
Sow	113-117
Ewe/Goat	150
Rabbit	28-32

Parturition

Act of giving birth called parturition. This time the foetus expelled through the birth canal.

When an animal is about to give birth, it shows signs:

- Distended udder which produces thick milky fluid called colostrums.
- Swollen vulva producing thick mucus like discharge.
- Loose and slackened pelvic girdle.
- Visible pin bones.
- General restlessness.

Animal parturates within 2-3 hours after this signs. The correct presentation is with the front feet first ,and the head outstretched and resting in between the feet.

Any other presentation called mal-presentation or breech presentation and requires assistance.

Reproduction in Poultry

The cock has no penis but a small opening near the vent through which sperms are emitted. Cock has testes within the body.

The hen has elongated oviduct for formation of an egg. Fertilization occurs internally.

During mating the cloaca of the hen and the vent of the cock fit into each other and then semen is poured into the cloaca ,then sucked to the oviducts.

The Reproductive System of a Hen

The reproductive system has the following parts;

i. Ovary
ii. Funnel(infundibulum).
iii. Magnum
iv. Ishtumus
v. Uterus/Shell gland
vi. Vaginal
vii. Cloaca

Ovary

Hen has two ovaries but one functional. Ova is formed in ovaries.

About 3500-4000 ova present inside ovary held by follicle. Mature ovum released via rapture of follicle. It moves into oviduct received by the funnel.

Funnel (infundibulum)

Fertilization occurs here. Chalazae also added to yolk.

It also collects the ovum and stores the sperm. Time here is 15 minutes and it is 11.6cm long.

Magnum

Thick albumen is added and stays for 3hrs. its 33cm long.

Isthmus

Its 10.6cm long, Shell membranes added and determines shape of egg.

Water, mineral salts and vitamins added and takes 15 minutes.

Uterus (shell gland)

Calcium deposits i.e.shell added around the egg. Pigments added.

Addition of albumin finished and stays here for 18-22hours.

Vagina

Short, 6.9cm long and for temporal storage of egg before laying

Cloaca

Egg moves out of cloaca through the vent and the cloaca extents out to prevent the egg from breaking.

NB; Egg formation not depended on fertilization. Egg formation takes 24-26hours.

The components of egg are obtained from body reserves of the hens body.

SELECTION OF BREEDING STOCK

Selection is used as a tool for livestock improvement. A breeding stock is a group of males and females which act as parents of future generations.

Selection is the process of allowing certain animals to be parents of future generations while culling others.

Culling is the removal of animals which do not perform to the desired level, from the herd. The animals retained have certain desirable characteristics which make them produce more.

Selected animals make up the breeding stock.

The breeding stock should pass the good qualities to their offsprings for better performance, to improve the livestock.

Selection process repeated for many generations increases chances of formation of desirable qualities in an animal.

Genetically termed as gene frequency(occurrence of the genes that carry desirable characteristics.) Selection increases occurrence of desirable genes and decreases occurance of undesirable genes.

During selection, the characteristics to be selected for are first studied closely to ascertain that it is not influenced by the environment, but mainly by the genetic make-up.

Selection helps improve characteristics which are highly heritable.

Heritability means the likelihood of a particular trait to be transmitted to the offspring and they are strongly inherited.

A character like milk yield is lowly heritable, i.e. it is weakly inherited and a bigger percentage of the character is affected by the environment.

The degree to which selection affects a character depends on the following factors;

The heritability of the character, The intensity with which the selection is done and the interval between generations and kind of selection being practiced.

Factors To Consider When Selecting A Breeding Stock.

- Age
- Level of performance
- Physical Fitness
- Health

- Body Conformation
- Temperament or Behaviour
- Quality of products
- Mothering Ability
- Adaptability
- Prolificacy

Age

- Young animals,
- Those that have not parturated for more than 3-times, should be selected.
- They have a longer productive life.
- Old animals are poor breeders and low producers.
- Production and breeding efficiency decline with age.

Level of performance

- Animals with highest production level selected.
- Performance best indicated by records.

Good performance of animal indicated by;

- High milk, wool and egg production,
- Good mothering ability
- High prepotency which is the ability of a parent to pass good qualities to their offsprings.
- The animals with poor performance should be culled.
- Good records kept and used by the farmer for this purpose.

Physical Fitness

Animals selected should be free from any physical defect e.g.

- mono-eyed,
- limping,
- irregular number of teats,
- scrotal hernia,
- defective and weak backline

Health

- Sick animals do not breed well and are expensive to keep.
- Animals that are resistant to diseases pass these characteristics to their offsprings

Body Conformation

- Animals for breeding to be selected according to proper body conformation.
- A dairy cow should be wedge-shaped with a large udder, thin legs, long neck.

Temperament or Behaviour

- Animals with bad behaviors should be culled. e.g Cannibalism, egg eating, aggressiveness, kicking

Quality of products

- Select animals that give products of high quality such as meat, wool, eggs, milk.

Mothering Ability

- Animals selected should have a good mothering ability,
- That is animals with good natural instinct towards their young ones.
- This will enable them to rear the young ones up to weaning.

Adaptability

Animals selected should be well adapted to the prevailing climatic condition in the area e.g Ardi and semi arid areas.

Prolificacy

- Animals selected should be highly prolific.
- That is, animals with the ability to give birth to many offsprings at a time(larger litter).
- This is a quality that should be considered when selecting pigs and rabbits.
- The ancestry records assist to choose the prolific breedsfor mating

SELECTION OF CATTLE AND SHEEP

Selection in cattle

Consider the following

Level of Performance Which Include:

- Milk Yield Buter Content.
- Length Of Lactation Period.
- Calving Intervals.

Age of the Animal, Fertility, physical Fitness, Health Of The Animal, Body Conformation and suitability of the enterprise-milk or beef

Selection in sheep

Consider the following:

Level of performance which includes;

- Mothering ability
- Growth rate
- Wool quality
- Carcass quality
- Twining rate Age

Selection in Pigs

Consider the following:

Carcass quality/dressing percentage

Suitability to the enterprise (bacon or pork)

Growth rate.

Health of the animal.

Mothering ability.

Prolificacy.

Number of teats

Temperament.

Body formation.

Age.

Heredity defects

Selection in Camels

Health of the animal.

Age.

Temperament.

Foraging ability.

Fertility.

Level of performance-milk, meat, fur and transport.

METHODS OF SELECTION

These include:

- **Mass selection** - Animals with superior characteristics (highly heritable breeds) are selected from a herd and then allowed to mate among each other at random.

The offsprings will show higher performance than their parents. This is because mass selection increases the occurrence of the desirable genes in a population.

- **Progeny testing** - is a offspring resulting from selected parents (Family selection). In this method a group of progenies (offrprings) are used as an aid to increase accuracy in the selection ofa breeding stock. This is method is used when the character to be selected is of low heritability and expressedby one sex only.

This method takes up to nine years for the results to be seen

Contemporary comparison

Contemporaries refers to other heifers in the herd sired by the same bull.

This is a progey tasting method which involves comparison of average production of daughters (Heifers) of each bull with that of the other heifer refered to as contemporaries.

In this methods it is assumed that the difference between the herds of the same breed are non-genetic in origin.

Advantages

- It is possible to compare heifers of different ages in different locations worldwide.
- It eliminates difference brought about by the environment.
- it is possible to make direct comparison of stut bulls at different artificial insemiation centres.
- It is accurate since we are using a large herd of animals.

Breeding

Process of mating selected males and females to produce offspring with the desired characteristics.

Reasons:

- To expand the inherited potential of the animal.
- To improve production by introducing new genes.
- To overcome production problems created by the environment.
- To satisfy consumers taste.
- For economic reasons e.g fast growth rate to reach the market early.

Terms Used in Breeding

Inheritance; Genetic transmission of characteristics from parents to offsprings.

The mechanism of inheritance is carried by the sex cells (gametes) and is controlled by genes found in the chromosomes.

Genes are very tiny units of inheritance carrying particular characteristics, such as colour, body shape and amount of milk production. Chromosomes are genetic materials which carry genes.

They exist in pairs paternal and maternal) in the nucleus f the body cells. They are always constant in number.

Dominant and Recessive Characteristics

A dominant gene is one that suppresses the other. It produces a dominant characteristic.

A recessive gene is one that is suppressed by the other. It produces a recessive characteristic.

Hybrid and Hybrid Vigour

A hybrid is an animal which is the product of crossing animals of two different breeds. It has both a dominant and recessive characters. A superior hybrid has %75 dominance and %25 recessive.

Hybrid vigour or heterosis is increased vigour and performance resulting from crossing two superior breeds. When two superior breeds e.g Pedigree friesian and Jersey breeds are mate the resultant offsprings have both the character of high milk yield and high butterfat content. Thus it is said the offsprings have hybrid figure whichis an increased perfomance and figure than both the two parents.

Epistasis

This is the masking of the effect of one gene (reccesive gene) by another gene(dominant) which is non-allelic, that is situated on different locus.

This is aimed at preventing the recesive gene from being expressed.

Mating in Livestock

Mating in Cattle

Heat signs occur every 21 days.

The heat period last for 18-30 hours on average 24 hours.

Cow should be served 12-18 hours after showing the first heat signs.

Heat Signs

Restlessness.

Mounting on others and when mounted on she stands still. Rise in body temperature.

Drop in milk production in lactating cows. Vulva swells and becomes reddish.

Clear or slimy mucus from the vulva.

Bellowing or mooing frequently.

Mating in Pigs

Heat signs in pigs occur after every 21 days. The heat lasts about 72 hours.

Sows or gilts should be served in 18- 36 hours of the heat period.

Signs of Heat

Restlessness.

Frequent urination.

Swelling and reddening of the vulva.

Clear or slimy discharge from the vulva.

Frequent mounting on others.

It responds very well to the 'riding test'.

Mating in Rabbits

Does are ready for mating 6-7 months of age. Heat signs occur every 14 days.

The doe should be taken to the buck and not vice versa.

Signs of Heat

Restlessness.

Frequent urination.

Swollen vulva.

The doe throws herself on the side.

The doe rubs herself against the wall or any other solid object.

The doe tries to contact other rabbits in the next hutch by peeping.

Methods of Service in Livestock

Natural Mating

Advantages:

It is more accurate.

It is less laborious.

Useful when heat signs of females cannot be easily detected.

Disadvantages

Inbreeding is not easily controlled.

Transmission of breeding diseases.

Extra feed for the male is required.

Large males can injure small females.

Wastage of semen.

It is cumbersome and expensive to transport a bull to remote areas.

Artificial insemination

Introduction of semen into the female reproductive tract by artificial means.

Advantages

There is economical use of semen.

It controls transmission of breeding diseases.

Sires that are unable to serve cows due to heavy weight or injury can produce semen to serve cows.

It prevents large bulls from injuring small cows. It reduces the expenses of keeping a male animal.

A small scale farmer who cannot afford to buy a superior bull can have the cows served at a low cost.

Semen can be stored for long. It helps to control inbreeding.

It eliminates the threat of keeping dangerous bulls from the farm.

It makes research work easier.

Disadvantages

Harmful characteristics can be spread quickly by one bull to the offsprings.

It requires skilled labour.

Low chance of conception due to death of semen during storage.

It is laborious:

Embryo Transplant

It is the implantation of an embryo (fertilized ova) from a high quality female (donor) in the uterus of a low grade female (recipient).

Advantages

Faster multiplication of an animal with superior characteristics . It is easier to transport embryos than the whole animal.

Embryos can be stored for a long period awaiting the availability by recipient females.

It stimulates milk production in a female (recipient) that was not ready to produce milk.

Low grade animals can be used in production and rearing of high quality animals. Offsprings of a superior female can spread quickly in an area.

Disadvantages

It is expensive.

It requires skilled personnel.

It requires special equipment for fertilization and storage of embryos.

Signs of Parturition in Livestock

Parturition is the act of giving birth in female animals.

Parturition in Cattle

The gestation period in cattle is 270-285 days averaging 280days.

Signs of Parturition

Restlessness

Enlarged or swollen vulva.

Clear mucus discharge from the vulva.

Slackening of the pelvic muscles.

Full and distended udder.

Thick milky fluid from the teats.

A water bag appears and bursts just before calving.

Parturition in Pigs

The gestation period in pigs is about 4 months or 3 months, 3 weeks and 3 days.

Signs of Parturition

Restlessness.

The vulva turns red and swells.

The udder becomes full with a milky fluid the sow starts to prepare a nest by collecting some beddings at one comer of the pen.

Parturition in Rabbits

The gestation period in rabbits is 28-32 days.

Signs of Parturition

Preparing a nest by plucking off hair from her belly.

Goes off feeding

Restlessness.

The udder distends.

12

CROSSBREEDING

A crossbreed is an organism borne out of purebred parents from two different breeds. Thus, crossbreeding refers to the process of mating two organisms from different breeds. Normally, the crossbred animals gain complementary traits that enhance their aesthetic or economic value.

Crossbreeding is usually done with the intention of producing offspring that share the traits of both parents, or to produce an organism with hybrid vigor. For the uninitiated, hybrid vigor (also called heterosis) is the increase in certain characteristics, such as growth rate, size, fertility, yield etc. of a particular crossbreed organism over its parents. To learn more about hybrid vigor, click here. Although crossbreeding is generally performed to improve the health and viability of organisms, irresponsible crossbreeding can also bring undesirable results—like animals of inferior quality—such as the dilution of a purebred gene pool towards extinction.

CROSSBREEDS ARE NOT 'HYBRIDS'

Many people posit that crossbreeds are the same as hybrids, but scientifically, this is not the case. Crossbreeds in animal breeding are crosses within a single species (but of a different breed), whereas hybrids are crosses between different species altogether. For example, a Ragamuffin is a crossbreed formed by mating the same species (cat), but different breeds (Ragdoll and Himalayan). A mule, on the other hand, is a hybrid animal formed by the mating of a donkey and a horse i.e. two different species.

When it comes to plant breeding, the term 'crossbreeding' is uncommonly used. Moreover, there is no universal term to distinguish hybridization from crossing in the case of plants.

Why Does Crossbreeding Occur?

Given the popular breeding strategies employed today, there has been a rise in inbreeding—therefore inbreeding depression within flocks and groups of livestock. When organisms with a very close genetical lineage mate, it is called inbreeding. Inbreeding depression refers to the reduction in levels of biological fitness in a given population as a result of inbreeding. To learn more about the perils of inbreeding, click here.

So, with inbreeding, the animals' reproductive capacity is hampered. One of the main benefits of crossbreeding is that there is a reduction in inbreeding, which also leads to hybrid vigor, as explained earlier. Many reports related to ruminants have observed that there are rising cases of infertility and calving ease amongst herds, especially in cattle like Holsteins. By using crossbreeding, a breeder can not only curb infertility, but also improve desired traits like calving ease, longevity and milk production.

CROSSBREEDING IN ANIMALS

Crossbreeding in Cats

The many cute and eccentric breeds of domestic cat that you see today are actually crossbreeds, and are produced by mating between existing, well-established breeds of cat, e.g., the American Lynx, Australian Tiffanie, Dwelf etc. Crossbreeding in cats is often done with the intention of combining selected traits from the foundation stock, or to propagate a rare mutation to curb excessive inbreeding. However, some new crossbreeds, like Aegean cats, are developed fully from a local landrace population. It must be noted that most experimental cat breeds are crossbreeds.

Crossbreeding in Dogs

Crossbreeding in dogs is getting much more popular, as crossbreed dogs are observed to develop hybrid vigor without losing their attractiveness. Certain planned crossbreeding between different breeds of purebred dogs are popularly called designer dogs. Designer dogs are more attractive and are high in demand in the pet market.

Crossbreeding in Horses

Creating a new breed of horse is often the main aim of crossbreeding in horses. One type of present-day horse crossbreeding technique is used to create many of the warmblood breeds of horses that we often see today at the horse track. Warmbloods are a type of horse that are increasingly used in popular equestrian events like dressage and charreada.

Common Concerns in Crossbreeding

One of the major concerns with crossbreeding is adding too much variability. At the start of the implementation of crossbreeding, the uniformity within a herd is likely to be disrupted. However, this lack of uniformity can turn costly to the producer (breeder), especially if they are unwilling to commit to the crossbreeding program over the long term. To get the maximum benefit out of crossbreeding, producers must be willing to commit to using the program for several generations. Producers, who often are farmers, do not usually have the time or money to do this. Perseverance and financing are needed for successful crossbreeding implementation, which makes crossbreeding an arduous task.

Research in Crossbreeding and Related Challenges

One of the major challenges in this field of academic research is in designing experiments to understand the effects and implications of crossbreeding. Most results are derived in the field without much rigorous experimental design, as a planned experiment in crossbreeding would be extremely costly, considering that many generations of animals and their offspring would need to be studied.

A recently concluded study conducted by a group of researchers in Germany attempted a comparative study of purebred producers and crossbred producers. They discovered that crossbreeding has manifested a significant improvement in functional traits, such as fecundity and survivability, but their study was restricted to first-generation animals only.

Presently, there is a need to conduct longer and more rigorous research studies to understand the effects of crossbreeding in subsequent generations. Moreover, most of the research in this domain specifically looks at European and North American conditions, so more research is also needed to acquire data from other parts of the world.

GENOMICS OF CROSSBRED FARM ANIMALS

Crossbreeding is a common strategy to promote animal production. In the past century, crossbreeding has been commonly conducted to produce commercial pigs and poultry as human food. In subtropical countries, crossbred cattle have been developed that combine the production performance of Taurine cattle with the tropical adaption of Zebu cattle. Composite cattle are developed by crossing two or more purebred breeds, aiming at exploiting breed complementarity and retaining some heterosis (hybrid vigor) in future generations. Dairy cattle are mostly purebred, but crossbred dairy cattle are becoming increasingly popular in recent years. Strategically, crossbreeding is a potential approach to improve sustainability in animal breeding by reducing inbreeding and enhancing fertility, survival, and other functional traits.

Genomics is an interdisciplinary field of biology focusing on the studies of genomes. A genome is an organism's complete set of DNA, including all of its genes. Unlike classic genetics, which focuses on individual genes and their roles in inheritance, genomics deals with the collective characterization and quantification of all of an organism's genes, their interrelations, and their influence on the organism. From the genomics perspective, crossbred animals differ considerably from purebred animals because their genome is a mosaic of genome regions inherited from their purebred ancestors. Thus, genomics solutions for crossbred animals need to be different. For example, ancestry estimation or genomic breed composition (GBC) in purebred animals is primarily motivated for breed registries and the identification of purebred animals when the pedigree is missing or incomplete. In contrast, the estimated GBC for crossbred animals are used to infer their genomic make-ups from their ancestors. Such information can help estimate heterozygosity, understand their breeding history, and make management decisions for crossbreeding programs. The breeding objective with purebred animals is to increase additive genetic gains, but non-addtive genetic effects such as dominance and epistasis effects are pivotal to produce crossbred animals of high-performance market values.

The past decades have witnessed many milestone discoveries in animal genomics which have fundamentally revolutionized many aspects of animal breeding and production. Nevertheless, there are far more questions still unanswered. This Research Topic represented an effort toward enhancing the understanding and applications of crossbred genomics. It included 25 papers, covering several aspects of the crossbred genomics in farm animals.

Interpretations of Genomic Breed Composition and "The Impure Purebred Paradox"

Genomic breed composition (GBC) of an individual animal refers to the partition of its genome according to the inheritance from its ancestors or ancestral breeds. The U.S. Council on Dairy Cattle Breeding (CDCB) uses an alternative term, namely Breed Base Representation (BBR), which is the adjusted genomic breed composition on each of five dairy breeds (Ayrshire, Brown Swiss, Guernsey, Holstein, and Jersey) as the potential parents (VanRaden and Cooper, 2015).

Interpretations of GBC depend on the estimation methods. For example, admixture model postulates that an observed genotype for a progeny is an instance of a multinomial distribution, with genotype probability being a mixture governed by allelic frequencies of the ancestors. Hence, GBC are estimated by the weights or admixture coefficients. Linear regression estimated GBC of to be adjusted regression coefficients of coded genotypes for a progeny on the ancestral allele frequencies, and bounded between 0 and 1.

A genomic prediction model estimates the SNP effects on candidate ancestry breeds as binary or categorical traits. GBC equals to the total genomic value for an animal pertaining to each ancestry breed. Researchers proposed a causal interpretation of GBC based on path theory, which decomposed the relationships between ancestors and their progenies into direct and indirect breed (path) effects. GBC was measured by relative ratio of direct (D-GBC) and combined (C-GBC) breed determination, respectively, from each putative ancestry breed to a progeny. C-GBC included direct breed effects and indirect breed effects due to genomic similarities. The estimated D-GBC and C-GBC were comparable when the ancestry breeds had a very distant relationship, and they corresponded well to the estimated GBC from linear regression and admixture model. However, large differences arose between D-GBC and C-GBC when ancestors were highly correlated. Overall, the estimated C-GBC was closer to the estimated GBC from linear regression and admixture models than D-GBC.

In reality, all the modern cattle breeds are correlated because they share common ancestors. The same is true with other farm animal species. The estimated GBC for a purebred animal is not always 100%. This phenomenon was referred to as "the Impure purebred Paradox". In the U.S. dairy genetic evaluation, for example, the reference population for a dairy breed consisted of animals with a BBR no e" 94% for that breed, and animals with BBR no e" 90% received single-breed genomic evaluation.

This was because the current methods tend to produce a small GBC value to a non-ancestry reference breed. The more significant the genomic similarity, the more noise. Statistically, this situation was an indication of increased false-negative error rates in the identification of purebred animals.

Researchers proposed applying regularization in admixture models to estimate GBC for purebred animals. Regularized admixture methods produced sparse solutions of admixture coefficients, thus effectively imposing penalties on small, non-essential components due to genomic similarity. The non-convex penalty outperformed the L1 norm penalty to suppress the noise in the estimated GBC.

Several issues are not addressed adequately. Firstly, accurately assessing GBC requires knowing or reliably estimating the allelic frequencies for the base population when the ancestor breeds were developed, because they are not observable. Secondly, while high-density SNP genotypes were used to estimate GBC, the impact of SNPs in high linkage disequilibrium on the estimated GBC has not been well-documented. In admixture models, for example, the likelihood is computed assuming mutual independence of SNP loci, but this assumption does not hold with high-density SNP arrays.

Finally, the current methods do not estimate GBC exactly based on genomic similarities identical-by-descend (IDB) between a progeny and the ancestry (reference) breeds. Rather, they reflect more of genomic similarities identical-in-statue (IIS).

Limited Efforts With Differential Gene Expression Profiling

Expression profiling is a logical next step after genome sequencing, which reveals the activity of genes in hundreds and thousands and depicts a global picture of cellular functions.

Expression profiling experiments involve measuring relative mRNA abundance in two or more experimental conditions. Altered gene expression suggests a change for the protein coded by the mRNA, probably indicating a homeostatic response or a pathological condition.

There were only three papers addressing differential gene expression in this Research Topic. Chen et al. compared the microRNA (miRNA) profiles of pectoral muscle in chickens at pre- to post-natal stages. Cui et al. identified differentially expressed miRNAs between cattle with high vs. low milk protein and fat percentages. A miRNA is a small single-stranded non-coding RNA molecule containing about 22 nucleotides in animals. It functions in RNA silencing and post-transcriptional regulation of gene expression.

First discovered in the early 1990s, miRNAs were not recognized as a distinct class of biological regulators until the early 2000s. Researchers investigated the expression pattern of pituitary-derived circular RNAs and their functions in Landrace × Yorkshire crossbred pigs. A circular RNA is a single-stranded RNA that forms a covalently closed continuous loop. Some circular RNAs have shown potential as gene regulators.

Conclusions and Prospects

Genomics focuses on the structure, function, evolution, mapping, and editing of genomes. Genomics studies also included studies of intragenomic phenomena such as epistasis, pleiotropy, heterosis, and other interactions between loci and alleles within the genome. Given such a broad spectrum of genomics domains, the coverage of this Research Topic is very limited.

The former used available genomic data to describe gene functions and interactions, whereas the latter attempts to predict the performance of individual animals based on low- to high-density genotype data. Studies in structural genomics, epigenomics, and metagenomics in crossbred livestock animals are essential, but they are not addressed in this collection.

Advances in genomics have triggered a revolution in discovery-based research and systems biology concerning complex biological systems. Driving genomics to practice, genomic prediction is at the core of enhancing animal breeding and farming management. We anticipate more efforts to specifically exploit genomic prediction models and cost-effective training strategies for crossbred animals. Innovative genomic mating and crossbreeding is appealing for improving commercial crossbreeding.

The objective for crossbreeding is to find optimal combinations which maximize the general combining ability (GCA) from the contributing parental lines and the special combining ability (SCA) between them, penalized by standard deviation of gamete breeding values passed from the parents to the offspring. This type of innovative mating or crossbreeding schemes is expected to produce high-performance and less-variable crossbred animals.

Finally, predicting heterosis remains a topic of interest. Heterosis is an old concept proposed by George Harrison Shull, American botanist and geneticist known as the father of hybrid corn, in 1914. In animal breeding, it refers to crossbred performance superiority relative to the parental average. Two competing but not mutually exclusive hypotheses, dominance hypothesis and dominance hypothesis, have been proposed to explain heterosis or hybrid vigor. Epigenetic components of hybrid vigor were established recently, pinpointing the involvement of small RNAs in the growth, vigor and adaptation of hybrids.

HETEROSIS

Heterosis is linearly related to heterozygosity, considered to be 100% in the first generation cross (F1) between two diverse parental breeds. In the following generations, it is measured as retained heterosis or heterozygosity relative to F_1. Genomic-estimated retained heterozygosity or heterosis (GRH) can be used to match parents to obtain optimized heterosis and produce progeny with improved performance and replacement females with better lifetime productivity. A silent feature is that GRH provides an additional metric for the existing purebred genomic evaluation systems, for example, in beef cattle to include crossbred predictions without any infrastructural change.

Heterosis is not new to the livestock industry and its benefits have been well documented. Heterosis comes in three different forms: individual, maternal, and paternal. Researchers explains that retained heterosis is the increase in performance of crossbred progeny relative to that of its purebred parents. Maternal heterosis is the increase in production of a cow above that of the average of her parent breeds. Advantages of maternal heterosis are seen in maternal ability, reproduction, longevity, calf survivability, pounds of calf weaned and younger age at puberty. Paternal heterosis is similar to maternal heterosis in that it is the genetic advantage provided by the sire; benefits are also seen as increased bull fertility.

Lowly Heritable Traits

Heterosis offers an array of advantages but its greatest impact is seen in lowly heritable traits. Heritability is the proportion of variation observed in animals due to genetics passed along generations and the phenotypic variation observed due to genetic and environmental effects.

Examples of lowly heritable traits are reproduction, longevity, maternal ability and health. Lowly heritable traits respond slowly to selection since the greatest amount of variation in the traits are due to environment rather than genetics. Heterosis is an effective way to improve these lowly heritable traits.

Breed Complementarity

Breeds are complementary to each other when one breed excels in certain traits the other breed does not and vice versa. If a successful mating is chosen the resulting progeny offer greater levels of performance in more traits than their straight-bred parents. Essentially, one would be using the strengths of one breed to offset the weaknesses of another. Researchers provide an example of the usefulness of breed complementarity in terms of matching cattle genetically to their environment and the resulting progeny to the marketplace. In the situation of a herd composed of crossbred Angus-Hereford cows mated to a Charolais bull, the crossbred cow offers the maternal capability along with carcass quality advantages while the Charolais bull will increase growth and carcass yield of his progeny. Thus, the maternally focused cow is a good fit for her environment and the high-growth calf can bring greater value to the marketplace.

System Considerations

There are a variety of breeding systems that can effectively capture the benefits of heterosis. To better illustrate these systems and their advantages see Table 1 below. The improvements in production associated with heterosis are substantial, which raises the question of why cross-breeding is not more widely adopted? One conclusion is that some of these crossbreeding systems do not fit a common-sense ranch management plan.

The average herd size in the United States is 40 cows which creates a barrier for many producers where herd size is limiting their ability to utilize a crossbreeding system.

Furthermore, management of breeding systems where multiple breeding pastures is required poses another obstacle. Another limiter, in an attempt to produce cattle that fall within the parameters of branded beef programs, many producers have trended toward straight-bred herds.

The shortcoming of operating with largely straight-bred cows is it overlooks the advantages of crossbreeding resulting in the cumulative effect of heterosis being lost. If the cows are crossbred, every animal on the ranch is impacted by heterosis, which is a value that can be captured every year regardless of how the calves are marketed.

The added value due to heterosis is not subject to change like other branded beef programs, which makes the "premium" for heterosis very impactful.

Table 1. Production improvements and management considerations associated with crossbreeding systems and heterosis

System	Increase in weight weaned/cow exposed, %	Number of breeding pastures	Minimum herd size
Straight-bred	0	1	Any
Two-breed rotation	16	2	50
Three-breed rotation	20	3	75
Rotational terminal	21	3	100
Composite	12-17	1	Any
Purchased crossbreds with terminal sire	24	1	Any

TYPES OF CROSSBREEDING STRATEGY

1. Two way Cross – Black Belly x Pelibuey
2. Criss-Cross(Two Breed Rotational cross) BB (male) x PB (female) then PB (male) x BB (female)
3. Three way Cross – BB x PB = 50% mix then crossed with Katahdin
4. Three-way Rotational – BBxPbXDP = F1XDP
5. Three-breed Roto-Terminal Crossing

Two Way Cross

In this case, rams of one breed are used to breed ewes of a second breed, resulting in crossbred lambs. This strategy takes advantage of hybrid vigour and/or complimentary breeding in the offspring. Breeding is relatively simple as you are only dealing with one breed of ewes and one breed of ram.

Two breed crossbeef cattle

The two breed cross system produces first cross, or F_1, progeny. In this system, the progeny resulting from the cross of two breeds are usually all sold for slaughter or to another commercial breeder. This system is frequently used in northern New South Wales where there are specific F_1 sales.

The system is most useful for situations in which females of a specific breed are well adapted to a given environment. These adapted females can be mated to a sire of another breed, resulting in heterosis for traits such as growth, improved carcase, feed conversion efficiency and vigour.

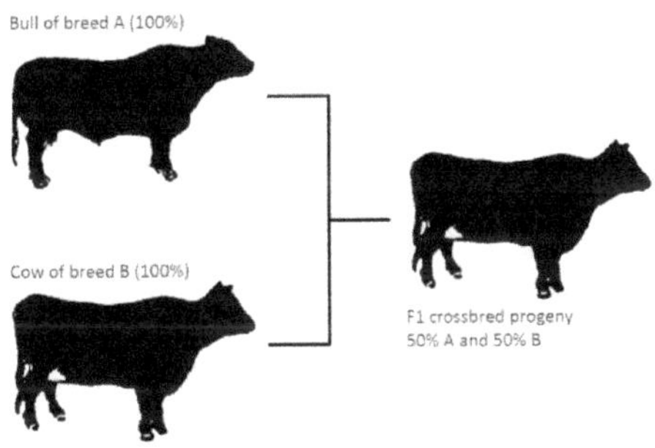

Fig. 1. Two breed cross occurs where breed A and breed B are two purebreds and the F1 progeny (AB) contains equal parts of the two breeds.

Backcross

In a backcross system, all male calves produced from the first cross are sold for slaughter. Female F_1 crossbred progeny are mated to males of one of the parental breeds and all progeny are sold for slaughter. This breeding system takes full advantage of heterosis for maternal traits such as fertility of the cow, and milking/mothering ability (as the mother expresses 100% of possible heterosis) and half of the possible heterosis for growth.

This approach is most useful where adaptation to a specific environment is required from a particular maternal breed but where characteristics from the other parental breed are desired for carcase or growth traits. The crossbred F1 female would also have satisfactory environmental adaptation.

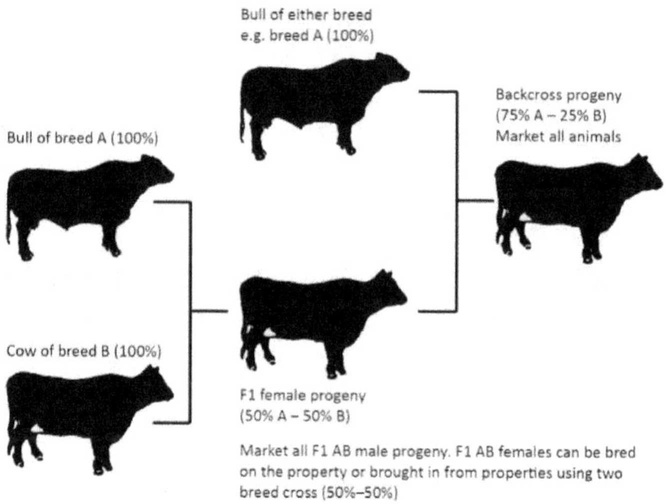

Fig 2. The backcross is obtained where all the females from a two breed cross are mated to a purebred bull of either of the original breeds. All the backcross progeny are marketed.

Continual backcrossing is the system used by producers to upgrade or change from one breed to another without having to buy purebred cows, such as in development of Brahman herds in Queensland.

Criss-Cross (Two breed rotational Cross)

The two-breed rotational cross or criss-cross is a relatively simple and popular form of crossbreeding. In this system, two breeds are mated and the resulting female (F_1) offspring are kept as replacements and mated back to one of the breeds. In following generations (F_2), females are bred to the opposite breed of their sire.

- A Dorper ewe is bred by a Katahdin ram and produce an offspring (F_1-female).
- That F1-female is then mated with a Dorper ram
- That is known as Criss-Cross Rotational Breeding

This strategy mates the two-way crossbred ewe lambs ('F_1' lambs) to a ram of a third breed. The resulting progeny are a mix of three different breeds. This strategy takes advantage of hybrid vigour in the crossbred ewe as well as in the three-way crossed lambs. However, all replacement ewes still need to be purchased. Some producers specialize in producing crossbred ewe lambs for this type of system.

Three way Cross(Three-breed terminal Cross)

In a terminal breeding system, a crossbred ewe (F1) is mated to a terminal purebred ram and all animals are sent to market. Replacement ewes are not kept for mating and therefore must either be purchased or produced separately. Purebreds can be used in a specialized role (i.e. to produce only females or only market sheep) and therefore the strong characteristics of each breed can be fully realized.

Advantages

- Maintain 100% heterosis in both the ewes and market animals.
- Can take full advantage of each purebred breeds strengths.

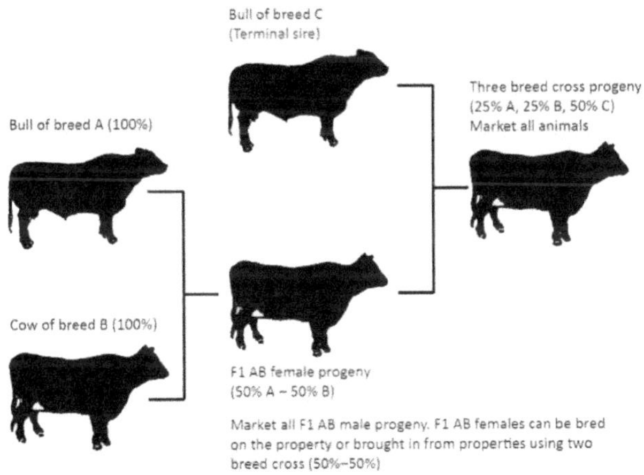

Fig. 3. The three breed cross is obtained when all the females from a two breed cross are mated to a bull of a third, unrelated breed. All the three breed cross progeny are marketed.

- Uniform market animal as every animal produced is the same genetically.
- System is easy to manage if replacement ewes are purchased and all animals produced go to market

Disadvantages

- If F1 female is purchased, this is an additional cost and disease could possibly be introduced into your flock.
- If F1 female is produced by you, it requires more management as two genetic pools must be maintained, one to produce replacement females and one to produce market animals.

Three-Way Rotational Crosses

Similar to the three-way cross, the three way rotational cross starts with mating a crossbred ewe to a ram of a third breed. The crossbred ewe lambs are kept as replacements rather than being sold. These three-way cross ewe lambs are then mated to one of the two breeds in the first cross, and the process continues in the same manner.

Rotational cross

Rotational crossbreeding, sometimes referred to as sequence breeding, is when males of two or more breeds are mated to crossbred females. Over a number of years, each breed will have contributed its strengths and weaknesses equally.

Variation seen in the progeny in early years of a rotational crossbreeding program may make it more difficult to consistently meet a specific market requirement in this production system. When the breeds used are similar, consistency of performance is less likely to be a problem, although levels of heterosis will also be lower if breeds or breed groupings are relatively closely related.

Levels of heterosis achieved in rotational crossbreeding depend on the number of breeds involved. Once stabilised after many crosses, with a number of breeds (n) contributing equally, the level of retained heterosis may be expressed as:

$(2n-2) / (2n-1)$

Rotational crosses express more heterosis than composites which use the same number of breeds. This increased heterosis in rotational systems is a result of close to maximum heterosis being achieved in each cross with the purebreed.

All animals in the herd benefit from heterosis for both growth and maternal traits in rotational crossbreeding. When three or more breeds are used, heterosis levels of 86% or greater may be achieved. These compare very favourably with self-replacing terminal cross systems in which only about half the progeny show heterosis for growth and only a third of progeny benefit from heterosis in their dam.

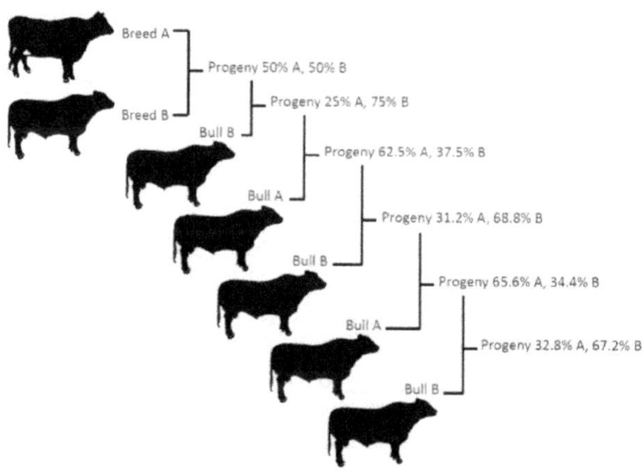

Fig. 4. Starting at 50 50, the rotation stabilises at 65 35 or 35 65, giving 65 from the last sire line used.

In rotational crossbreeding, replacement females are generated for the enterprise from the mating program. All females are potentially available for selection as replacements, whereas in self replacing terminal cross systems, about a third of the heifers are not available for selection. This means a reduced possibility for genetic improvement through heifer selection, placing that pressure on bull selection.

Because in rotational crossbreeding the mating involves several groups of females of different breed combinations with bulls of different breeds, this system has specific management requirements.

Composite breed

Development of a composite or synthetic breed results from the crossing of two or more existing breeds. There are many examples of this in Queensland: Santa Gertrudis, Droughtmaster, Braford, Charbray, Brangus and Belmont Red.

The primary advantage of forming composite breeds is that after the initial crosses are made, management requirements are the same as for straight breeding. Should a market signal indicate a change to the characteristics of the composite, there is opportunity to change direction by incorporating another breed or crossbreed.

The initial choice of breeds must be based on those which have desirable traits for a particular environment and for the target market.

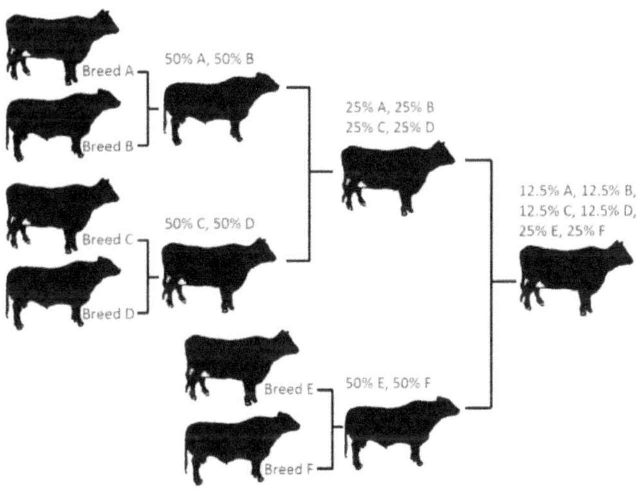

Fig. 5. One simple approach to a composite breed

The percentage of heterosis increases as more breeds contribute in the initial mating program. While the heterosis will not be as high as that achieved with a rotational crossbreeding program with the same number of breeds, the management requirements will be reduced.

For instance, if there are three breeds in a given composite, the amount of retained heterosis would be expected to be (3-1) ÷ 3 or two-thirds or 67%.

Inbreeding is not usually significant when numbers are greater than 200 or 300 breeders. However, in smaller herds inbreeding can be a problem. In the extreme case where a herd uses only one bull all heterosis is lost after approximately eight generations or 40 years.

GLOSSARY

Additive genetic relationship: The additive genetic relationship between two animals is the amount of DNA they share due to the fact that they are related

Additivity: is the assumption that each allele influencing a trait does so independently of the other allele present at that locus and all other alleles at all other loci, e.g. if alleles G and g are worth 1 and -1 respectively then additivity assumes GG is worth 2, Gg is worth 0, and gg is worth –2.

Albumen firmness: Quality description of the albumen (egg white) of an egg. Albumen is judged on the basis of clarity and firmness or thickness. A clear albumen is defined as being free from discolorations or from any foreign bodies.

Animal Model: Mathematical approach to determine the genetic and environmental factors which may affect animal performances. This system allows an accurate prediction of the breeding values of future reproducers. The Animal Model simultaneously evaluates dams (@&) and sires (B&) using all their ancestor relationships. This means that every animal known in a given pedigree is used to evaluate both the dam and sire. This increases the accuracy of evaluation and should be a major step in breeder acceptance of the new evaluation system.

Artificial fertilisation: The bringing together of semen and eggs under laboratory conditions.

Artificial insemination: Collecting semen from a male and bringing this into the genital tract of a female. The advantages of AI are 1) genetic improvement: superior animals can be used more often and more efficiently, 2) control of diseases: a) instead of males, their semen is transported b) semen can be tested for several diseases c) no transmission of venereal diseases.

Atresia ani: Hereditary genetic defect: animals are born without anus.

Allele: An is a version of the sequence of DNA nucleotides at a locus. Not all individuals carry exactly the same sequence of DNA nucleotides at the same locus. This allelic variation is the source of genetic variation

Balanced breeding: Breeding for a combination of characteristics, concerning animal biology, animal health, efficiency, environment, animal welfare and economy.

Bovine Leukocyte Adhesion Deficiency (BLAD): is a hereditary genetic disease (detected in the Holstein breed), an adhesion deficiency of bovine leukocytes to antigens, which shows in calves as not being able to recover after an illness. A DNA-test is available to detect animals that are carriers of the defect allele.

Best Linear Unbiased Prediction (BLUP): A statistical method, that gives the estimation of Breeding Values. This is a rating or breeding quality number and is a prediction of the breeding potential of the individual animal and how likely it is that that animal will improve (or not improve) its offspring. BLUP calculations are used to predict the genetic make-up of an animal for all kinds of traits. With BLUP it is possible to track and predict the different inherited traits through complicated mathematical and statistical calculations.

Bovine Spongiform Encephalopathy (BSE): sometimes known as "mad cow" disease, is a prion disease of cattle first identified in 1986. BSE occurs in adult animals in both sexes, typically in four and five year olds. It is a neurological disease involving pronounced changes in mental state, abnormalities of posture and movement and of sensation. The clinical disease usually lasts for several weeks. Only a small proportion of affected cattle show what would be considered typical "mad cow" signs. Possibly, when humans eat meat from an infected animal, they develop a similar disease. Creutzfeldt-Jacob Disease (CJD) is a rare and fatal neurodegenerative disease of unknown cause.

Breeding organisation (BO): Organisation involved in the breeding of farm animals.

Breeding value: The estimated genetic value of an individual. The part of an individual's genotypic value that is due to independent and therefore transmittable gene effects.

Broiler: A type of chicken bred for meat production.

Breeding goal: is the specification of the traits to be improved including the emphasis given to each trait. It gives the direction in which the population should improve.

Breeding program: is a program aiming at defined breeding objectives for the production of a next generation of animals. It is the combination of recording selected traits, the estimation of breeding values, the selection of potential parents and a mating programme for the selected parents including appropriate (artificial) reproduction methods.

Breeding value: is the mean genetic value of an individual as a parent for a trait. It is estimated as twice the average superiority of the individual's progeny relative to all other progeny under conditions of random mating

Challenge test: Tests designed to identify differences between individuals, families, lines or strain crosses in their ability to cope with diseases or stress factors likely to be encountered in practice. Results from challenge tests are used to select relatives for improved resistance. In case of transmittable diseases, test farms are operated with maximal bio-security.

Cloning (Somatic): Producing offspring with the same genetic information, e.g. embryonic cloning, identical twins.

Complex Vertebral Malformation (CVM): Genetic defect in cattle associated with the disorder range from earlier embryonic death to late term stillborn calves with neck and leg deformities. A DNA-test is available to detect animals that are carrier of the defect allele.

Congenital defects: Defects present at birth.

Cryopreservation: Preservation by means of freezing, e.g. semen, embryos.

Cryptorchism: Hereditary genetic disease (genetic defect) in which testicles are not descended.

Chromosome: A is a discrete block of DNA and is one of the basic structures of the genome. All nuclear DNA is organized into chromosomes with the number varying between animal species. Genes on a chromosome are linked and tend to be inherited.

Co-dominance: is a situation in which a heterozygote shows the phenotypic effects of both alleles equally. See 'Additivity'.

DNA: is Deoxyribonucleic Acid, which is a macromolecule in the form of a doublestranded helix that carries the genetic information in all cells in higher organisms

Dominant allele: A dominant allele is an allele which has an effect on the phenotype not only when it is homozygous but also when it is heterozygous. When allele E is dominant over e, EE and Ee have the same phenotypic value.

Embryo transfer: Recovering embryos from a donor animal and transferring these embryos to a recipient animal.

Environment: The can be defined as anything that influences the animal's performance that is not related to the genetic makeup of the animal, starting at the earliest possible moment in life, even before conception.

Epistasis: is when loci are non-additive. The genotypic value of a locus on a trait depends upon the genotypes at other loci or a situation in which the differential phenotypic expression of a genotype depends on the genotype at another locus.

Farm Animal Breeding: Strategies applied by specialized farmers to increase desirable traits selecting the appropriate animals as ancestors of the new generations.

Fry: Young fish at an early stage.

Gene: A is the hereditary unit, a region of DNA on a chromosome containing genetic information which is transcribed into RNA and is translated into a polypeptide chain with a physiological function. A gene can mutate to various forms called alleles

Genome wide selection (genomic selection): Use of total breeding values for juvenile animals, predicted from a large number of estimated marker haplotype effects across the whole genome. Single Nucleotide Polymorphisms (SNPs) are used as high density markers in genome wide selection.

Genetic diversity: High variety of alleles of genes within a population.

Genomics: Study of an organism's genome and the use of the genes (the genes of a cell, or tissue, at the DNA (genotype), mRNA (transcriptome), or protein (proteome) levels). It deals with the systematic use of genome information, associated with other data, to provide answers in biology, medicine and industry. The field includes intensive efforts to determine the entire DNA sequence of organisms and fine-scale genetic mapping efforts, and also includes studies of intragenomic phenomena such as heterosis, epistasis, pleiotropy and other interactions between loci and alleles within the genome. The major tools and methods related to genomics are bioinformatics, genetic analysis, measurement of gene expression, and determination of gene function. Such identified genes can be called major genes located at Quantitative Trait Loci (QTL). Although the term QTL strictly applies to genes of any effect, in practice it refers only to major genes, as only these will be large enough to be detected and mapped on the genome. Following the pattern of inheritance at such QTL might assist in selection.

Haugh Units: A measure of the firmness of albumen in the eggs, correcting albumen height for variable egg weight (layer chicken).

Hermaphrodism: Biological mode of reproduction in which an individual presents alternatively or simultaneously male and female territory in its gonad.

Heritability: Always is estimated for a specific population in a specific environment because it reflects the genetic variation for a trait in that specific population relative to the phenotypic population

Heterozygote: Heterozygote is an individual carrying two distinct alleles at a locus, e.g. Ee.

Homozygote: Homozygote is an individual carrying two copies of the same allele at a locus, e.g. ee or EE.

IMF: Intramuscular fat or marbling of muscle meat.

Inbreeding: genes that two animals have in common due to common anchestors. Inbreeding can be used to increase genetic variation between families in order to increase response to selection. In commercial breeding programmes, inbreeding is seldom used. Loss of genetic diversity due to inbreeding depends on effective population size and selection intensity.

Interbull: International breeding value estimation in dairy cattle. Interbull is a non-profit organisation, responsible for the standardisation of international genetic evaluations for cattle. In practice this means, that a French farmer may use semen from a South American bull with known breeding value for French conditions, because the international breeding value is comparable globally. There is an extensive international trade of bull semen, globally.

In vitro embryo production: The production of embryos outside an animals' body using sperm and unfertilised eggs.

infinitesimal model: The infinitesimal model assumes that all traits are determined by an infinite number of genes, each with an infinitely small effect. This assumption results in a smooth bell-shaped distribution that can be described by the Normal Distribution. This distribution implies a number of rules that animal breeding theory is built on.

Layer: A type of chicken bred for efficient egg production.

Leucosis: A malignant disease of the lymphatic system in chickens, caused by a virus.

Locus: A is a position on a chromosome, for example of a gene. The plural is loci

Marker assisted selection (MAS): Selection using genomic markers. The idea behind marker assisted selection is that there may be genes with significant effects that may be targeted specifically in selection. Some traits are controlled by single genes (e.g. hair colour) but most traits of economic importance are quantitative traits that most likely are controlled by a fairly large number of genes. However, some of these genes might have a larger effect.

Mass selection: A form of selection in which only individuals with phenotypic values greater or less than a threshold level are used for breeding. It involves no use of family information. (Compare with pedigree selection).

Mastitis: Mammary gland or udder inflammation caused by various species of bacteria.

MF: Mule Foot is a genetic defect in cattle expressed as fused hoofs. A marker-test is available to detect animals that are carriers of the defect allele.

Monofactorial genetic effects: One gene being responsible for a certain genetic effect, e.g. halothane gene, BLAD, CVM.

Monosex population: production of population of animals of only one phenotypic sex by gamete management (sperm sexing, gynogenesis, sex inversion) or by the control of environmental factors as grading or for example in fish by the application of hot or cold temperature during the sexual differentiation period.

Muscle hypertrophy: Extreme growth of skeletal muscle as in some breeds of cattle, sheep, pigs (double muscling).

Mycoplasma: Pathogenic bacteria causing many diseases of humans, plants and animals. Due to their specific structure they have low sensitivity to the effect of antibiotics. In addition, the majority of mycoplasms are capable of evading the hosts' immune system; therefore, they can exist in an animal for a long time, often for the entire lifespan.

Meiosis: is the process carried out in the germ cells by which gametes are formed. In diploids this involves the creation of haploid cells (sperm, oocytes) from the diploid progenitor cells

Mendelian Sampling: The Mendelian Sampling term indicates the chance factor in distributing half the genetic material from each parent to their offspring.

Mendelian: sampling is the random sampling of parental genes caused by segregation and independent assortment of genes during germ cell formation, and by random selection of gametes in the formation of the embryo

N and P emission: All animals require Nitrogen and Phosphorus in their feed and when they produce manure it will contain some N and P. This is brought into the environment, e.g. grassland or arable land. If the growth period and need of the crop are not consistent with the amount of N (Nitrogen) or P (Phosphorus) brought on the land, N and P may leak into the air, lakes, rivers or ground water. Animals digesting their feed efficiently will pollute the environment less.

Oestrus induction: Hormonal stimulation of oestrus at desired moment to ensure a better control and care of reproducers and offspring.

Osteoporosis: Osteoporosis is a disease in which bones become fragile and more likely to break.

Overdominance: occurs when the heterozygote has a genotypic value higher than either parent.

Polledness: An animal born without the potential to grow horns.

Production system: The production system represents a set of decisions and activities by which the improvement, reproduction, maintenance, breeding and feeding of animals are organized and conducted, their health is ensured, the forms of organization of breeders are conceived. All this in correlation with biological and production requirements, in terms of economic efficiency, environmental sustainability and social acceptance.

Recessive allele: A is an allele which only has an effect on the phenotype when it is homozygous. Therefore if allele e is recessive, ee yields a different phenotype from Ee and EE, which have the same phenotype.

RYR-1 gene: Also known as halothane gene, is a gene that encodes for the skeletal muscle rynodine receptor in pigs. The locus RYR-1 has two alleles (N: normal, dominant and n: halothane sensitivity, recessive). Pigs with nn or Nn genotype are more susceptible to stressful stimuli. This pork gene causes the pork to be pale, soft, and exudative. A DNA-test has been developed to detect this gene in pigs, so that the pigs carrying this gene are not used for selection. It was the first genome test in farm animal breeding.

Salmonella: Salmonella is a bacterium. There is a widespread occurrence in animals, especially in poultry and swine. Environmental sources of the organism include water, soil, insects, factory surfaces, kitchen surfaces, animal faeces, raw meats, raw poultry, and raw seafoods. Humans infected with Salmonella bacteria can get nausea, abdominal cramps, diarrhea, fever, headache or vomit.

Somatic cell count: The somatic cell count (SCC) is commonly used as a measure of milk quality. Somatic cells are simply animal body cells present at low levels in normal milk. High levels of these cells in milk indicate abnormal, reduced-quality milk that is caused by an intramammary bacterial infection (mastitis).

Sperm sexing: Separation of male and female spermatozoa. After the sexing procedure, the semen can be used to produce predominantly male or female offspring.

Splayleg: Sows sometimes sit on their unwary offspring and kill them, and any degree of locomotor impairment in baby pigs increases this risk. Splayleg is a condition in which the hindlimbs and sometimes the forelimbs of a newborn pig temporarily are unable to support the body. If affected pigs are nursed through the period of high risk just after farrowing, they may compensate by enhanced synthesis of muscle proteins and then may grow normally. Slippery floors make the splayleg problem worse. Affected pigs may be helped with a loose coupling between the hindlimbs to prevent the limbs splaying outwards.

Sudden death syndrome: Birds (broiler chickens) which have died suddenly are found on their backs with no other obvious pathology. The cause is probably metabolic. It can be induced by lactic acidosis and about 70% of birds affected are males.

Sustainability: Sustainability in farm animal breeding and reproduction means the extent to which animal breeding and reproduction, as managed by professional organisations, contribute to maintenance and good care of animal genetic resources for present and future generations (www.sefabar.org).

Traceability: Organisation of a production process in such a way that all the steps can be 'traced'. E.g. when a piece of meat is bought in a supermarket, it should be possible to 'trace' back to the farm where it was produced, and to the parents of the animal .

Transgenic: Animals with an artificially modified gene or a gene of another species introduced into their genome, e.g. a gene that can produce milk causing no allergic reactions in humans. Introducing such a different gene into an organism is called 'genetic modification': GM

Triploidy: biological mechanism happening in which an individual developed with 3 sets of chromosomes (i.e.: 2 of its mother and 1 from his father) instead of 2 in diploids (1 from each of its parents).

True breeding value (A): The true breeding value (A) of an animal is its additive genetic component, half is which is inherited by the offspring

Variance component: Variation in a population is `expressed in a variance component. The symbol for a variance component is s_2 and the subscript indicates what type of variance component it is: P, G, or E. The genetic component consists of three underlying effects: 1. The epistatic effect: interaction between genes 2. The dominance effect: interaction between alleles of the same gene 3. The additive effect: everything that is left over after correcting for the interacting effects

Weaning: Accustom animals to do without the mother's milk (mammals) or leaving prey (fish).

Yolk/albumen ratio: Amount of yolk compared to amount of albumen in an egg. It can be used as a measure of egg quality in layer breeding programmes.

Zoonotic disease: Disease that can be transmitted from animals to humans.

Zoonotic risk: Risk that an animal disease will be transmitted to humans.

BIBLIOGRAPHY

Abplanalp, H. 1990. Inbreeding. In Poultry breeding and genetics (ed. Crawford, R.D.), pp. 955–984. Elsevier, Amsterdam.

Adkison, L.R., Skow L.C., Thomas T.L., Petrash M., Womack J.E. (1988). Somatic cell mapping and restriction fragment analysis of bovine genes for fibronectin and gamma crystallin. Cytogenet. Cell. Genet. 47: 155–159.

Alison, VE, Davis UC (2009) Potential effects of biotechnology on animal health and well-being. Applications of Animal Biotechnology in Animal Health, Department of Animal Science, University of California, California 1-5.

Andersen, B.B., Jensen, B., Nielsen, A., Christensen, L. G. and Liboriussen, T. 2003. Rød Dansk Malkerace - avlsmæssigt og kulturhistorisk belyst. Report no. 50 in animal husbandry from the Danish Institute of Agricultural Sciences.

Anderson, V.L. and Kempthorne, O. 1954. A model for the study of quantitative inheritance. Genetics 9: 883–898.

Areal, F, Riesgo L, Gómez-Barbero M, Rodríguez-Cerezo E (2012) Consequence of a coexistence policy on the adoption of GMHT crops in the European Union. Food Policy 37(4): 401-411.

Asaye, M, Biyazen H, Girma M (2014) Genetic engineering in animal production: Applications and prospects. Biochem Biotechnol Res 2(2): 12-22.

Ayana, E, Fentahun G, Gizachew, Negash A, Mitku F, et al. (2017) Review on Applications of Genetic Engineering and Cloning in Farm animal 4(1)

Ballou, J.D. 1997. Ancestral inbreeding only minimally affects inbreeding depression in mammalian populations. Journal of Heredity 8: 169–178.

Belonsky, G.M. and Kennedy, B.W. 1988. Selection on individual phenotype and best linear unbiased predictor of breeding value in a closed swine herd. Journal of Animal Science 66: 1124–1131.

Bijlsma, R., Bundgaard, J. and Boerema, A.C. 2000. Does inbreeding affect the extinction risk of small populations?: predictions from Drosophila. Journal of Evolutionary Biology 3: 502–514.

Bijlsma, R., Bundgaard, J. and Van Putten, W.F. 1999. Environmental dependence of inbreeding depression and purging in Drosophila melanogaster. Journal of Evolutionary Biology 12: 1125–1137.

Blasco, A (2007) The role of genetic engineering in livestock production Livestock Science 113(2-3): 191-201.

Bohren, B.B., Hill, W.G. and Robertson, A. 1966. Some observations on asymmetrical correlated responses to selection. Genetical Research 7: 44–57.

Boichard D (2016) Genomic selection in domestic animals: Principles, applications and perspectives compte rendus biologies 339(7-8): 274-277.

Bolormaa S (2010) Multivariate analysis of a genome wide association study in dairy cattle. Journal of dairy science 93(8): 3818-3833.

Brem, G., Brenig, B., Muller, M., Springmann, K., (1989) Ex situ cryoconservation of genomes and genes of endangered cattle breeds by means of modern biotechnological methods. FAO Animal Production and Health Paper No.76

Briskie, J.V. and Mackintosh, M. 2004. Hatching failure increases with severity of population bottlenecks in birds. Proceedings of the National Academy of Sciences of the United States of America 101: 558–561.

Bruce, A.B. 1910. The Mendelian theory of heredity and the augmentation of vigor. Science 32: 627–628.

Bryant, E.H. and Meffert, L. M. 1988. Effect of an experimental bottleneck on morphological integration in the housefly. Evolution 42: 698–707.

Bryant, E.H., McCommas, S.A. and Combs, L.M. 1986. The effect of an experimental bottleneck upon quantitative genetic variation in the housefly. Genetics 114: 1191–1211.

Buri, P. 1956. Gene frequency in small populations of mutant Drosophila. Evolution 10: 367–402.

Charlesworth, B. 1998. The effect of synergistic epistasis on the inbreeding load. Genetical Research 71: 85–89.

Charlesworth, B. and Charlesworth, D. 1999. The genetic basis of inbreeding depression. Genetical Research 74: 329–340.

Charlesworth, D. and Charlesworth, B. 1987. Inbreeding depression and its evolutionary consequences. Annual Review of Ecology and Systematics 18: 237–268.

Christensen, L. G. and Pedersen, J. 1988. [Crossbreeding of dairy cattle.] Report no. 650 from the National Institute of Animal Science, Denmark, Copenhagen.

Clayton, G.A., Morris, J.A. and Robertson, A. 1957. An experimental check on quantitative genetical theory. I. Short-term responses to selection. Journal of Genetics 55: 131–151.

Clutton-Brock, Juliet. Domesticated Animals from Early Times. Austin: University of Texas Press, 1981.

Cockerham, C.C. 1984. Additive by additive variance with inbreeding and linkage. Genetics 108: 487–500.

Cockerham, C.C. and Weir, B.S. 1973. Descent measures for two loci with some applications. Theoretical Population Biology 4: 300–330.

Cockerham, C.C. and Weir, B.S. 1983. Variance of actual inbreeding. Theoretical Population Biology 23: 85–109.

Cockerham, C.C. and Weir, B.S. 1984. Covariances of relatives stemming from a population undergoing mixed self and random mating. Biometrics 40: 157–164.

Conrad G, Harold C (2009) Acceptable Genes. Religious, Traditional and Genetically Modified Foods State University of New York Press, Albany, pp 135-140.

Crnokrak, P. and Barrett, S.C.H. 2002. Purging the genetic load: a review of the experimental evidence. Evolution 56: 2347–2358.

Crnokrak, P. and Roff, D.A. 1999. Inbreeding depression in the wild. Heredity 83: 260–270.

Crow, J.F. 1993. Mutation, mean fitness, and genetic load. In Oxford surveys in evolutionary biology (ed. Futuyma, D. and Antonovics, J.), pp. 3–42. Oxford University Press, NY.

Crow, J.F. and Kimura, M. 1970. An introduction to population genetics theory. Harper and Row, NY.

Curran G, Koszarycz Y (2004) Genetic engineering: Creating an ethical framework. Australian Journal of Theology 2: 1-6.

Darwin, Charles. The Variation of Animals and Plants under Domestication. Washington Square: New York University Press, 1988.

Darwin, C. 1868. The variation of animals and plants under domestication. John Murray, London.

Darwin, C. 1876. The effects of cross and self-fertilization in the vegetable kingdom. Appleton, NY.

Davenport, C.B. 1908. Degeneration, albinism, and inbreeding. Science 28: 454–455.

Davis L.G., Dibner M.D., and Battey J.F., (1986). "Basic Methods In Molecular Biology", Elsevier Science Publishing Co, Inc., New York.

Day, S.B., Bryant, E.H. and Meffert, L.M. 2003. The infuence of variable rates of inbreeding on fitness, environmental responsiveness, and evolutionary potential. Evolution 57: 1314–1324.

Denning C, Priddle H (2003) New frontiers in gene targeting and cloning: success, application and challenges in domestic animals and human embryonic stem cells. Reproduction 126(1): 1-11.

DeRose, M.A. and Roff, D.A. 1999. A comparison of inbreeding depression in life-history and morphological traits in animals. Evolution 53: 1288–1292.

Drinkwater R.D., Hediger R., Hetzel D.J.S., (1990). "Polymorphism and location of minisatellite sequences in sheep", Proc. 13th World Congr. on Genetics Applied to Livestock Production, Edinburgh 129–132.

Dudash, M.R. 1990. Relative fitness of selfed and outcrossed progeny in a self-compatible, protandrous species, Sabatia angularis L. (Gentianaceae): A comparison in three environments. Evolution 44: 1129–1139.

Edwards M.D., Stuber C.W., Wendel J.F., (1987). Molecular - marker - facilitated investigations of quantitative - trait loci in maize. I. Numbers, genomic distribution and types of gene action. Genetics 116: 113–125.

Ehiobu, N.G., Goddard, M.E. and Taylor, J.F. 1989. Effect of rate of inbreeding on inbreeding depression in Drosophila melanogaster. Theoretical and Applied Genetics 77: 123–127.

Ellegren, H., Hartman, G., Johansson, M. and Andersson, L. 1993. Major histocompatibility complex monomorphism and low levels of DNA fingerprinting variability in a reintroduced and rapidly expanding population of beavers. Proceedings of the National Academy of Sciences of the United States of America 90: 8150–8153.

Falconer D.S., (1981). Introduction to quantitative genetics, Second edition Longman, London and New York.

Falconer, D.S. and Mackay, T.F.C. 1996. Introduction to quantitative genetics. Longman, Harlow.

Fernández, A., Toro, M.A. and López-Fanjul, C. 1995. The effect of inbreeding on the redistribution of genetic variance of fecundity and viability in Tribolium castaneum. Heredity 75: 376–381.

Fowler, K. and Whitlock, M.C. 1999a. The distribution of phenotypic variance with inbreeding. Evolution 53: 1143–1156.

Fowler, K. and Whitlock, M.C. 1999b. The variance in inbreeding depression and the recovery of fitness in bottlenecked populations. Proceedings of the Royal Society of London, series B 266: 2061–2066.

Frankel, O.H. and Soulé, M.E. 1981. Conservation and evolution. Cambridge University Press, Cambridge.

Frankham, R. 1999. Resolving conceptual issues in conservation genetics: the roles of laboratory species and meta-analysis. Hereditas 130: 195–201.

Frankham, R., Ballou, J.D. and Briscoe, D.A. 2002. Introduction to conservation genetics. Cambridge University Press, Cambridge.

Frankham, R., Gilligan, D.M., Morris, D. and Briscoe, D.A. 2001. Inbreeding and extinction: effects of purging. Conservation Genetics 2: 279–285.

Franklin, I.R. 1980. Evolutionary change in small populations. In Conservation biology: an evolutionary-ecological perspective (ed. Soulé, M.E. and Wilcox, B.A.), pp. 135–150. Sinauer, Sunderland, MA.

Franklin, I.R. and Frankham, R. 1998. How large must populations be to retain evolutionary potential? Animal Conservation 1: 69–70.

Frewer L van der Lans I, Fischer A, Reinders M, Menozzi D, et al. (2013) Public Perceptions of Agri-food Applications of Genetic Modification A Systematic Review and Meta-Analysis. Trends in Food Science and Technology 30(2): 142-152.

Fu, Y.-B., Namkoong, G. and Carlson, J.E. 1998. Comparison of breeding strategies for purging inbreeding depression via simulation. Conservation Biology 12: 856–864.

García, N., López-Fanjul, C. and García-Dorado, A. 1994. The genetics of viability in Drosophila melanogaster: effects of inbreeding and artificial selection. Evolution 48: 1277–1285.

Georges M., Mishra A., Sargent L., Steele N., Zhao X., (1990). "Progress toward a primary DNA marker map in cattle", Proc. 13th World Congr. on Genetic Applications to Livestock Production, Edinburgh 107–112.

Gething, M.-J. and Sambrook, J. 1992. Protein folding in the cell. Nature 355: 33–45.

Good, R.L. and Hallauer, A.R. 1977. Inbreeding depression in maize by selfing and self-sibbing. Crop Science 17: 935–940.

Goodnight, C.J. 1987. On the effect of founder events on epistatic genetic variance. Evolution 41: 80–91.

Goodnight, C.J. 1988. Epistasis and the effect of founder events on the additive genetic variance. Evolution 42: 441–454.

Hallauer, A.R. and Sears, J.H. 1973. Changes in quantitative traits associated with inbreeding in a synthetic variety of maize. Crop Science 13: 327–330.

Hediger, R., Ansari H.A., Stranzinger G.F., (1991). Chromosome banding and gene localizations support extensive conservation of chromosome structure between cattle and sheep. Cytogenetics and Cell Genetics. 57: 127–134.

Hediger, R., Johnson, S.E., Barendse, W., Drinkwater, R., Moore, S. and Hetzel, D.J.S., (1990). Assignment of the growth hormone gene locus to 19q26-qter in cattle and to 11q25-qter in sheep by in situ hybridization, Genomics 8: 171–174.

Hedrick, P.W. 1994. Purging inbreeding depression and the probability of extinction: full-sib mating. Heredity 73: 363–372.

Hedrick, P.W. and Kalinowski, S.T. 2000. Inbreeding depression in conservation biology. Annual Review of Ecology and Systematics 31: 139–162.

Hetzel D.J.S., (1991). The Use of Reference Families For Genome Mapping in Domestic Livestock. In a Gene-Mapping Techniques and Applications, ed Schook L.B., Lewin H.A., McLaren D.G., Marcel Dekker Inc. New York, p51–64.

Hetzel D.J.S., Drinkwater R.D., Aspden W.J., (1989). Towards an RFLP marker for Pompe's disease in cattle, Anim. Genet. 20: 25.

Hilbert, P., et al., (1989). Analysis of genetic variation in the Belgian Blue cattle breed using DNA sequence polymorphism at the growth hormone, low density lipoprotein receptor, alpha-subunit of glycoprotein hormones and thyroglobulin loci, Anim. Genet. 20: 383–394.

Hill, W.G. and Robertson, A. 1966. The effects of linkage on limits of artificial selection. Genetical Research 8: 269–294.

Hoelzel, A.R., Halley, J., O'Brien, S.J., Campagna, C., Arnbom, T., Le Boeuf, B., Ralls, K. and Dover, G.A. 1993. Elephant seal genetic variation and the use of simulation models to investigate historical population bottlenecks. Journal of Heredity 84: 443–449.

Hoeschele, I. 1991. Additive and nonadditive genetic variance in female fertility of Holsteins. Journal of Dairy Science 74: 1743–1752.

Hollis D, Chapman R, Panaretto B, Moore G (2004) Morphological changes in the skin and wool fibers of Merino sheep infused with mouse epidermal growth factor. Aust J BiolSci 36(4): 419-34.

Hugon HM (2006) Genetic engineering applications in animal breeding. Elect J Biotechnol, 9: 158-162.

Ibtisham F, Zhang L, Xiao M, Lilong A, Muhammad B, et al. (2017) Genomic selection and its application in animal breeding. 47(3): 301-310.

Izquierdo, Marta (2001) Genetic engineering transference engineering. 2nd Madrid, Edicione Pirámide, pp. 344.

Jacob H.J., Lindpaintner K., et al (1991). Genetic Mapping of a Gene Causing Hypertension in the Stroke-Prone Spontaneously Hypertensive Rat. Cell. 213–224.

James DM, Gary BA (2000) Genetic engineering and cloning may improve milk, livestock production. California Agric 54: 62-63.

Jeffreys A.J., Wilson V., Thein S.L., (1985). Hypervariable 'minisatellite' regions in human DNA, Nature 314: 65–73.

Jiang L (2010) Genome wide association studies for milk production traits in Chinese Holstein PLoS One 5(10): e13661.

Jonas E, Koning D (2015) Genomic selection needs to be carefully assessed to meet specific requirements in livestock breeding programs. Frontiers in Genetics 6: 49.

Jones, D.F. 1917. Dominance of linked factors as a means of accounting for heterosis. Genetics 2: 466–479.

Joron, M. and Brakefield, P.M. 2003. Captivity masks inbreeding effects on male mating success in butterflies. Nature 424: 191–194.

Karkkainen, K., Kuittinen, H., Treuren, R. van Vogl, C., Oikarinen, S. and Savolainen, O. 1999. Genetic basis of inbreeding depression in Arabis petraea. Evolution 53: 1354–1365.

Karp, Gerald (2008) Cell and Molecular Biology: concepts and Experiments. 3rd New York, Willey, 785 p. ISBN04-714-6580.

Kashi Y., Soller M., Hallerman E., Beckmann J.S., (1986). Restriction Fragment Length Polymorphisms in Dairy Cattle Genetic Improvement. In Proc. of the Third World Congress on Genetics Applied to Livestock Production, Nebraska, 12: 57–63.

Keeble, F. and Pellew, C. 1910. The mode of inheritance of stature and of time of flowering in peas Pisum sativum. Journal of Genetics 1: 869–876.

Keller, L.F. and Waller, D.M. 2002. Inbreeding effects in wild populations. Trends in Ecology and Evolution 17: 230–241.

Kolmodin, R., Strandberg, E., Jorjani, H. and Danell, B. 2003. Selection in the presence of a genotype by environment interaction: response in environmental sensitivity. Animal Science 76: 375–385.

Kristensen, T.N., Dahlgaard, J. and Loeschcke, V. 2002. Inbreeding affects Hsp 70 expression in two species of Drosophila even at benign temperatures. Evolutionary Ecology Research 4: 1209–1216.

Kristensen, T.N., Dahlgaard, J. and Loeschcke, V. 2003. Effects of inbreeding and environmental stress on fitness-using Drosophila buzzatii as a model organism. Conservation Genetics 4: 453–465.

Kristensen, T.N., Sørensen, A.C., Sorensen, D., Pedersen, K.S., Sørensen, J.G. and Loeschcke, V. 2005. A test of quantitative genetic theory using Drosophila – effects of inbreeding and rate of inbreeding on heritabilities and variance components. Journal of Evolutionary Biology In press.

Laikre, L., Ryman, N. and Thompson, E.A. 1993. Hereditary blindness in a captive wolf (Canis lupus) population. Conservation Biology 7: 592–601.

Lande, R. 1979. Quantitative genetic analysis of multivariate evolution, applied to brain: body size allometry. Evolution 33: 402–416.

Lande, R. 1995. Mutation and conservation. Conservation Biology 9: 782–791.

Lander, E.S., Botstein, D., (1989) Mapping mendelian factors underlying quantitative traits using RFLP linkage maps. Genetics 121: 185–199

Latter, B.D.H., Mulley, J.C., Reid, D. and Pascoe, L. 1995. Reduced genetic load revealed by slow inbreeding in Drosophila melanogaster. Genetics 139: 287–297.

Latter, R. and Robertson, A. 1962. The effects of inbreeding and artificial selection on reproductive fitness. Genetical Research 3: 110–138.

Lerner, I.M. 1954. Genetic homeostasis. Oliver and Boyd, Edinburgh.

Lewontin, R.C. 1974. The analysis of variance and the analysis of causes. American Journal of Human Genetics 26: 400–411.

Li H., Gyllensten U.B., Cui X., Saiki R.K., Erlich H.A., Arnheim N., (1988). Amplification and analysis of DNA sequences in single human sperm and diploid cells. Nature 335: 414–417.

Li, Z.K., Luo, L.J., Mei, H.W., Wang, D.L., Shu, Q.Y., Tabien, R., Zhong, D.B., Ying, C.S., Stansel, J.W., Khush, G.S. and Paterson, A.H. 2001. Overdominant epistatic loci are the primary genetic basis of inbreeding depression and heterosis in rice.I. Biomass and grain yield. Genetics 158: 1737–1753.

LibreTexts Libraries (LTL) (2019) Genetically Engineered Vaccines.

López-Fanjul, C. and Villaverde, A. 1989. Inbreeding increases genetic variance for viability in Drosophila melanogaster. Evolution 43: 1800–1804.

López-Fanjul, C., Fernández, A. and Toro, M.A. 1999. The role of epistasis in the increase in the additive genetic variance after population bottlenecks. Genetical Research 73: 45–59.

López-Fanjul, C., Fernández, A. and Toro, M.A. 2000. Epistasis and the conversion of non-additive genetic variance at population bottlenecks. Theoretical Population Biology 58: 49–59.

López-Fanjul, C., Fernández, A. and Toro, M.A. 2002. The effect of epistasis on the excess of the additive and nonadditive variances after population bottlenecks. Evolution 56: 865–876.

López-Fanjul, C., Guerra, J. and García, A. 1989. Changes in the distribution of the genetic variance of a quantitative trait in small populations of Drosophila melanogaster. Genetics, Selection, Evolution 21: 159–168.

Lund M (2011) A common reference population from four European Holstein populations increases reliability of genomic predictions. Genetics Selection Evolution evolution/ 43(1): 43.

Luty, J.A., et al., (1990). Five polymorphic microsatellite VNTR's on the human X chromosome, Am. J. Hum, Genet. 46: 776–783.

Lynch, M. 1988. Design and analysis of experiments on random drift and inbreeding depression. Genetics 120: 791–807.

Lynch, M. and Walsh, B. 1998. Genetics and analysis of quantitative traits. Sinauer Associates, Sunderland, MA.

MacLennan D.H., Duff C., Zorzato F., Fujii J., Phillips M., Korneluk R.G., Frodis W., Britt B.A., and Worton R.G. (1990). Nature 343: 559–562.

Madsen, T., Shine, R., Olsson, M. and Wittzell, H. 1999. Restoration of an inbred adder population. Nature 402: 34–35.

Malécot, P. 1948. Les mathématiques de l'hérédité. Masson, Paris.

Man, W.Y.N., James, J.W. and Nicholas, F.W. 2002. Effect of inbreeding contribution from particular ancestors: a preliminary analysis of first lactation milk yields from Holstein Friesians in Australia. Proceedings of the seventh world congress on genetics applied to livestock production,Montpellier, CD-ROM communication[23–01].

Martin B., Nienhuis J., King G., Schaeffer A. (1989). Restriction fragment length polymorphisms associated with water use efficiency in tomato. Science 243: 1725–1727.

Mason I.L., (1988). Evolution of Domesticated Animals. Longman. Harlow. U.K.

Meagher, S., Penn, D.J. and Potts, W.K. 2000. Male-male competition magnifies inbreeding depression in wild house mice. Proceedings of the National Academy of Sciences of the United States of America 97: 3324–3329.

Mega EA, Shoemaker CF, Rowe JD, BonDurant RH, Anderson GB, et al. (2006) Production and processing of milk from transgenic goats expressing human lysozyme in the mammary gland. J Dairy Sci 89(2): 518-524.

Melo E, Canavessi A, Franco M, Rumpf R (2007) Animal trangenesis: state of the art and applications. J Appl Genet 48(1): 47-61.

Meuwissen, T.H.E. 1997. Maximizing the response of selection with a predefined rate of inbreeding. Journal of Animal Science 75: 934–940.

Meuwissen, T.H.E. and Woolliams, J.A. 1994. Effective sizes of livestock populations to prevent a decline in fitness. Theoretical and Applied Genetics 89: 1019–1026.

Miglior, F., Burnside, E.B. and Hohenboken, W.D. 1994. Heterogeneity among families of Holstein cattle in inbreeding depression for production traits. Proceedings of the fifth world congress on genetics applied to livestock production, Guelph, vol. 18, pp. 479–482.

Miglior, F., Burnside, E.B. and Kennedy, B.W. 1995. Production traits of Holstein cattle: estimation of nonadditive genetic variance components and inbreeding depression. Journal of Dairy Science 78: 1174–1180.

Misztal, I., Lawlor, T.J. and Gengler, N. 1997. Relationships among estimates of inbreeding depression, dominance and additive variance for linear traits in Holsteins. Genetics, Selection, Evolution 29: 319–326.

Mitton, J.B. 1993. Enzyme heterozygosity, metabolism, and developmental stability. Genetica 89: 47–65.

Mora C, Menozzi D, Kleter G, lusine H, Ara M, et al. (2012) Factors Acting the Adoption of Genetically Modifed Animals in the Food and Pharmaceutical Chains, Bio-based and Applied Economics 1(3): 313-329.

Muller M, Brem G (1998) Transgenic approaches to the increase of disease resistance in farm animals. Revue Scientifique et Technique-Office International Des Epizooties 17: 365-373.

Murray J, Mohamad-Fauzi N, Cooper C, Maga E (2010) Current status of transgenic animal research for human health applications. Acta Scientiae Veterinariae 38(Suppl 2): 627-632.

Nadeau J.H., (1989). Maps of linkage and synteny homologies between mouse and man. Trends in Genet 5: 82–86.

Neim, M. (1972). American Naturalist 106: 283–292.

Nicholas, F.W. and Smith, C. 1983. Increased rates of genetic change in dairy cattle by embryo transfer and splitting. Animal Production 36: 341–353.

Nyerhovwo J (2004) Fostering biotechnology entrepreneurship in developing countries. Afr J Biotechnol 3: 291-300.

O'Brien S.J., and Marshall-Greaves J.A. (1992). Report of the Committee on Comparative Gene Mapping, Human Gene Mapping Workshop 10.5, Cytogenet. Cell. Genet. (in press).

Orita, M., Iwahana, H., Kanazawa, H., Hayashi, K., and Sekiya, T. (1989) Detection of Polymorphisms of Human DNA by Gel Electrophoresis as Single-strand Conformational Polymorphisms. Prog. Nat. Acad. Sci., 86: 2766–2770

Orita, M., Suzuki, Y., Sekiya, T., and Hayashi, K. (1989) "Rapid and Sensitive Detection of Point Mutations and DNA Polymorphisms using the Polymerase Chain Reaction." Genomics, 5, 874–879

Ott J., (1985). Analysis of Human Genetic Linkage. Johns Hopkins University. Baltimore.

Park F (2007) Lent viral vectors: are they the future of animal Transgenesis Physiology Genomics 31(2): 159-173. population. PloS one 5(10): e13661.

Paterson A.H., Lander E.S., Hewitt J.D., Peterson S., Lincoln S.E., Tanksley S.D. (1989). Resolution of quantitative traits into Mendelian factors by using a complete linkage map of restriction fragment length polymorphisms. Nature 335: 721–726.

Pedersen, K.S., Kristensen, T.N. and Loeschcke, V. 2005. Effects of inbreeding and rate of inbreeding in Drosophila melanogaster – Hsp70 expression and fitness. Journal of Evolutionary Biology In press.

Phillips, P.C., Whitlock, M.C. and Fowler, K. 2001. Inbreeding changes the shape of the genetic covariance matrix in Drosophila melanogaster. Genetics 158: 1137–1145.

Pirchner, F. 1985. Genetic structure of populations.I. Closed populations or matings among related individuals. In General and quantitative genetics (ed. Chapman, A.B.), pp. 227–250. Elsevier, Amsterdam.

Plotsky, Y., Cahener, A., Haberfeld, A., Lavi, U., Hillel, J. (1990) "Analysis of genetic association between DNA fingerprint bands and quantitative traits using DNA mixes." Proceedings of World Congress on Genetics Applied to Livestock Production. 13: 133–136

Prakash C (2002) Look Mom! No Antibiotic Resistance Marker Genes.

Pusey, A. and Wolf, M. 1996. Inbreeding avoidance in animals. Trends in Ecology and Evolution 11: 201–206.

Queitsch, C., Sangster, T.A. and Lindquist, S. 2002. Hsp90 as a capacitor of phenotypic variation. Nature 417: 618–624.

Ralls, K. and Ballou, J. 1983. Extinction: lessons from zoos. In Genetics and conservation: a reference for managing wild animal and plant populations (ed. Schonewald-Cox, S.M. Chambers, B. MacBryde, B. and Thomas, L.), pp. 164–184. Benjamin/Cummings, Menlo Park, CA.

Ralls, K., Ballou, J.D. and Templeton, A. 1988. Estimates of lethal equivalents and the cost of inbreeding in mammals. Conservation Biology 2: 185–193.

Reed, D.H. and Bryant, E.H. 2000. Experimental tests of minimum viable population size. Animal Conservation 3: 7–14.

Reed, D.H., Briscoe, D.A. and Frankham, R. 2002. Inbreeding and extinction: the effect of environmental stress and lineage. Conservation Genetics 3: 301–307.

Reed, D.H., Lowe, E.H., Briscoe, D.A. and Frankham, R. 2003. Inbreeding and extinction: effects of rate of inbreeding. Conservation Genetics 4: 405–410.

Reynolds J., Weir B.S., Cockerham C.C., (1983). Genetics 105: 767–779.

Robertson, A. 1952. The effect of inbreeding on the variation due to recessive genes. Genetics 37: 189–207.

Royale N.J., Clarkson R.E., Wong Z., Jeffreys A.J., (1988). Clustering of hypervariable minisatellites in the proterminal regions of human autosomes, Genomics 3: 352–360.

Rutherford, S.L. and Lindquist, S. 1998. Hsp90 as a capacitor for morphological evolution. Nature 396: 336–342.

Rye, M. and Mao, I.L. 1998. Nonadditive genetic effects and inbreeding depression for body weight in Atlantic salmon (Salmo salar L.). Livestock Production Science 57: 15–22.

Saiki R.K., et al., (1988). Primer directed enzymatic amplification of DNA with a thermostable DNA polymerase, Science 239: 487–491.

Sambrook J., Frisch E.F., and Maniatis T., (1989). "Molecular Cloning - A Laboratory Manual", 2nd Edition. Cold Spring Harbor Laboratory Press, USA.

Sánchez, L., Bijma, P. and Woolliams, J.A. 2003. Minimizing inbreeding by managing genetic contributions across generations. Genetics 164: 1589–1595.

Sanger F., Nicklen S., Coulson A.R., (1977). DNA sequencing with chain terminating inhibitors, Proc. Natl. Acad. Sci. U.S.A. 74: 5463–5467.

Scott G, Mattew B (2011) Genetically engineered animals and public health. Compelling Benefits for Health Care, Nutrition, the Environment, and Animal Welfare 22-30.

Sinclair A.H., Berta P., Palmer M.S. et al (1990). A gene from the human sex-determining region encodes a protein with homology to a conserved DNA-binding motif. Nature 346: 240–244.

Smith J.C., et al., (1990). Highly polymorphic minisatellite sequences: Allele frequencies and mutation rates for five locus-specific probes in a caucasian population, J. Forensic Sci. Soc. 30: 19–32.

Smith M, Asche F, Guttormsen A, Wiener J (2010) Genetically modified salmon and full impact assessment. Science 330: 1052-1053.

Smith, L.A., Cassell, B.G. and Pearson, R.E. 1998. The effects of inbreeding on the lifetime performance of dairy cattle. Journal of Dairy Science 81: 2729–2737.

Soller M., (1991). Mapping Quantitative Trait Loci Affecting Traits of Economic Importance in Animal Populations using Molecular Markers. In Gene Mapping Techniques and Applications' ed Schook L.B., Lewin H.A., McLaren D.G., Marcel Dekker Inc. New York.

Soller, M. (1990) "Strategies and opportunities for mapping QTL in agriculturally important animals." Womack J.E. ed., New York, Cold Spring Harbor Laboratory Press, p53–60

Sonesson, A.K., Grundy, B., Woolliams, J.A. and Meuwissen, T.H.E. 2000. Selection with control of inbreeding in populations with overlapping generations: a comparison of methods. Animal Science 70: 1–8.

Sørensen, J.G., Kristensen, T.N. and Loeschcke, V. 2003. The evolutionary and ecological role of heat shock proteins. Ecology Letters 6: 1025–1037.

Stearns, S.C., Kaiser, M. and Kawecki, T.J. 1995. The differential genetic and environmental canalization of fitness components in Drosophila melanogaster. Journal of Evolutionary Biology 8: 539–557.

Sullivan E, Pommer J, Robl J (2008) Commercializing genetically engineered animal biomedical products. Reprod Fertil Dev 20: 61-65.

Sussan E, and Asa M (1998) The Merck veterinary manual. 8th Merck and Co. Inc. W hite House station, New York, Pp 187-1880.

Tassabehji M., Read A.P., Newton V.E., Harris R., Ballings R., Gruss P., Strachan T., (1992). Waardenburg's syndrome patients have mutations in the human homologue of the PAX-3 paired box gene. Nature. 355: 635–636.

Templeton, A.R. and Read, B. 1984. Factors eliminating inbreeding depression in a captive herd of Speke's gazelle (Gazella spekei). spekei Zoo Biology 3: 177–199.

Templeton, A.R. and Read, B. 1994. Inbreeding: one word, several meanings, much confusion. In Conservation genetics (ed. Loeschcke, V., Tomiuk, J. and Jain, S.K.), pp. 91–105. Birkhäuser, Basel.

Threadgill D.W., Womack J.E., (1991). Synteny mapping of human chromosome 8 loci in cattle. Animal Genetics. 22: 117–122.

Trask B.J., (1991). Fluorescence in situ hybridization: applications in cytogenetics and gene mapping. Trends in Genetics 7: p149–154.

Vàzquez-Salat N, Salter B, Smets G, Houdebine L (2012) The current state of GMO governance: Are we ready for GM animals? Biotechnology Advances 30(6): 1336-1343.

Vermeulen, C.J. and Bijlsma, R. 2004. Characterization of conditionally expressed mutants affecting age-specific survival in inbred lines of Drosophila melanogaster: Lethal conditions and temperature sensitive periods. Genetics 167: 1241–1248.

Verrier, É., Colleau, J.J. and Foulley, J.-L. 1993. Long-term effects of selection based on the animal model BLUP in a finite population. Theoretical and Applied Genetics 87: 446–454.

Vigilant L., Stoneking M., Harpending H., Hawkes, K., Wilson A. (1991) "African Populations and the Evolution of Human Mitochondrial DNA" Science 253: 1503–1507

Visscher, P.M., Smith, D., Hall, S.J.G. and Williams, J.L. 2001. A viable herd of genetically uniform cattle. Nature 409: 303.

Waddington, C.H. 1942. Canalization of development and the inheritance of acquired characters. Nature 150: 563–565.

Wallace M.R. et al (1990). Science 249: 181–186.

Waller, D.M. 1993. The statics and dynamics of mating systems. In The natural history of inbreeding and outbreeding: theoretical and emperical perspectives (ed. Thornhill, N.W.), pp.97–117. University of Chicago Press, Chicago.

Walsh, B. and Lynch, M. 1998. Evolution and selection of quantitative traits. http: //nitro.biosci.arizona.edu/zbook/volume_2/chapters/vol2_03.html

Wang, J., Caballero, A., Keightley, P.D. and Hill, W.G. 1998. Bottleneck effect on genetic variance: a theoretical investigation of the role of dominance. Genetics 150: 435–447.

Wang, J., Hill, W.G., Charlesworth, D. and Charlesworth, B. 1999. Dynamics of inbreeding depression due to deleterious mutations in small populations: mutation parameters and inbreeding rate. Genetical Research 74: 165–178.

Wang, S., Hard, J.J. and Utter, F. 2002. Salmonid inbreeding: a review. Reviews in Fish Biology and Fisheries 11: 301–319.

Weber J.L., May P.E., (1989). Abundant class of DNA polymorphisms which can be typed using polymerase chain reaction, Am. J. Hum. Genet. 44: 388–396.

Weir, B.S. and Cockerham, C.C. 1969. Group inbreeding with two linked loci. Genetics 63: 711–742.

Weir, B.S., Avery, P.J. and Hill, W.G. 1980. Effect of mating structure on variation in inbreeding. Theoretical Population Biology 18: 396–429.

Weller, J.I., Kashi, Y., Soller, M., (1990) Power of "daughter" and "granddaughter" designs for genetic mapping of quantitative traits in dairy cattle using genetic markers. J. Dairy Sci 73: 2525–2532

White, J.M. 1972. Inbreeding effects upon growth and maternal ability in laboratory mice. Genetics 70: 307–317.

Whitelaw C, Lillico S, King T (2008) Production of transgenic farm animals by viral vector-mediated gene transfer. Reprod Domest 2: 355-358.

Whitlock, M.C. and Fowler, K. 1996. The distribution among populations in phenotypic variance with inbreeding. Evolution 50: 1919–1926.

Whitlock, M.C. and Fowler, K. 1999. The changes in genetic and environmental variance with inbreeding in Drosophila melanogaster. Genetics 152: 345–353.

Whitlock, M.C., Phillips, P.C. and Fowler, K. 2002. Persistence of changes in the genetic covariance matrix after a bottleneck. Evolution 56: 1968–1975.

Whitlock, M.C., Phillips, P.C. and Wade, M.J. 1993. Gene interaction affects the additive genetic variance in subdivided populations with migration and extinction. Evolution 47: 1758–1769.

Wiener, G., Lee, G.J. and Woolliams, J.A. 1992a. Effects of rapid inbreeding and of crossing of inbred lines on the body weight growth of sheep. Animal Production 55: 89–99.

Wiener, G., Lee, G.J. and Woolliams, J.A. 1992b. Effects of rapid inbreeding and of crossing of inbred lines on the growth of linear body dimensions of sheep. Animal Production 55: 101–114.

Wiener, G., Lee, G.J. and Woolliams, J.A. 1992c. Effects of rapid inbreeding and of crossing of inbred lines on conception rate, prolificacy and ewe survival in sheep. Animal Production 55: 115–121.

Wiener, G., Lee, G.J. and Woolliams, J.A. 1994. Consequences of inbreeding for financial returns from sheep. Animal Production 59: 245–249.

Wiggans G, VanRaden P, Cooper T (2011) The genomic evaluation system in the United States: Past, present, future. Journal of Dairy Science 94(6): 3202-3211.

Willis, J.H. and Orr, H.A. 1993. Increased heritable variation following population bottlenecks: the role of dominance. Evolution 47: 949–957.

Womack J.E., (1987). Comparative gene mapping: a valuable new tool for mammalian development studies. Dev. Genet. 8: 281–293.

Womack J.E., (1990). Status of the Bovine Gene Map. In "Mapping the genomes of agriculturally important animals". Womack J.E., ed. New York. Cold Spring Harbour Laboratory Press, p115–121

Woolliams, J.A. and Bijma, P. 2000. Predicting rates of inbreeding in populations undergoing selection. Genetics 154: 1851–1864.

Wray, N.R. and Goddard, M.E. 1994. Increasing long-term response to selection. Genetics, Selection, Evolution 26: 431–451.

Wright, S. 1951. The genetical structure of populations. Annals of Eugenics 15: 323–354.

Yum, S, Youn, K, Choi, W (2018) Development of genome engineering technologies in cattle: from random to specific. J Animal Sci Biotechnol 9.

INDEX

D

E

F

www.ingramcontent.com/pod-product-compliance
Lightning Source LLC
LaVergne TN
LVHW062117200926
848484LV00007B/1694
* 9 7 8 1 7 8 7 1 5 0 5 1 5 *